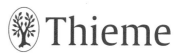

Complications in Vascular Interventional Therapy: Case-Based Solutions

Stefan Mueller-Huelsbeck, MD, PhD, EBIR, FICA
Professor of Radiology, Board Certified Neuroradiologist
Department of Diagnostic and Interventional Radiology and Neuroradiology
Diakonissen Hospital Flensburg
Flensburg, Germany

Thomas Jahnke, MD, PhD, EBIR, FICA, FSIR
Professor of Radiology
Department of Diagnostic and Interventional Radiology and Nuclear Medicine
Friedrich-Ebert-Hospital Neumuenster
Neumuenster, Germany

With contributions from
Fabrizio Fanelli, Timothy I. Joseph, Sanjoy Kundu, Keigo Osuga, Kenneth Robert Thomson,
Dimitrios Tsetis, Raman Uberoi

540 illustrations

Thieme
Stuttgart • New York • Delhi • Rio de Janeiro

Library of Congress Cataloging-in-Publication Data

Names: Mueller-Huelsbeck, Stefan, author. | Jahnke,
    Thomas, author.
Title: Complications in vascular interventional therapy:
    case-based solutions/Stefan Mueller-Huelsbeck,
    Thomas Jahnke.
Description: Stuttgart; New York: Thieme, [2016] | Includes
    bibliographical references and index.
Identifiers: LCCN 2016011336 | ISBN 9783131758316
    (hardcover)
Subjects: | MESH: Endovascular Procedures—adverse
    effects | Case Reports
Classification: LCC RD593 | NLM WG 170 | DDC
617.48—dc23 LC record available at http://lccn.loc.
gov/2016011336

© 2016 by Georg Thieme Verlag KG

Thieme Publishers Stuttgart
Rüdigerstrasse 14, 70469 Stuttgart, Germany
+49 [0]711 8931 421, customerservice@thieme.de

Thieme Publishers New York
333 Seventh Avenue, New York, NY 10001 USA
+1 800 782 3488, customerservice@thieme.com

Thieme Publishers Delhi
A-12, Second Floor, Sector-2, Noida-201301
Uttar Pradesh, India
+91 120 45 566 00, customerservice@thieme.in

Thieme Publishers Rio, Thieme Publicações Ltda.
Edifício Rodolpho de Paoli, 25ª andar
Av. Nilo Peçanha, 50 – Sala 2508,
Rio de Janeiro 20020-906 Brasil
Tel: +55 21 3172-2297 / +55 21 3172-1896

Cover design: Thieme Publishing Group
Typesetting by Thomson Digital, India

Printed in India by Manipal Technologies Ltd   5 4 3 2 1

ISBN 978-3-13-175831-6

Also available as an e-book:
eISBN 978-3-13-175841-5

Important note: Medicine is an ever-changing science undergoing continual development. Research and clinical experience are continually expanding our knowledge, in particular our knowledge of proper treatment and drug therapy. Insofar as this book mentions any dosage or application, readers may rest assured that the authors, editors, and publishers have made every effort to ensure that such references are in accordance with **the state of knowledge at the time of production of the book.**

Nevertheless, this does not involve, imply, or express any guarantee or responsibility on the part of the publishers in respect to any dosage instructions and forms of applications stated in the book. **Every user is requested to examine carefully** the manufacturers' leaflets accompanying each drug and to check, if necessary in consultation with a physician or specialist, whether the dosage schedules mentioned therein or the contraindications stated by the manufacturers differ from the statements made in the present book. Such examination is particularly important with drugs that are either rarely used or have been newly released on the market. Every dosage schedule or every form of application used is entirely at the user's own risk and responsibility. The authors and publishers request every user to report to the publishers any discrepancies or inaccuracies noticed. If errors in this work are found after publication, errata will be posted at www.thieme.com on the product description page.

Some of the product names, patents, and registered designs referred to in this book are in fact registered trademarks or proprietary names even though specific reference to this fact is not always made in the text. Therefore, the appearance of a name without designation as proprietary is not to be construed as a representation by the publisher that it is in the public domain.

Contents

Foreword

Endovascular procedures for treating arterial, venous, and also various oncological diseases have become an integral part of modern medicine. Although these procedures may be enormously beneficial for the patients, in some cases things may go wrong—technical problems may occur and complications may happen. However, in most of these situations, the interventionist should be able to solve the problem or even treat a complication by interventional means. To accomplish this, it is indispensable to be able to recognize a potential problem and analyze the situation meticulously. And even more importantly, by knowing what can happen, problems and complications can be avoided. There is a common saying in radiology: "You only see what you know" and, to adapt this to interventional radiology: "You can only avoid what you expect to happen."

This compendium gives a case-based overview of the most common and important complications that may occur during endovascular procedures. The authors not only describe the complications and how they arose, they also provide practical tips and techniques on how to manage complications—be it by endovascular means or with the help of partners from other disciplines.

By reading this book the reader will be confronted with a large variety of undesired events and situations that may occur during daily routine. Although they may not have experienced some of these situations personally, by having read about them in this book the reader will be well prepared to recognize and handle them.

Klaus Hausegger, MD, FCIRSE
Founder of the International Conference on
Complications in Interventional Radiology
Poertschach and Klagenfurt, Austria

Preface

Almost 50 years ago, Charles Dotter performed the first successful angioplasty on an 85-year-old woman suffering from gangrene of the forefoot. The procedure was reported as uneventful, resulting in wound healing after minor amputation. Since then, interventional procedures have developed into a widespread instrument for treatment of vascular and nonvascular diseases.

These procedures are uneventful in the vast majority of the cases and are reported as technically successful for treatment of the symptoms of underlying disease. However, in a small number of cases, unexpected events will occur and any physician actively performing endovascular procedures will eventually encounter complications while treating his or her patients. Complications can occur at any point in or during the procedure, and they may happen regardless of the training level of the physician, although type and severity of complications do vary depending on the complexity of procedures performed.

The value of conferences on morbidity and mortality is well known. By discussing cases where something went wrong, a physician will be able to enhance his or her own skills. For adequate management of a complication it can be crucial if a similar case has been heard of before.

We use a case-based format in this book so that the reader will benefit from real-life events, collected over the 20 years of experience in endovascular therapy.

This first edition of the textbook is focused on vascular disease complications and their management. It is addressed to interventionists like radiologists, neuroradiologists, cardiologists, angiologists, and vascular surgeons performing interventional vascular procedures.

The case selection in this book does not claim to be complete in terms of finding the ideal solution to manage a dedicated complication. It is difficult to represent the great variety of options in interventional therapy. However, we try to offer representative complications covering most vascular procedures. The presentation of similar cases underlines the fact that these complications seem to happen more often during daily routine.

We hope you will find this compendium an interesting and useful contribution to your daily practice.

Stefan Mueller-Huelsbeck, MD, PhD, EBIR, FICA
Thomas Jahnke, MD, PhD, EBIR, FICA, FSIR

Contributors

Fabrizio Fanelli, MD, EBIR
Professor of Radiology
Vascular and Interventional Radiology Unit
Department of Radiological Sciences
Sapienza University of Rome
Rome, Italy

Thomas Jahnke, MD, PhD, EBIR, FICA, FSIR
Professor of Radiology
Department of Diagnostic and Interventional
    Radiology and Nuclear Medicine
Friedrich-Ebert-Hospital Neumuenster
Neumuenster, Germany

Timothy I. Joseph, FRANZCR, MBBS, BSc (Life Sci)
Interventional Radiologist
The Alfred Hospital
Melbourne, Victoria, Australia

Sanjoy Kundu, BSc, MD, FRCPC, RVT, RPVI, FSIR, FCIRSE, FACPh, FASA; Diplomate of the American Board of Phlebology
Medical Director
The Vein Institute of Toronto
Active Staff
Scarborough Hospital-General Campus
Medical Director, Quality Assurance Advisor
Toronto Vascular Ultrasound
Toronto, Ontario

Stefan Mueller-Huelsbeck, MD, PhD, EBIR, FICA
Professor of Radiology, Board Certified
    Neuroradiologist
Department of Diagnostic and Interventional
    Radiology and Neuroradiology
Diakonissen Hospital Flensburg
Flensburg, Germany

Keigo Osuga, MD, PhD
Associate Professor of Radiology
Department of Diagnostic and Interventional
    Radiology
Osaka University Graduate School of Medicine
Osaka, Japan

Kenneth Robert Thomson, MD, FRANZCR, EBIR
Professor of Radiology
Radiology Department
The Alfred Hospital
Melbourne, Victoria, Australia

Dimitrios Tsetis, MD, PhD, FCIRSE, EBIR
Associate Professor of Interventional Radiology
Unit of Interventional Radiology
Department of Radiology
University Hospital of Heraklion
Faculty of Medicine
University of Crete
Crete, Greece

Raman Uberoi, BMScPath, MBBchir, MRCP, FRCR, EBIR
Honorary Senior Lecturer
Consultant Interventional Radiologist
John Radcliffe Hospital
University of Oxford
Oxford, United Kingdom

1 Introduction

Any physician actively performing endovascular procedures has experienced complications at some point or another. Some of us have even lost patients to complications encountered during treatments. The lively and emotional discussions at morbidity and mortality (M&M) sessions show that in many cases it just needs a good idea from someone else to overcome an acute problem.

Thomas Edison once said, "Experience is merely the sum of all our mistakes." To some extent this holds true for physicians. In medicine, however, we should also be able to learn from mistakes that others have made in order to prevent harm to our own patients.

Complications in endovascular therapy may result in an intensification of therapy, prolonged morbidity, and even death. Several factors can influence the occurrence of and the severity of complications. These include the operator's experience, the patient's condition, including his or her co-morbidities, and the lesion that needs to be treated. Typical complications are bleeding, pseudoaneurysm formation, arteriovenous fistulae, infection, distal embolization, perforations, flow-limiting dissection, and foreign body embolization.[1] Editors and contributing authors have selected cases with educational benefit, in order to strengthen the readers' vigilance and knowledge for both avoiding and solving complications during endovascular therapy.

References

1. Yadav JS, Sachar R, Casserly IP. Manual of peripheral vascular intervention. Philadelphia: Lippincott Williams & Wilkins; 2005:344–360

2 Minor and Major Complications

2.1 Definitions

Minor complication is defined as a treatment-related adverse event requiring nominal therapy or no treatment with or without overnight hospitalization for observation.

1. No therapy, no consequence. Or,
2. Nominal therapy, no consequence; includes overnight admission for observation only.

Major complication is defined as a treatment-related adverse event requiring further therapy with increase in the level of care or prolonged hospitalization.

1. Requires therapy, minor hospitalization (< 48 h).
2. Requires major therapy, unplanned increase in level of care, prolonged hospitalization (> 48 h).
3. Has permanent adverse sequelae. Or,
4. Results in death.

2.2 Avoiding Complications

2.2.1 Intervention Confusion

Endovascular therapy on the wrong body part, performing inadequate procedures, or even treating the wrong person are all examples of intervention confusion. With regard to all performed procedures, treating the wrong person or body part is rare. When they occur, however, the impact on the patient and on all individuals involved in the care process is momentous. Intervention confusion is generally considered preventable.

The aim of standard operation procedure (SOP) is to prevent confusion by implementing and *consistently* applying the following three complementary steps in the preparation of each patient for endovascular interventions:

1. Preoperative verification process (including patient identification, procedures, site[s], laterality and level, confirmed by source documents, consent form, medical records, and discussion with the patient).
2. Marking the intervention site(s) on the patient.
3. "Team time-out" just prior to the start of the intervention, involving verbal communication by all the professionals involved.

It is essential that all members of the pre- and perioperative teams are actively involved and effectively communicate with each other. In addition, it is important to involve the patient as much as possible.

A Patient Safety Checklist and knowledge of how to deal with impaired renal function and allergic reactions to contrast media will also help avoid complications.[1,2]

2.2.2 Patient Safety Checklist

It is strongly recommended that the patient is prepared according to the Cardiovascular and Interventional Radiological Society of Europe (CIRSE) IR Patient Safety Checklist (**Fig. 2.1**). The essential points on the checklist will minimize problems of communication and misinformation or any further confusion before starting the procedure.

2.2.3 Periprocedural Documentation

It is of utmost importance to document and store all procedural steps, including fluoroscopic images, especially when they make a significant contribution to the progress of a procedure. In this way, the operator can later highlight these steps in the report after storing the images in the picture archiving and communication system (PACS).

The importance of adequate image documentation is emphasized in the following case example:

A 48-year-old woman had been undergoing hemodialysis for many years. The patient suffered from recurrent swelling of her face and left arm (the arm with the Brescia-Cimino shunt). Repeated percutaneous transluminal angioplasty (PTA) was performed and the final stent (self-expanding 14 × 40 mm, open-cell design) at the level of the left brachiocephalic vein was placed 6 months ago. A moderate stenosis of the unstented part of the brachiocephalic vein close to the vena cava superior (VCS) was assumed to be responsible for the current symptoms (**Fig. 2.2**). A direct stenting procedure of the stenosed venous part was performed (self-expanding stent 16 × 40 mm). Unfortunately, the correct stent position was not documented. The

Patient Name		CIRSE IR Patient Safety Checklist		CIRSE
Patient ID				
Date of Birth		Procedure:		
Male ☐ Female ☐				
Ward:		Date:		
Referring Physician				Cardiovascular and Interventional Radiological Society of Europe

PROCEDURE PLANNING	YES	NO	N/A	SIGN IN	YES	NO	N/A	SIGN OUT	YES	NO	N/A
Discussed referring Physician/MDT	☐	☐	☐	All team members introduced	☐	☐		Post-op Note Written	☐	☐	
Imaging Sss Reviewed	☐	☐	☐	All Records with Patient	☐	☐	☐	Vital signs normal during procedure	☐	☐	☐
Relevant Medical History	☐	☐	☐	Correct patient/side/site	☐	☐		Medication and CM Recorded	☐	☐	☐
Informed Consent	☐	☐		Patient Fasting	☐	☐	☐	Lab Tests Ordered	☐	☐	☐
CIN Prophylaxis	☐	☐	☐	IV Access	☐	☐	☐	All Samples Labelled and Sent to Lab	☐	☐	☐
Specific Tools Present/Ordered	☐	☐	☐	Monitoring Equipment Attached	☐	☐	☐	Procedure Results discussed with Patient	☐	☐	☐
Fasting Order Given	☐	☐	☐	Coagulation screen/Lab Tests checked	☐	☐	☐	Post-discharge instruction given	☐	☐	☐
Relevant Lab Tests Ordered	☐	☐	☐	Allergies and/or Phrophylaxis Checked	☐	☐		Follow-up tests/imaging ordered	☐	☐	☐
Anaesthesiologist Necessary	☐	☐	☐	Antibiotics/other drugs administered	☐	☐	☐	Follow-up OPD appointment made	☐	☐	☐
Anticoagulant Medication Stopped	☐	☐	☐	Consent/Complications Discussed	☐	☐		Procedure results communicated to referrer	☐	☐	
Postinterventional (ICU) Bed Required	☐	☐	☐								
Contrast Allergy Prophylaxis Necessary	☐	☐	☐								

Name: _____   Name: _____   Name: _____

Signature: _____   Signature: _____   Signature: _____

Fig. 2.1 CIRSE IR Patient Safety Checklist. CIN, contrast-induced neuropathy; CM, contrast media; ICU, Intensive Care Unit; MDT, multidisciplinary team member; OPD, Outpatient Department. Reproduced with permission from CIRSE.

stent (closed-cell design) migrated into the VCS (**Fig. 2.3**) during the removal of the PTA balloon, which was carefully deflated. The patient was asymptomatic and the swelling of the face and arm disappeared completely. However, the operator would have been more satisfied if at least one stored image had documented the initial correctly placed stent.

Adequate documentation is also vital for legal and forensic reasons.[3,4]

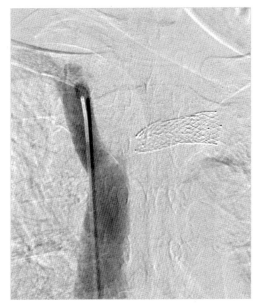

Fig. 2.2 Severely stenosed left brachiocephalic vein close to the VCS. The previously implanted self-expanding, open-cell stent seems compressed at the proximal end.

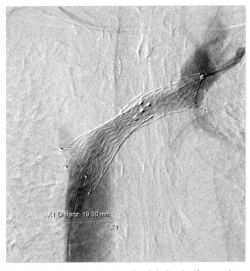

Fig. 2.3 Angiography showing the dislodged self-expanding, closed-cell stent (16 × 40 mm) after successful PTA with a 12 × 40-mm over-the-wire balloon. During balloon removal via a stiff Amplatz wire (Boston Scientific), the stent migrated.

References

1. http://www.cirse.org/files/files/Profession/IR_Checklist_new.pdf
2. Lee MJ, Fanelli F, Haage P, Hausegger K, Van Lienden KP. Patient safety in interventional radiology: a CIRSE IR checklist. Cardiovasc Intervent Radiol 2012;35(2):244–246
3. Durack JC. The value proposition of structured reporting in interventional radiology. AJR Am J Roentgenol 2014;203(4):734–738
4. Omary RA, Bettmann MA, Cardella JF, et al; Society of Interventional Radiology Standards of Practice Committee. Quality improvement guidelines for the reporting and archiving of interventional radiology procedures. J Vasc Interv Radiol 2002;13(9 pt 1):879–881

3 Patient-Related Complications

3.1 General Complications Related to Endovascular Procedures

3.1.1 Impaired Renal Function

In the case of impaired renal function, patients should be treated according to the current European Society of Urogenital Radiology (ESUR) guidelines (http://www.esur.org/esur-guidelines/). Following these guidelines will minimize problems related to uncontrolled iodized contrast media application.[1]

3.1.2 Known Allergic Reactions to Contrast Material

Patients with known allergic reactions to contrast material should be prepared according to international guidelines.[2] The *ACR Manual on Contrast Media, Version 10.1, 2015* from the ACR Committee on Drugs and Contrast Media will help in both prevention and treatment of acute reactions to contrast media (http://www.acr.org/quality-safety/resources/~/media/37D84428BF1D4E1B9A3A2918DA9E27A3.pdf/).

3.1.3 Radiation Exposure

Practitioners should have extensive knowledge of dose management protocols during endovascular therapy in order to avoid excessive radiation exposure to both the patient and staff.[3,4]

3.1.4 Infection

Strategies for preventing infections during endovascular procedures include general, preoperative, intraoperative, and postoperative regimes. These strategies are important because vascular patients are prone to infection (i.e., in cases of diabetes, chronic wounds, renal impairment, and malignancies responsible for an impaired immunity).[5] The *Joint Practice Guideline for Sterile Technique during Vascular and Interventional Radiology Procedures* from the Society of Interventional Radiology, Association of Perioperative Registered Nurses and the Association for Radiologic and Imaging Nursing, is a particularly useful reference work (http://www.sirweb.org/clinical/cpg/QI35.pdf).

3.2 Management of Vascular Complications

Major periprocedural complications are uncommon in interventions, but they may manifest suddenly and require swift and orderly response. Although the experience of the surgeon, nursing, and technical staff is important, the relative rarity of serious events makes the use of a checklist a valuable practice, helping to ensure organized implementation of a preplanned response.

"Planning for failure" is a strategy used by effective teams that perform procedures with significant risks. Patel et al (2012) report improved endovascular outcomes with a preprocedural "mental rehearsal" in hybrid aortic cases.[6] In 2013, Chen developed a checklist for response to a cerebral artery aneurysm perforation and a separate checklist for thrombosis in neurosurgical interventions.[7] These listed expected responses from the surgeon, anesthesiologist, nursing and technologist staff, each with specific roles and responsibilities.

In the case of thrombosis, the interventionist should record the activated clotting time (ACT) and request an empiric bolus of heparin based on the patient's weight and predetermined dose. If vasospasm is detected at the site of the sheath, intra-arterial nitroglycerin should be given. Nursing staff should administer fluids, and the technologist should prepare aspiration or thrombolysis devices.

For bleeding complications, the interventionist should clearly communicate details of the complication to the staff and his or her plans for correction. Serious bleeding from a superficial femoral artery (SFA) intervention is rare, but a high femoral artery puncture or concomitant iliac artery intervention can lead to rapid blood loss into the pelvis. A retroperitoneal hemorrhage can quickly result in shock. Clearly and succinctly articulating the problem and the anticipated next steps is critical, and it is important to verbally confirm that team members have heard and understood what was said.

Arterial access should be maintained. Required equipment, such as a covered stent, tourniquet, or occlusion balloon should be requested. The nurse should maintain fluids and blood products as necessary and request an anesthesiologist to assist if the patient is in extremis. The technologist should alert the operating room staff of the potential need for open conversion, and the operating room should be prepared if endovascular solutions are limited or if there is hemodynamic instability.

3.2.1 Thrombosis

Recognition: Team member recognizes the angiographic finding, pulse deficit, or other evidence of thrombosis and verbally states the problem.

Consider contributing factors: Evaluate hemodynamic status, arterial access potentially obturating the sheath, and angiography to confirm the cessation of bleeding.

Medical treatment: Bolus with heparin, check ACT, maintain therapeutic anticoagulation, consider vasodilator administration (intra-arterial nitroglycerin).

Interventional treatment: Review options as follows: treat inflow stenosis, repeat angioplasty, additional stent implantation, thrombectomy, catheter-directed thrombolysis, mechanical or rheolytic thrombectomy.

Repeat angiography to evaluate the result.

Preventing Thrombosis

Anticoagulation with heparin by inhibiting cofactors that promote proper thrombin formation, using a typical measurement of heparin in ACT with a target ranging from 200 to 350 seconds depending on type of endovascular therapy. In addition, aspirin and clopidogrel were administered in the majority of the patients, whereas glycoprotein IIb/IIIa inhibitors were used less frequently.[8]

3.2.2 Arterial Hemorrhage

Recognition: Team member recognizes abnormal bleeding by hemodynamic instability and verbally states the problem. Call for help if needed. Ensure hemodynamic monitors are attached and functional. Evaluate access site or site of suspected vascular injury, if accessible.

Hemorrhage control: Apply manual direct pressure if bleeding is from an accessible, compressible site. Maintain arterial access, but consider exchanging for a larger-diameter sheath, if needed. Position an occlusion balloon, with angiography to confirm cessation of bleeding.

Resuscitation: Large-bore intravenous line (consider more than one) with crystalloid solution (saline or Plasma-Lyte). Notify blood bank, send blood specimen, and request for transfusion. Consider reversal of anticoagulation (protamine 1 mg to reverse 100 units of heparin). Notify vascular surgeon if endovascular therapy is not practical or if the patient is unstable. Notify the operating room staff.

Treatment: Prolonged balloon occlusion,[9] covered stent, coiling and glue injection,[10,11] external compression, reversal of anticoagulation, surgical treatment including vessel repair and fasciotomy for suspected compartment syndrome.[12]

Communication: Inform family members of situation and plans.

Preventing Arterial Hemorrhage

Control coagulation status carefully before starting the procedure and check ACT during the procedure.

3.2.3 Vessel Perforation

Recognition: Team member recognizes contrast extravasation on angiogram and/or abnormal bleeding by hemodynamic instability and verbally states the problem. Further steps in terms of hemorrhage control, resuscitation, and treatment are covered in 3.2.2 Arterial Hemorrhage.

Balloon tamponade at low pressure for 2–4 minutes can be particularly helpful.[9]

Preventing Vessel Perforation

Prevent guidewire perforations by obtaining high–image quality angiograms, following all guidewire manipulations using overlay/roadmap techniques, always keeping the distal wire's end stable and under control. If possible, visualize the distal wire's end during the entire procedure to avoid inadvertent selection of downstream vessel branches. Be aware of this especially during catheter exchange over the wire.

Preventing vessel perforation is directly related to vessel size and degree of vessel wall calcification. Balloon sizing and inflation pressure should be appropriate: start with a smaller balloon and low inflation pressure. If the patient complains of pain at the treatment site, the balloon size and/or inflation pressure might be too high.

3.2.4 Distal Embolization

Recognition: Recognize typical predictors like total occlusions, long and irregular lesions, as well as thrombotic occlusion.[13,14] Mechanical thrombectomy and atherectomy procedures are prone to distal embolization.[15,16]

Interventional treatment: Consider basic syringe aspiration via large inner lumen catheters, and advanced mechanical aspiration.

Preventing Distal Embolization

Evaluate the use of embolic protection devices in dedicated procedures.[17–20]

3.2.5 Device Malfunction

Carefully read instructions for use and request training for complex devices. Proctoring services as well as attending workshops and learning centers will help with familiarization.

Preventing Device Malfunction

For percutaneous transluminal angioplasty (PTA) balloons, be aware of rated burst pressure. For stents, evaluate the delivery mechanism. With regard to embolic agents and embolization material, be mindful of the application and delivery process.

References

1. Stacul F, Van der Molen AJ, Reimer P, et al; Contrast Media Safety Committee of the European Society of Urogenital Radiology (ESUR). Contrast induced nephropathy: updated ESUR Contrast Media Safety Committee guidelines. Eur Radiol 2011;21(12):2527–2541

2. Bush WH Jr. Treatment of acute contrast reactions. In: Bush WH Jr, Krecke KN, King BF Jr, Bettmann MA, eds. Radiology life support (RAD-LS). London/New York: Hodder Arnold; 1999:31–51

3. Finch W, Shamsa K, Lee MS. Cardiovascular complications of radiation exposure. Rev Cardiovasc Med 2014;15(3):232–244

4. Ketteler ER, Brown KR. Radiation exposure in endovascular procedures. J Vasc Surg 2011;53(1 suppl):35S–38S

5. Reddy P, Liebovitz D, Chrisman H, Nemcek AA Jr, Noskin GA. Infection control practices among interventional radiologists: results of an online survey. J Vasc Interv Radiol 2009;20(8):1070–1074

6. Patel SR, Gohel MS, Hamady M, Albayati MA, Riga CV, Cheshire N. Reducing errors in combined open/endovascular arterial procedures: influence of a structured mental rehearsal before the endovascular phase. J Endovasc Ther 2012;19(3):383–389

7. Chen M. A checklist for cerebral aneurysm embolization complications. J Neurointervent Surg 2013;5(1):20–27

8. Adjunctive pharmacotherapy: unfractionated heparin. In: Manual of Interventional Cardiology. Available at: http://www.jbpub.com/physicianspress/iscarufh.pdf. Accessed September 5, 2014.

9. Hayes PD, Chokkalingam A, Jones R. Arterial perforation during infrainguinal lower limb angioplasty does not worsen outcome: results from 1409 patients. J Endovasc Ther 2002;9(4):422–427

10. Lopera J. Embolization in trauma: principles and techniques. Semin Interv Radiol 2010;27(1):14–28

11. Ponnuthurai FA, Ormerod OJ, Forfar C. Microcoil embolization of distal coronary artery perforation without reversal of anticoagulation: a simple, effective approach. J Invasive Cardiol 2007;19(8):E222–E225

12. Davaine J, Lintz F, Cappelli M, Chaillou P, Gouin F, Patra P. Acute compartment syndrome of the thigh secondary to isolated common femoral vessel injury: an unusual etiology. Ann Vasc Surg 2013;27(6):802.e1–e4

13. Shammas NW, Shammas GA, Dippel EJ, Jerin M, Shammas WJ. Predictors of distal embolization in peripheral percutaneous interventions: a report from a large peripheral vascular registry. J Invasive Cardiol 2009;21(12):628–631

14. Shrikhande GV, Khan SZ, Hussain HG, Dayal R, McKinsey JF, Morrissey N. Lesion types and device characteristics that predict distal embolization during percutaneous lower extremity interventions. J Vasc Surg 2011;53(2):347–352

15. Roberts D, Niazi K, Miller W, et al; DEFINITIVE Ca(++) investigators. Effective endovascular treatment of calcified femoropopliteal disease with directional atherectomy and distal embolic protection: final results of the DEFINITIVE Ca(++) trial. Catheter Cardiovasc Interv 2014;84(2):236–244

16. Shammas NW, Weissman NJ, Coiner D, Shammas GA, Dippel E, Jerin M. Treatment of subacute and chronic thrombotic occlusions of lower extremity peripheral arteries with the excimer laser: a feasibility study. Cardiovasc Revasc Med 2012;13(4):211–214

17. Lookstein RA, Lewis S. Distal embolic protection for infrainguinal interventions: how to and when? Tech Vasc Interv Radiol 2010;13:54–58

18. Mueller-Huelsbeck S, Schaefer PJ, Huemme TH, et al. Embolic protection devices for peripheral application: wasteful or useful? J Endovasc Ther 2009;16(1 suppl):I163–I169

19. Dippel EJ, Parikh N, Wallace KL. Use of SpiderFX embolic protection device vs. distal embolic event: hospital length of stay, operating room time, costs and mortality. J Am Coll Cardiol 2013;62(18_S1):B161

20. Zeller T, Schmidt A, Rastan A, et al. New approach to protected percutaneous transluminal angioplasty in the lower limbs. J Endovasc Ther 2013;20(3):409–419

4 Case-Based Procedure-Related Complications

4.1 Systemic Complication

Fatal retroperitoneal hemorrhage after antegrade locoregional thrombolysis

Patient History

A 64-year-old woman with peripheral vascular disease presented with acute limb ischemia of her left leg. Cardiovascular risk factors were hypertension, coronary heart disease, and smoking. She had mild rest pain; the leg was still viable (Rutherford IIa). It was decided to treat the patient endovascularly by locoregional lysis.

Initial Treatment Received

Antegrade puncture of the left common femoral artery was performed. Selective angiography revealed acute occlusion of the superficial femoral artery (SFA) without visible reconstitution of flow in popliteal and infragenual arteries (**Fig. 4.1**).

The patient was heparinized and a 10-cm side-hole catheter was placed into the proximal aspect of the SFA (**Fig. 4.2**). A bolus of 5 mg of recombinant tissue plasminogen activator (rtPA) was applied and long-term locoregional thrombolysis was initiated with 1 mg rtPA per hour. After 24 hours of lysis there was still significant thrombus burden; thus, locoregional treatment was continued for another 12 hours (total cumulative dose ca. 35 mg). Angiography after 36 hours showed residual thrombus in the below-the-knee (BTK) arteries (**Fig. 4.3**). In addition, there was wall-adherent clot present in the SFA. Residual clot was treated by aspiration and intra-arterial bolus application of 5 mg rtPA. Control angiography now showed an acceptable result with unobstructed flow in the SFA and a single infragenual artery reaching the foot (**Fig. 4.4**).

Thrombolysis was stopped and the patient was continued on IV heparin (target partial thromboplastin time [PTT] 60–80 s). The sheath in the left groin was left in place for another 2 hours. It was then removed and the groin was manually compressed. After hemostasis was achieved a pressure bandage was applied and the patient transported to the clinical ward for further observation.

Problems Encountered during Treatment

During the first 24 hours of treatment the patient developed mild groin hematoma that started oozing from the puncture site. This problem was managed by changing the 4F sheath to a 6F standard sheath after 24 hours of lysis (**Fig. 4.5**). The remainder of the locoregional treatment time was clinically unremarkable.

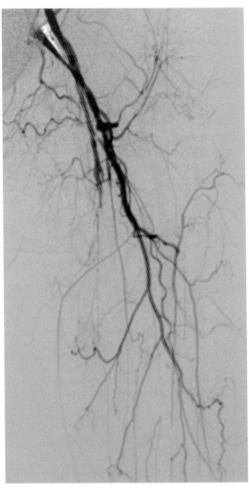

Fig. 4.1 Acute occlusion of the left SFA.

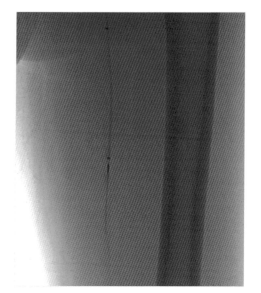

Fig. 4.2 Side-hole lysis catheter in place in the left SFA.

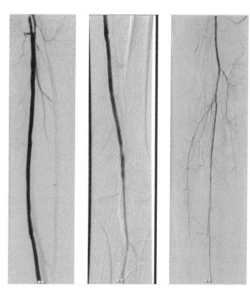

Fig. 4.4 Final result after 36 hours of locoregional lysis, bolus application of rtPA, and aspiration thrombectomy.

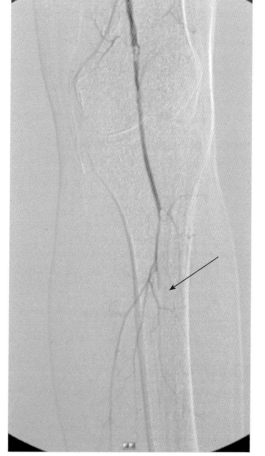

Fig. 4.3 Angiography after 36 hours of locoregional lysis showing residual thrombus in the BTK arteries (*arrow*).

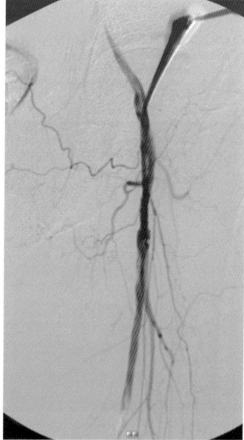

Fig. 4.5 Following exchange of a 4F sheath with a 6F standard sheath no extravasation of contrast material was detected.

Imaging Plan

Angiographic controls after 24 and 36 hours.

Resulting Complication

Two hours after final sheath removal the patient was found lying unresponsive in her bed. There was only mild groin hematoma, which appeared to be unchanged from the previous episode of mild subcutaneous bleeding. Cardiopulmonary resuscitation was performed immediately and it was possible to stabilize the patient with a sinus rhythm. However, she remained in a coma and needed ventilation. Subsequently performed cranial MRI showed diffuse cortical hyperintensities indicating global hypoxemic damage to the brain (**Fig. 4.6**). The patient died 3 days after treatment. Autopsy showed a moderate retroperitoneal hematoma.

Possible Strategies for Complication Management

- Evaluate alternatives for local fibrinolysis therapy as mechanical thrombectomy, eventually combined with low-dose fibrinolysis, especially in older patients.

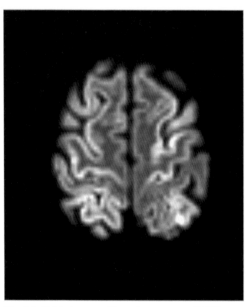

Fig. 4.6 Fluid-attenuated inversion-recovery (FLAIR) magnetic resonance imaging (MRI) shows cortical hyperintensities consistent with diffuse hypoxemic grey matter damage.

- In case of local fibrinolysis therapy, check the patient carefully for potential bleeding complications.
- All patients undergoing long-term fibrinolysis must be referred to an ICU.
- Additional imaging, such as ultrasound and even native CT in clinical unclear situations, should be indicated immediately.

Final Complication Management

An approach to control local bleeding was performed by upsizing the sheath from 4F to 6F. However, the retroperitoneal hematoma was unrecognized. Control of vital parameters as possible in an ICU is of utmost importance.

Complication Analysis

There was unrecognized retroperitoneal bleeding leading to hypovolemia and consecutive cardio-respiratory arrest. This type of complication can only be managed by close clinical surveillance. In case of suspected retroperitoneal bleeding computed tomography (CT) should be performed. Signs of retroperitoneal bleeding in patients on locoregional lysis should prompt termination of the procedure.

Prevention Strategies and Take-home Message

- Avoid antegrade punctures in patients with acute limb ischemia. Locoregional lysis should be performed preferably using a retrograde crossover approach, which limits the likelihood of significant bleeding complications.
- Limit peripheral thrombolysis in terms of dose and time of treatment. Bleeding complications are more likely to occur the longer the patients are treated.
- Use active closure device after local thrombolysis treatment.

Further Reading

Rajan DK, Patel NH, Cardella JF et al. Quality improvement guidelines for percutaneous management of acute limb ischemia. J Vasc Interv Radiol 2009;20(7 suppl):208–218

Working Party on Thrombolysis in the Management of Limb Ischemia. Thrombolysis in the management of lower limb peripheral arterial occlusion—a consensus document. Am J Cardiol 1998;81(2):207–218

4.2 Access-Related Complications

4.2.1 Access Creation

Sudden groin swelling after successful 4F retrograde puncture

Patient History

A 76-year-old patient suffered from lifestyle-limiting claudication (walking < 200 m). Noninvasive diagnostic imaging presented a moderate stenosis of the proximal right-side external iliac artery. She was scheduled for angioplasty via an ipsilateral retrograde groin approach for percutaneous transluminal angioplasty (PTA) or even stenting, if warranted.

Initial Treatment Received

Ipsilateral retrograde groin (common femoral artery [CFA]) puncture under local anesthesia; successful insertion of a 4F 10-cm-long standard sheath.

Problems Encountered during Treatment

Development of ipsilateral groin swelling!

Imaging Plan

Angiography of the right groin in an oblique projection to detect an underlying vessel injury.

Resulting Complication

Mild contrast media extravasation was depicted, probably at the posterior wall of the CFA (**Fig. 4.7**).

Possible Strategies for Complication Management

- Manual compression (MC) of the groin for at least 5 minutes, while leaving the sheath in place.
- When MC fails, creation of contralateral access with crossover balloon tamponade at the level of the bleeding site; preparation of consecutive endovascular procedures, for example, coiling of side branches (if they seem to be the source of bleeding).
- MC of the groin for at least 10 minutes after sheath removal.

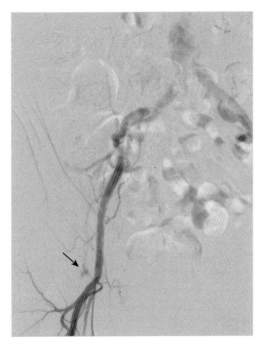

Fig. 4.7 Digital subtraction angiography (DSA). Contrast injection through the side port of the 4F sheath. DSA shows mild lateral contrast media extravasation (*arrow*) at the level of the lower third of the CFA. The source of bleeding was suspected to be at the lateral aspect of posterior wall.

- Upsizing of 4F sheath until hemostasis (if leakage at the arteriotomy).
- Surgery (if an endovascular approach fails).

Final Complication Management

MC (5 minutes) of the groin with the sheath left in place. Control angiography showed no further bleeding (**Fig. 4.8**).

Complication Analysis

Retrograde puncture of the CFA resulted in vessel wall damage. There was penetration of the posterior lateral side of the CFA wall resulting from the initial puncture with an open Seldinger needle.

Prevention Strategies and Take-home Message

- In case of unclear anatomy of the CFA (i.e., obese patients, nonpalpable pulse), ultrasound should be used in order to gather further anatomical information.

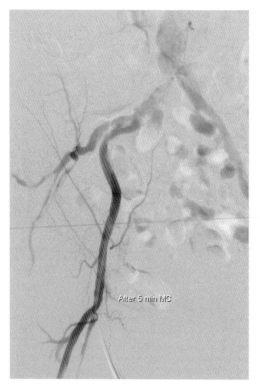

Fig. 4.8 No further contrast extravasation visible during follow-up angiography. The planned endovascular procedure was continued.

- Sufficient groin compression, even after failed puncture is of utmost importance!
- Perform every vessel puncture, even retrograde access to the CFA, with great care even if it appears simple!
- Be aware of groin swelling and hematoma formation at the puncture site; do not hesitate to look for a potential bleeding source, especially prior to further anticoagulation!
- Prefer "anterior stick" puncture to classical Seldinger technique with intentional penetration of posterior femoral wall. Posterior vessel wall injuries may lead to significant bleeding complications and impair thrombolysis treatment for cases of distal embolization.

Further Reading

Kalish J, Eslami M, Gillespie D, et al; Vascular Study Group of New England. Routine use of ultrasound guidance in femoral arterial access for peripheral vascular intervention decreases groin hematoma rates. J Vasc Surg 2015;61(5):1231–1238

Lo RC, Fokkema MT, Curran T, et al. Routine use of ultrasound-guided access reduces access site-related complications after lower extremity percutaneous revascularization. J Vasc Surg 2015;61(2):405–412

Superficial femoral artery pseudoaneurysm and arteriovenous fistula

Patient History

A 79-year-old patient presented with right groin hematoma and groin swelling 2 days after percutaneous coronary intervention via retrograde access to the right common femoral artery (CFA). Apart from his coronary heart disease no further comorbidities were reported. After coronary angiography a vascular closure device was used successfully and immediate hemostasis of the puncture site was achieved. The patient now presented in a hemodynamically stable condition. Clinical inspection of the right groin showed significant hematoma and swelling with a pulsating tumor.

Initial Treatment Received

Percutaneous coronary intervention (PCI).

Problems Encountered during Treatment

Unremarkable procedure, no complications reported!

Imaging Plan

Color duplex ultrasound of the right groin.

Resulting Complication

There was a pseudoaneurysm located in the proximal aspect of the superficial femoral artery (SFA); in addition, an arteriovenous fistula (AVF) was depicted (**Fig. 4.9**).

Possible Strategies for Complication Management

- Endovascular treatment via contralateral retrograde access to the CFA.
- Catheterization of the feeder channel to the femoral vein, for example using a microcatheter and followed by selective microcoil embolization; however, the small aneurysm remains untreated.

- Placement of a covered self-expanding stent (stent graft).
- Surgery (if an endovascular approach fails).

Final Complication Management

Endovascular treatment via contralateral retrograde access to the CFA (7F sheath, 45 cm long).

A 0.035-inch guidewire placement in the SFA and stent graft placement covering both the fistula and the aneurysm (**Figs. 4.10** and **4.11**).

Complication Analysis

Suspected (possibly repeated) retrograde puncture of the SFA resulted in vein and vessel wall penetration. Anticoagulation after the procedure and insufficient compression of the groin might have contributed to the development of this complication.

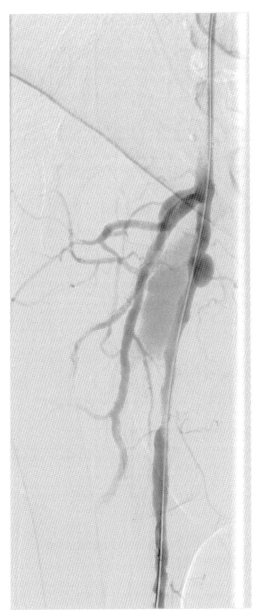

Fig. 4.9 Angiography of the femoral artery bifurcation in crossover technique. A pseudoaneurysm is located in the proximal aspect of the SFA; initial femoral vein opacification is consistent with an AVF.

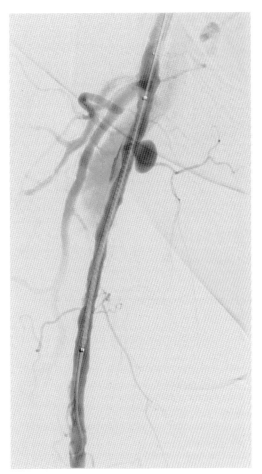

Fig. 4.10 Oblique view during angiography showing the neck of the pseudoaneurysm, a nonflow-limiting dissection of the SFA, and the contrast filling of the femoral vein. A 6 × 10-mm e-PTFE (expanded polytetrafluoroethylene)-covered stent is already in place.

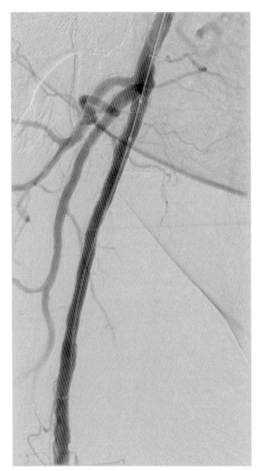

Fig. 4.11 Final angiography after stent placement and balloon angioplasty. Neither the small aneurysm nor the AVF is depicted.

Prevention Strategies and Take-home Message

- Avoid groin access with direct puncture of the SFA.
- Sufficient groin compression, even after failed puncture, is of utmost importance!
- If the location of the CFA is uncertain (i.e., obese patients, nonpalpable pulse), ultrasound should be used in order to gather further anatomical information.
- Use the contralateral groin or an alternative access route (radial or brachial approach).

Further Reading

Kendrick AS, Sprouse LR II. Repair of a combined femoral pseudoaneurysm and AVF using a covered stent graft. Am Surg 2007;73(3):227–229

Bleeding after failed antegrade groin access and PTA-related embolic event

Patient History

A 65-year-old patient suffered from peripheral arterial occlusive disease (PAOD) with lifestyle-limiting walking distance of less than 150 m. Due to obesity, a right groin antegrade puncture of the common femoral artery (CFA) was chosen (part 1). Unfortunately, access failed and the patient developed minor groin hematoma resistant to manual compression. It was decided to finalize the procedure via crossover technique from a contralateral retrograde groin access (part 2).

Initial diagnostic angiography (DA) showed some minor contrast extravasation at the recent puncture site. On top of that a distal embolic event occurred after initially planned PTA.

Initial Treatment Received

Failed ipsilateral antegrade groin access (part 1).
PTA of the femoropopliteal artery (part 2).

Problems Encountered during Treatment

Repeated failed CFA puncture (part 1).
PTA of the femoropopliteal artery via crossover technique (part 2).

Imaging Plan

Angiography.

Resulting Complication

Mild contrast extravasation at the mid-part of the right CFA (**Fig. 4.12**).

Acute occlusion of the posterior tibial artery located at the level of the medial malleolus (**Figs. 4.13** and **4.14**).

Possible Strategies for Complication Management

Bleeding:
- Endovascular treatment via contralateral retrograde access to the CFA.
- Long-term PTA at the level of bleeding site.
- Placement of a covered self-expanding stent (stent graft), which is usually not indicated at the CFA level.

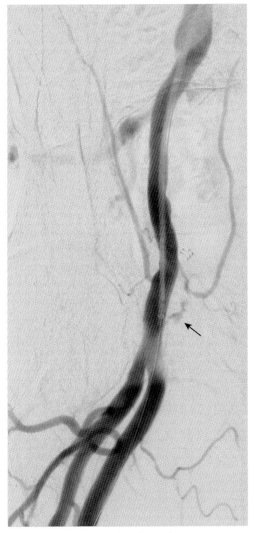

Fig. 4.12 Angiography of the femoral artery bifurcation using crossover technique. A moderate contrast extravasation (*arrow*) medial to the CFA is depicted. Suspected stenosis or thrombus formation at the origin of the SFA.

• Surgery (if an endovascular approach fails).
Embolization:
• Percutaneous aspiration thrombectomy (PAT).
• Admission of local short-term fibrinolysis.
• Surgery (rather unlikely at this distal level).

Final Complication Management

Bleeding: Endovascular treatment via contralateral retrograde access to the CFA (6F sheath, 45 cm long). Long-term PTA for about 180 seconds at

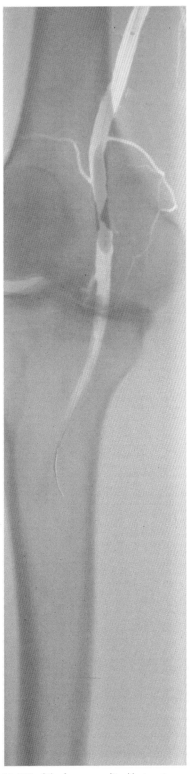

Fig. 4.13 PTA of the femoropopliteal lesion—image overlay technique.

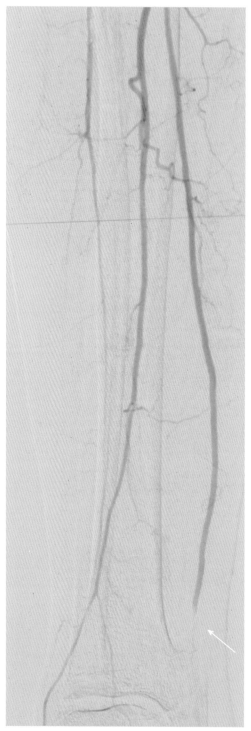

Fig. 4.14 Sudden stoppage of contrast media opacification at the level of the distal posterior tibial artery (*arrow*), originally the most important feeder artery to the foot.

the bleeding level of the CFA using a 6 × 40-mm balloon (**Figs. 4.15** and **4.16**). Bleeding stopped after long-term PTA.

Embolization: Four repetitions of PAT using a rapid-exchange (RX) 0.014-inch-compatible monorail catheter. The thromboembolism was sucked out successfully (**Figs. 4.17–4.19**).

Complication Analysis

Bleeding: Repeated antegrade groin puncture caused vessel injury, which resulted in significant

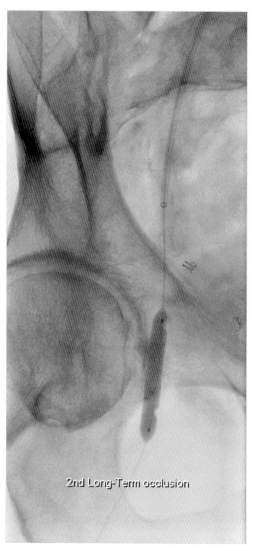

2nd Long-Term occlusion

Fig. 4.15 Long-term PTA at the CFA level.

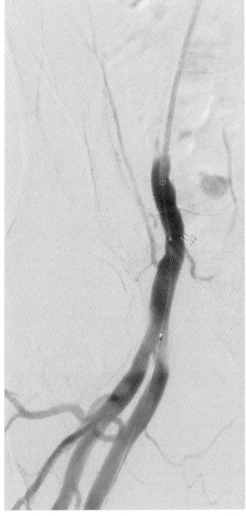

Fig. 4.16 No further bleeding at the CFA level was visible.

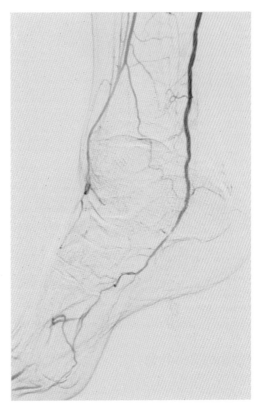

Fig. 4.17 Complete thromboembolism removal after successful PAT.

be used in order to gather further anatomical information.
- Sufficient groin compression, even after failed puncture, is of utmost importance!
- Use the contralateral groin or an alternative access route (radial or brachial approach).

bleeding. Insufficient external compression during puncture might have contributed to the development of this complication.

Embolization: Thromboembolism might have resulted from thrombus formation at the CFA and proximal superficial femoral artery (SFA), which is embolized down during PTA procedure.

Prevention Strategies and Take-home Message

Bleeding:
- Where the location of the CFA is uncertain (i.e., obese patients, nonpalpable pulse), a Doppler probe or B-mode ultrasound should

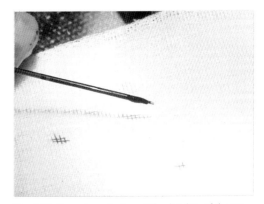

Fig. 4.18 Thromboembolism at the distal tip of the RX PAT catheter.

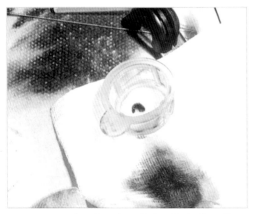

Fig. 4.19 Complete thromboembolism flushed in a filter.

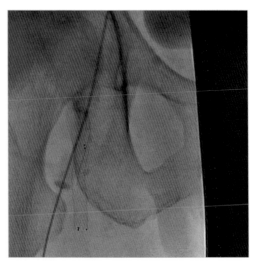

Fig. 4.20 Scaled wire (Terumo) coating at the level of the origin of the superficial femoral artery (SFA). Note: a self-expanding stent is located in the proximal SFA.

- If ipsilateral access is essential, ask a colleague to assist you.

Embolization:

- Thromboembolism can be very unpredictable.

Further Reading

Stone PA, Campbell JE. Complications related to femoral artery access for transcatheter procedures. Vasc Endovasc Surg 2012;46(8):617–623

Wu W, Hua S, Li Y, et al. Incidence, risk factors, treatment and prognosis of popliteal artery embolism in the superficial femoral artery interventions. PLoS One 2014;9(9):e107717

Hydrophilic-coated wire scaling during puncture needle manipulation (case 1)

Patient History

A 60-year-old patient suffering from recurrence of peripheral arterial occlusive disease (PAOD) was scheduled for diagnostic angiography (DA). During retrograde groin puncture there were problems inserting the atraumatic 0.035-inch sheath wire. A 0.035-inch hydrophilic wire was used to cannulate the artery through a Seldinger needle in order to establish access to the external iliac artery (EIA). The guidewire could be inserted but it could not easily be pulled back to correct the position. Despite considerable resistance the guidewire was removed through the needle, which was left in place. During this procedure scaling of the hydrophilic coating occurred, and the foreign material separated from the wire and remained inside the common femoral artery (CFA) (**Fig. 4.20**).

Initial Treatment Received

Failed retrograde groin access.

Problems Encountered during Treatment

Placement of a sheath wire prior to retrograde sheath placement failed. Attempts were made to insert a sheath over a hydrophylic-coated guidewire. During removal of the wire, parts of the coating were scaled from the wire and remained in the vessel.

Imaging Plan

Angiography from the contralateral groin.

Resulting Complication

Iatrogenic foreign body in the CFA.

Possible Strategies for Complication Management

- Endovascular treatment via contralateral retrograde access to the CFA.
- Placement of a snare to engage the foreign body.
- Surgery (if an endovascular approach fails).

Final Complication Management

Endovascular treatment via contralateral retrograde access to the CFA was attempted (6F sheath,

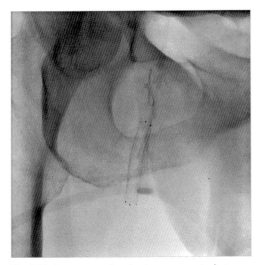

Fig. 4.21 A snare was placed using crossover technique distally to the foreign body. The scaled wire fragment can be caught best by slightly rotating the open snare. Once the fragment is engaged and fixed, safe removal into the (crossover) sheath can be performed.

45 cm long). Using a suture it was possible to grab the foreign body, which was finally removed (**Figs. 4.21** and **4.22**).

Complication Analysis

Uncontrolled manipulation of a hydrophilic guidewire in combination with a sharp, beveled stainless steel puncture needle resulted in scaling of the coating.

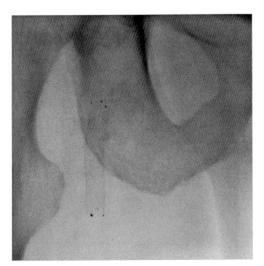

Fig. 4.22 Fluoroscopy after complete removal of the foreign body.

Prevention Strategies and Take-home Message

- Never pull a wire in an uncontrolled fashion through a beveled Seldinger needle.
- If, during retrieval of a hydrophylic guidewire, resistance is felt, the wire should be removed together with the puncture needle.
- Rotation of a deployed snare using a torque device might help catch a foreign body.

Further Reading

Capuano F, Simon C, Roscitano A, Sinatra R. Percutaneous transluminal coronary angioplasty hardware entrapment: guidewire entrapment. J Cardiovasc Med (Hagerstown) 2008;9(11):1140–1141

Collins N, Horlick E, Dzavik V. Triple wire technique for removal of fractured angioplasty guidewire. J Invasive Cardiol 2007;19(8):E230–E234

Kang JH, Rha SW, Lee DI, et al. Successful retrieval of a fractured and entrapped 0.035-inch Terumo wire in the femoral artery using biopsy forceps. Korean Circ J 2012;42(3):201–204

Martí V, Markarian L. Angioplasty guidewire entrapment after stent implantation: report of two cases and review of the literature. Arch Cardiol Mex 2007;77(1):54–57

Ozkan M, Yokusoglu M, Uzun M. Retained percutaneous transluminal coronary angioplasty guidewire in coronary circulation. Acta Cardiol 2005;60(6):653–654

Rossi M, Citone M, Krokidis M, Varano G, Orgera G. Percutaneous retrieval of a guidewire fragment with the use of an angioplasty balloon and an angiographic catheter: the sandwich technique. Cardiovasc Interv Radiol 2013;36(6):1707–1710

Hydrophilic-coated wire scaling during puncture needle manipulation (case 2)

Patient History

An 83-year-old man was scheduled for diagnostic angiography (DA) for further evaluation of lower limb claudication. Both limbs were symptomatic.

Initial Treatment Received

Failed ipsilateral retrograde groin access, therefore switching to right-side contralateral retrograde groin puncture for performing DA (**Fig. 4.23**).

Problems Encountered during Treatment

Due to failed placement of a sheath wire through the open Seldinger needle for further retrograde sheath placement, the operator switched to a

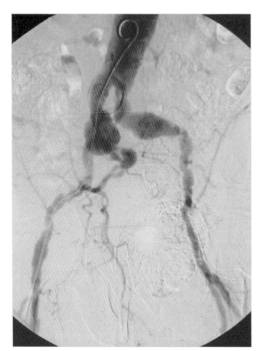

Fig. 4.23 DA from the right groin after failed retrograde access via the left groin. The left common femoral artery is not narrowed.

hydrophilic-coated wire. Slight advancement of the wire was possible, but access to the true vessel lumen failed and the attempt to remove the wire back through the needle was only successful under considerable force. On examination, it was noticed that the coating was torn from the wire core (Fig. 4.24).

Imaging Plan

Angiography from the contralateral groin in crossover technique to visualize any ripped-off hydrophilic coating potentially compromising blood flow.

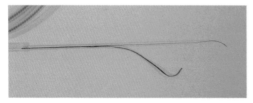

Fig. 4.24 Photograph of the retrieved wire after failed placement. Note the separation of hydrophilic coating and wire core. Parts of the distal hydrophilic coating are missing.

Resulting Complication

Intramural iatrogenic foreign body displacement of parts from hydrophylic coating.

Possible Strategies for Complication Management

- No action was undertaken due to the extraluminal position of the torn coating and the uncompromised flow verified by DA.
- In the case of an intraluminal position of the torn-off coating, attempts at placement of a snare to engage the foreign body would be recommended.
- Surgery (if an endovascular approach fails).

Final Complication Management

Everything was left as it was due to the uncompromised flow and the extraluminal position of the coating (Figs. 4.25 and 4.26). The patient was informed of the problem.

Complication Analysis

An uncontrolled manipulation of a hydrophilic guidewire in combination with a sharp stainless steel Seldinger needle resulted in snarling of the coating.

Prevention Strategies and Take-home Message

- Never remove a wire in an uncontrolled manner back through a Seldinger needle.
- If during guidewire manipulation a resistance is noticed, the wire with the entire

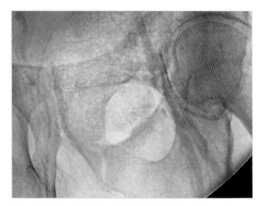

Fig. 4.25 Magnified angiography indicating the extraluminal position of the separated hydrophylic wire coating.

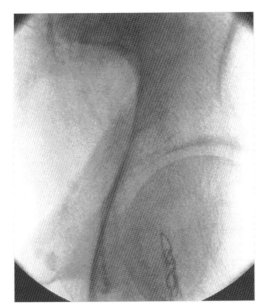

Fig. 4.26 Fluoroscopy in oblique projection showing the torn-off wire coating.

needle needs to be removed in order to avoid any damage of the hydrophilic coating with resulting ripping and potential compromise of blood flow or embolization.

Further Reading

Kang JH, Rha SW, Lee DI, et al. Successful retrieval of a fractured and entrapped 0.035-inch Terumo wire in the femoral artery using biopsy forceps. Korean Circ J 2012;42(3):201–204

Patel T, Shah S, Pandya R, Sanghvi K, Fonseca K. Broken guidewire fragment: a simplified retrieval technique. Catheter Cardiovasc Interv 2000;51:483–486

Rossi M, Citone M, Krokidis M, Varano G, Orgera G. Percutaneous retrieval of a guidewire fragment with the use of an angioplasty balloon and an angiographic catheter: the sandwich technique. Cardiovasc Interv Radiol 2013;36(6):1707–1710

Van Gaal WJ, Porto I, Banning AP. Guidewire fracture with retained filament in the LAD and aorta. Int J Cardiol 2006;112:e9–e11

Complex iatrogenic femoral arterial access injury

Patient History

A 48-year-old man suffered from severe upper thigh pain that developed immediately after diagnostic coronary angiography via retrograde access to the right common femoral artery (CFA). Apart from his coronary heart disease no further comorbidities were reported.

Hemostasis of the puncture site was achieved with manual compression. Clinical inspection showed right groin and upper thigh swelling, while clinical examination revealed a deep palpating mass and an upper thigh bruit.

Initial Treatment Received

Diagnostic coronary angiography.

Problems Encountered during Treatment

Multiple punctures in order to gain right femoral artery access. Otherwise no obvious complications were encountered during the procedure.

Imaging Plan

Color Doppler ultrasonography, followed by computed tomography angiography (CTA) if necessary. Reservation of digital subtraction angiography (DSA) through a contralateral femoral approach in case endovascular repair was considered.

Resulting Complication

Deep femoral artery (DFA) pseudoaneurysm (PA) with extensive mural thrombus and small residual lumen (**Fig. 4.27**) in combination with ipsilateral arteriovenous fistula (AVF) between superficial femoral artery (SFA) and common femoral vein (CFV) (**Fig. 4.28**) verified by color Doppler ultrasound.

Possible Strategies for Complication Management

- Close observation for smaller PAs and AVFs as there is a possibility of spontaneous closure.
- Noninvasive procedures such as prolonged pressure bandaging and ultrasound-guided compression.
- Percutaneous ultrasound-guided thrombin injection for the treatment of PAs.
- Stent graft implantation mostly through percutaneous contralateral retrograde access to the CFA.
- Catheterization of the feeder vessel, for example using a microcatheter and followed by selective microcoil embolization.
- Alternative agents for embolization: glue, large particles, gelfoam.
- Surgery (if endovascular approach fails).

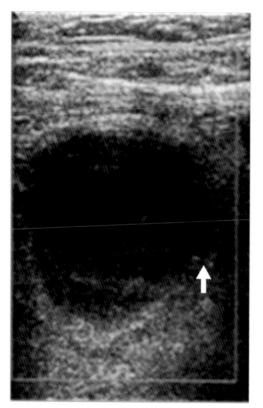

Fig. 4.27 Color ultrasonography shows a 3-cm right DFA pseudoaneurysm mostly occupied by mural thrombus and small residual lumen (*arrow*).

Final Complication Management

Compression to the right groin using the ultrasound probe for 30 minutes failed to seal both the AVF and the PA. Endovascular treatment via contralateral retrograde access to the CFA (8F

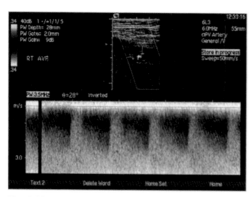

Fig. 4.28 Color Doppler ultrasound depicts a fistulous track between right SFA and CFV verified by a mixture of colors and increased Doppler waveform velocities.

45-cm-long sheath) was attempted next. Selective right CFA and SFA angiograms confirmed the presence of a PA originating from a DFA branch in combination with an AVF between proximal SFA and CFV (**Figs. 4.29** and **4.30**).

Initially a 6 × 40-mm self-expandable covered stent (Fluency, Bard PV) (**Fig. 4.31**) was deployed at the site of the AVF (**Fig. 4.32**), and subsequently the DFA branch from which the PA originated was superselectively catheterized with a 2.4F 130-cm-long coaxial microcatheter (Progreat, Terumo) (**Fig. 4.33**) and embolized with a 4-mm microcoil (**Fig. 4.34**).

Complication Analysis

Before gaining proper femoral arterial access, multiple unsuccessful low femoral punctures were made, which resulted in perforation (with subsequent pseudoaneurysm development) of a DFA branch as well as AVF development between the SFA and CFV.

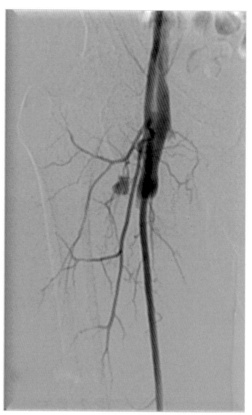

Fig. 4.29 Selective right common femoral angiogram demonstrates the pseudoaneurysm originating from a DFA branch and the AVF between proximal SFA and CFV.

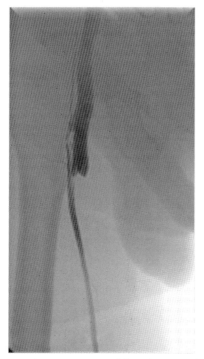

Fig. 4.30 Selective angiogram of the right proximal SFA demonstrates the precise site of the AVF.

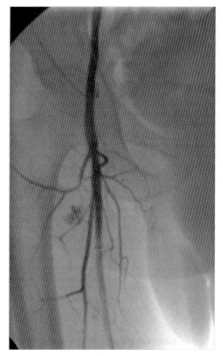

Fig. 4.32 A 6 × 40-mm self-expandable Fluency covered stent was deployed that successfully sealed the AVF.

Prevention Strategies and Take-home Message

- Avoid low femoral puncture, especially in obese patients in whom external landmarks for puncture (e.g., inguinal crease) can be misleading.

- Ultrasound guidance for CFA access is strongly recommended in obese patients, in patients with weak femoral pulse, and following initial "blind" unsuccessful puncture attempts.
- Color Doppler ultrasound should be the first imaging modality to detect all types of femoral arterial access complications in symptomatic patients.

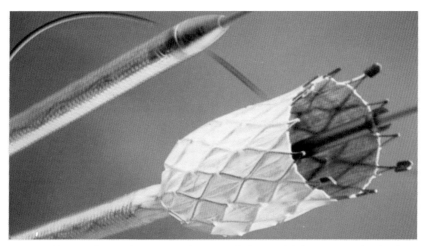

Fig. 4.31 Fluency self-expanding stent graft composed of a nitinol skeleton encapsulated with two ultrathin e-PTFE (expanded polytetrafluoroethylene) layers.

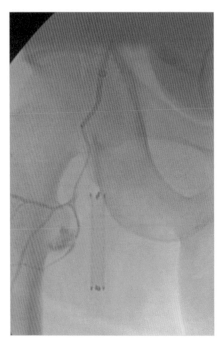

Fig. 4.33 Superselective catheterization with a 2.4F 130-cm-long coaxial microcatheter of the DFA branch from which the pseudoaneurysm originates.

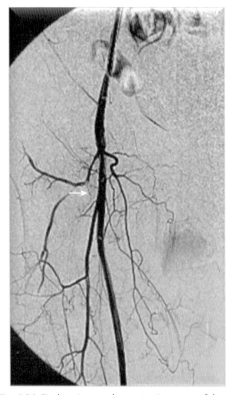

Fig. 4.34 Final angiogram demonstrating successful sealing of both the pseudoaneurysm with a microcoil (*arrow*) and AVF by a stent graft.

Further Reading

Deitch SG, Gupta R. Radioembolization complicated by dissection of the common femoral artery. Semin Interv Radiol 2011;28(2):133–136

Merriweather N, Sulzbach-Hoke LM. Managing risk of complications at femoral vascular access sites in percutaneous coronary intervention. Crit Care Nurs 2012;32(5):16–29

Tavris DR, Wang Y, Jacobs S, et al. Bleeding and vascular complications at the femoral access site following percutaneous coronary intervention (PCI): an evaluation of hemostasis strategies. J Invasive Cardiol 2012;24(7):328–334

Bleeding complication due to an unrecognized side-branch perforation during retrograde groin access for PCI

Patient History

An 82-year-old woman suffered from mild right groin hematoma and groin swelling, and onset of abdominal pain several hours after retrograde groin access for percutaneous coronary intervention (PCI) and final vascular closure with a 6F StarClose device (Abbott Vascular). Red blood cell count showed a significant decrease. The clinical condition of the woman declined significantly and contrast-enhanced computed tomography (CT) was initiated.

Initial Treatment Received

PCI.

Problems Encountered during Treatment

Unremarkable procedure, no complications reported!

Imaging Plan

Contrast-enhanced CT.

Resulting Complication

A huge retroperitoneal hematoma was depicted in CT, reaching to the liver (**Fig. 4.35**) and showing contrast media extravasation at the right-side abdominal wall as an indicator of an active source of bleeding (**Fig. 4.36**). Questioning the operator for any problems during the recent PCI revealed that the patient had experienced an episode of heavy flank pain during hydrophilic guidewire advancement, which was self-limiting (after guidewire removal)!

Possible Strategies for Complication Management

- Endovascular treatment via contralateral or ipsilateral retrograde access to the common

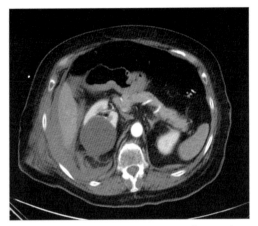

Fig. 4.35 Axial contrast-enhanced CT scan showing the retroperitoneal hematoma reaching to the liver and the pararenal space.

femoral artery (CFA); angiography via the sheath/catheter to evaluate the exact origin of the bleeding. Preparation of selective catheterization of the feeder vessel, for example using a microcatheter, and followed by selective microcoil embolization distally and proximally to the bleeding source.
- Alternatives for embolization: glue, large particles, gelfoam.
- Surgery (if an endovascular approach fails).

Final Complication Management

Endovascular treatment via an ipsilateral retrograde access to the CFA (4F sheath, 10 cm long)

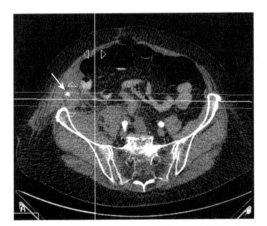

Fig. 4.36 Axial contrast-enhanced CT scan at the level of the anterior superior spine. A focal area of hyperdensity (*arrow*) is located at the inner side of the anterior oblique abdominal muscle.

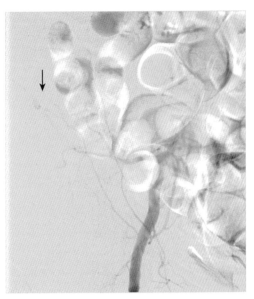

Fig. 4.37 Angiography of the right CFA and external iliac artery via the 4F sheath. The early phase depicts the deep circumflex iliac artery as the source of bleeding (*arrow*).

was performed. After placement of a 2.7F microcatheter, the deep circumflex iliac artery was cannulated; contrast injection verified the bleeding source (**Figs. 4.37** and **4.38**). The microcatheter was placed beyond the bleeding source and two 4-mm coils were implanted (0.018-inch compatible). The coiling was completed by implanting

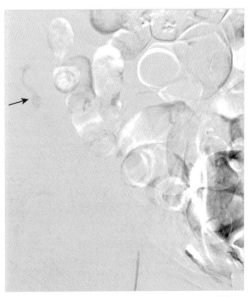

Fig. 4.38 Angiography of the right CFA and external iliac artery via the 4F sheath. The later phase depicts a large area of contrast extravasation (*arrow*).

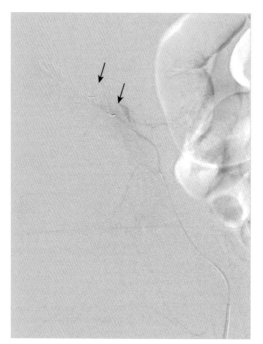

Fig. 4.39 Angiography after endovascular placement of a 2.7F microcatheter positioned in the deep circumflex iliac artery. Coils (4 mm, 0.018-inch compatible) were placed proximally and distally to the source of hemorrhage to rule out "back-door" bleeding (*arrows*).

additional coils proximally to the source of bleeding (**Fig. 4.39**).

Complication Analysis

Unrecognized hydrophilic-coated guidewire advancement into a hypogastric side branch resulted in vessel perforation and hemorrhage. Anticoagulation following the PCI procedure might have aggravated the extent of the bleeding. However, the fact that the operator ignored the sudden onset of self-limiting flank pain also contributed to the development of this complication.

Prevention Strategies Take-home Message

- Always visually control endovascular tools. Especially when using guidewires with a hydrophilic-coated tip, the distal position of the wire should be controlled by fluoroscopy and advanced with care.

- If the patient reports sudden and unexpected pain, the operator should check his or her tools and rule out any complication; the patient is always right until proven otherwise!
- Follow up your patients clinically; in case of any uncertainty, indicate further diagnostics!

Further Reading

Kiviniemi T, Puurunen M, Schlitt A, et al. Performance of bleeding risk-prediction scores in patients with atrial fibrillation undergoing percutaneous coronary intervention. Am J Cardiol 2014;113(12):1995–2001

Lee MS, Applegate B, Rao SV, Kirtane AJ, Seto A, Stone GW. Minimizing femoral artery access complications during percutaneous coronary intervention: a comprehensive review. Catheter Cardiovasc Interv 2014;84(1):62–69

Mamas MA, Anderson SG, Carr M, et al. Baseline bleeding risk and arterial access site practice in relation to procedural outcomes after percutaneous coronary intervention. J Am Coll Cardiol 2014;64(15):1554–1564

Stone PA, Campbell JE, AbuRahma AF. Femoral pseudoaneurysms after percutaneous access. J Vasc Surg 2014;60(5):1359–1366

Rupture of a deep femoral artery side branch during diagnostic angiography

Patient History

A 75-year-old patient with suspected bilateral carotid artery stenosis was referred for diagnostic angiography (DA). The patient was on low-dose aspirin and had received a loading dose of 300 mg of clopidogrel before the diagnostic procedure.

Initial Treatment Received

None.

Problems Encountered during Treatment

Multiple attempts were made to puncture the right common femoral artery (CFA). However, access was created in the proximal aspect of the superficial femoral artery (SFA). Shortly after placement of a 5F standard sheath the patient presented clinical signs of hypovolemia (hypotension, dizziness, cold sweats). He also complained about pain in his right groin, which appeared tender and swollen.

Imaging Plan

Angiography via the sheath in the right femoral artery was performed in order to detect possible vascular injury.

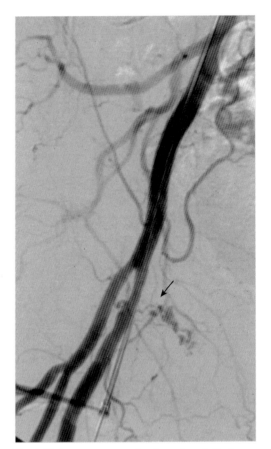

Fig. 4.40 Contrast extravasation (*arrow*) medial to the SFA after sheath insertion.

Resulting Complication

There was active contrast extravasation close to the access site; however, the exact source was unclear (**Fig. 4.40**).

Possible Strategies for Complication Management

- Upsizing sheath to account for possible leakage from sheath entry point.
- Removal of the sheath and manual compression of the groin.
- Antegrade access from contralateral groin in crossover technique; balloon tamponade, detection of bleeding source and further techniques (stent graft, embolization).
- Surgery (if endovascular approach fails).

Final Complication Management

Endovascular treatment via a left retrograde femoral access with crossover cannulation of the right iliac artery was initiated. Following a crossover manoeuver with a curved diagnostic catheter and a hydrophilic 0.035-inch guidewire, a 6F, 45-cm-long sheath was positioned with its tip in the external iliac artery. The guidewire was advanced into the SFA, the sheath was removed, and the proximal aspect of the vessel occluded for 5 minutes with a 6 × 40-mm standard balloon catheter.

Control angiography via the crossover sheath detected continuous bleeding and identified a side branch of the deep femoral artery as the actual bleeding source (**Fig. 4.41**). The deep femoral artery was cannulated using a diagnostic catheter and a hydrophilic 0.035-inch guidewire. A 2.7F microcatheter was advanced through the diagnostic catheter into the bleeding side branch, which was embolized with platinum microcoils (**Fig. 4.42**).

Postintervention no remaining extravasation was detected (**Fig. 4.43**).

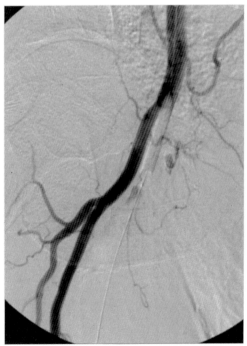

Fig. 4.41 Continuous contrast extravasation despite balloon tamponade of the arteriotomy, apparently due to injury of a side branch of the deep femoral artery.

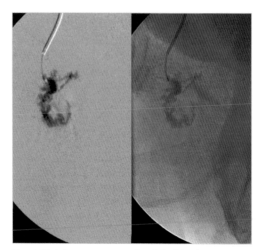

Fig. 4.42 Selective angiography of the bleeding side branch via a 2.7F microcatheter.

Complication Analysis

Multiple attempts to puncture the right CFA resulted in injury to a side branch of the deep femoral artery. Initial angiography via the sheath was misinterpreted and the actual injury was revealed after balloon tamponade of the arteriotomy was performed. Management of the complication was done endovascularly by microcoil embolization.

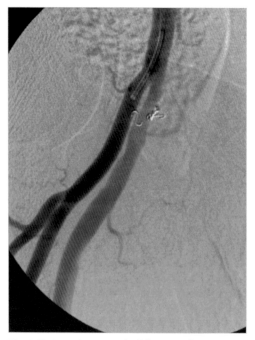

Fig. 4.43 Control angiography following coil embolization of the bleeding side branch of the deep femoral artery. No extravasation is visible.

Prevention Strategies and Take-home Message

- Limit the number of attempts to puncture the CFA.
- When encountering difficulties use ultrasound guidance to gather further anatomical information and enable proper puncture.
- Be aware of groin swelling and hematoma formation at the puncture site; do not hesitate to look for active bleeding, especially prior to further interventions.

Further Reading

Bates MC, Campbell JE. Technique for ipsilateral rescue embolization of common femoral side branch vessel injury. Catheter Cardiovasc Interv 2007;70(6):791–794

High common femoral artery puncture with sheath kinking

Patient History

A 63-year-old patient with right lower extremity intermittent claudication was referred to endovascular therapy for a distal stenosis of the right superficial femoral artery (SFA). Due to tortuous iliac artery anatomy an antegrade approach was chosen to address the lesion.

Initial Treatment Received

SFA intervention.

Problems Encountered during Treatment

Initial puncture of the CFA was uneventful and a 6F standard sheath could be inserted without any problems. A few minutes after sheath placement the patient complained about dizziness, sweating, and nausea. There was no bleeding or hematoma visible; however, blood pressure measurements showed a significant pressure drop, indicating acute volume loss.

Imaging Plan

Angiography via the sheath in the right femoral artery was performed in order to detect possible vascular injury.

Resulting Complication

Angiography revealed a high common femoral puncture close to the origin of the inferior epigastric artery. There was contrast extravasation from the sheath entry point due to kinking of the sheath (**Fig. 4.44**). Apparently the bleeding was into the retroperitoneum, not the groin, due to the high entry point of the sheath.

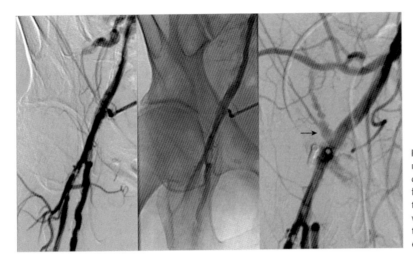

Fig. 4.44 Angiography revealed retroperitoneal contrast extravasation from the entry point of the kinked sheath, which was located close to the origin of the inferior epigastric artery (*arrow*).

Possible Strategies for Complication Management

- Upsizing the sheath to seal leakage at the entry point.
- Removal of the sheath and manual compression of the groin (least preferred option because bleeding was into the retroperitoneal space).
- Antegrade access from contralateral groin using crossover technique and balloon tamponade.
- Further endovascular treatment (stent graft, embolization).
- Surgery (if an endovascular approach fails).

Final Complication Management

To facilitate endovascular treatment of this complication the left femoral artery was punctured and retrograde femoral access was established. Following a crossover maneuver with a curved diagnostic catheter and a hydrophilic 0.035-inch guidewire, a 6F, 45-cm-long sheath was positioned with its tip in the external iliac artery. The guidewire was advanced into the SFA (**Fig. 4.45**), the kinked sheath was removed, and the puncture side occluded for 10 minutes with a 7 × 40-mm standard balloon catheter (**Fig. 4.46**). Control angiography via the crossover sheath did not show further bleeding (**Fig. 4.47**).

Complication Analysis

High puncture of the right common femoral artery (CFA) in combination with vessel calcification led to kinking of the sheath. The arteriotomy was not sufficiently sealed, which resulted in retroperitoneal hemorrhage. Balloon tamponade was performed and hemostasis was reached without the need for further interventions.

Prevention Strategies and Take-home Message

- With challenging groin anatomy, ultrasound guidance should be used to establish safe access to the CFA.

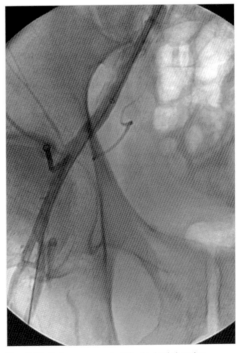

Fig. 4.45 Before removal of the kinked sheath a guidewire was advanced into the SFA.

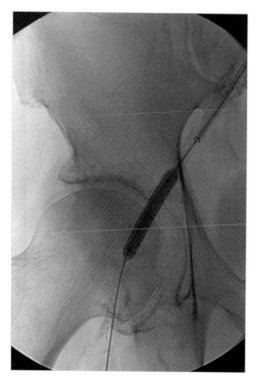

Fig. 4.46 Internal balloon tamponade at the puncture site using a 7 × 40-mm standard balloon catheter.

- The puncture should aim at the mid-level of the CFA over the femoral head.
- The puncture should aim at least 1 cm below the origin of the inferior epigastric artery to maintain a safe distance from the inguinal ligament and avoid retroperitoneal bleeding.
- Significant and life-threatening hemorrhage can arise from the groin access even if there is no swelling or hematoma formation at the puncture site.

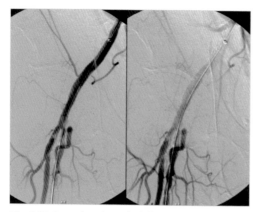

Fig. 4.47 Control angiography following sheath removal and 10 minutes balloon tamponade does not show signs of ongoing bleeding.

Further Reading

Seto AH, Abu-Fadel MS, Sparling JM, et al. Real-time ultrasound guidance facilitates femoral arterial access and reduces vascular complications: FAUST (Femoral Arterial Access With Ultrasound Trial). JACC Cardiovasc Interv 2010;3(7):751–758

Vavuranakis M, Kalogeras K, Vrachatis D, et al. Inferior epigastric artery as a landmark for transfemoral TAVI. Optimizing vascular access? Catheter Cardiovasc Interv 2013;81(6):1061–1066

Injury to the inferior epigastric artery during puncture

Patient History

A 43-year-old patient with lifestyle-limiting claudication was referred for endovascular treatment of TASC (TransAtlantic Inter-Society Consensus) B-type lesion in the left superficial femoral artery (SFA). The patient was obese and had typical risk factors of peripheral vascular disease with hypertension, nicotine use, and hypercholesterolemia.

Initial Treatment Received

None.

Problems Encountered during Treatment

Following local anesthesia the antegrade puncture of the left common femoral artery (CFA) was attempted. However, access to the artery was not reached and multiple punctures were tried. Before vessel access with wire insertion for sheath placement was established the patient started to complain of pain in the left groin. There was rapid development of tenderness and swelling in the left infrainguinal region. The patient also developed physiological signs of blood loss with development of hypotension and tachycardia, successfully controlled by leg elevation and fluid resuscitation. Injection of contrast medium through the puncture needle showed extravasation (**Fig. 4.48**).

Imaging Plan

Retrograde puncture of the contralateral CFA, crossover cannulation, and sheath placement to the left iliac artery to locate the suspected bleeding source.

Resulting Complication

There was active bleeding arising from the inferior epigastric artery due to a laceration (**Fig. 4.49**).

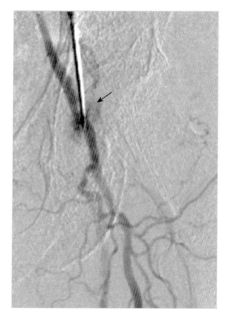

Fig. 4.48 Angiography via the puncture needle showed contrast medium extravasation.

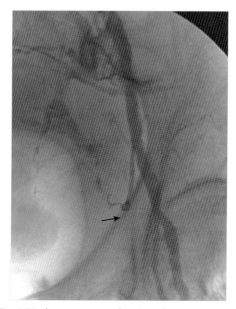

Fig. 4.50 Fluoroscopy view showing a diagnostic catheter in the bleeding artery.

Possible Strategies for Complication Management

- Manual compression of the groin.
- Balloon tamponade.
- Selective embolization.
- Surgery (if an endovascular approach fails).

Final Complication Management

Cannulation of the inferior epigastric artery and coil embolization (**Figs. 4.50** and **4.51**).

Complication Analysis

In obese patients the skin entry point for an antegrade puncture often has to be above the inguinal ligament in order to establish high enough access to the CFA, which is needed for intubation of the SFA. In this case multiple attempts to puncture the left CFA failed and one of the high punctures

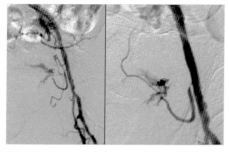

Fig. 4.49 Digital subtraction angiography showed laceration of the inferior epigastric artery and active bleeding.

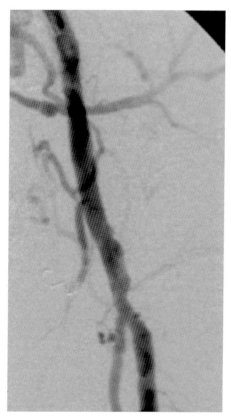

Fig. 4.51 Selective angiography showing the successfully embolized artery. No signs of continuous bleeding were present.

resulted in laceration of the inferior epigastric artery. Manual compression was performed initially; however, it could not control the bleeding. A diagnostic catheter tracked over a hydrophylic guidewire using the crossover technique could easily cannulate the bleeding vessel. A single 3-mm platinum coil was sufficient to seal the lacerated artery and led to hemostasis.

Prevention Strategies and Take-home Message

- If the anatomy of the CFA is uncertain (i.e., obese patients, nonpalpable pulse), a Doppler probe or B-mode ultrasound should be used in order to gather further anatomical information.
- When performing antegrade punctures, start as distally as possible and aim at the segment of the CFA over the femoral head.
- Be aware of groin swelling and hematoma formation at the puncture site. Do not hesitate to look for potential bleeding sources, and be prepared for contralateral access.

Further Reading

Park SW, Ko SY, Yoon SY, et al. Transcatheter arterial embolization for hemoperitoneum: unusual manifestation of iatrogenic injury to abdominal muscular arteries. Abdom Imaging 2011;36(1):74–78

Park YJ, Lee SY, Kim SH, Kim IH, Kim SW, Lee SO. Transcatheter coil embolization of the inferior epigastric artery in a huge abdominal wall hematoma caused by paracentesis in a patient with liver cirrhosis. Korean J Hepatol 2011;17(3):233–237

Sanchez CE, Helmy T. Percutaneous management of inferior epigastric artery injury after cardiac catheterization. Catheter Cardiovasc Interv 2012;79(4):633–637

Sobkin PR, Bloom AI, Wilson MW, et al. Massive abdominal wall hemorrhage from injury to the inferior epigastric artery: a retrospective review. J Vasc Interv Radiol 2008;19(3):327–332

Yalamanchili S, Harvey SM, Friedman A, Shams JN, Silberzweig JE. Transarterial embolization for inferior epigastric artery injury. Vasc Endovasc Surg 2008;42(5):489–493

Retrograde groin access complicated by external iliac artery dissection (case 1)

Patient History

In a 65-year-old man with buttock claudication, color duplex ultrasound detected common iliac artery (CIA) stenosis. The patient presented for interventional treatment. Apart from hypertension no further cardiovascular risk factors were present.

Initial Treatment Received

None.

Problems Encountered during Treatment

Following local anesthesia in the left groin, retrograde puncture of the common femoral artery (CFA) was performed. During insertion of the introducer wire, resistance was felt; however, the guidewire was further advanced. During the maneuver the patient complained of moderate pain in the left pelvis/groin area. A standard 4F vascular sheath was inserted.

Imaging Plan

Angiography.

Resulting Complication

There was extensive dissection of the external iliac artery (EIA) reaching into the CFA (**Fig. 4.52**). Angiography revealed the position of the sheath to be subintimal (**Fig. 4.53**). The femoral pulse was still palpable and the patient did not present with any clinical signs of acute limb ischemia.

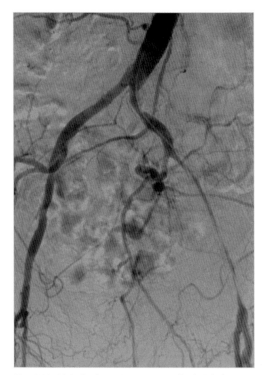

Fig. 4.52 Digital subtraction angiography (DSA) showing extensive dissection of the left EIA.

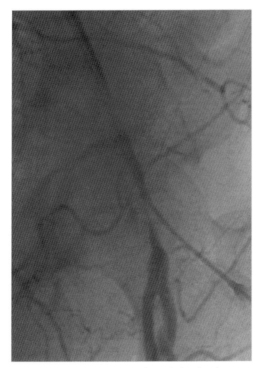

Fig. 4.53 DSA of the left groin through the sheath showing a subintimal position of the device.

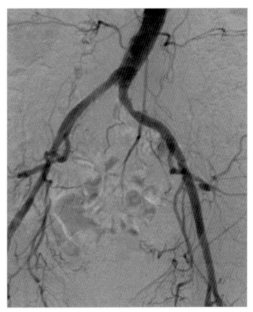

Fig. 4.54 DSA 2 days after failed access and dissection showing restitution of the lumen and realignment of the intimal flap.

Possible Strategies for Complication Management

- Crossover recanalization of the true lumen; angioplasty and consecutive stent placement (not preferred because of extension of the dissection into the CFA).
- Abort procedure. Removal of the sheath and manual compression of the groin. Clinical re-evaluation.
- Surgery (if endovascular approach fails).

Final Complication Management

Because the femoral pulse in the left groin was palpable and no clinical signs of acute limb ischemia were present, it was decided to abort the procedure and remove the sheath. Manual compression was performed and hemostasis achieved. The patient was heparinized and re-scheduled for angiography from the contralateral groin 2 days later. This follow-up study showed total restitution of the EIA lumen without need for further treatment (**Fig. 4.54**). The stenosis in the left CIA was successfully stented during this procedure.

Complication Analysis

Guidewire advancement through the puncture needle was performed despite resistance. Apparently the sheath wire had entered the subintimal space and was further introduced, which dissected the EIA. Antegrade blood flow in the iliac artery was sufficient to realign the intimal flap to the vessel wall. Stent placement was not necessary.

Prevention Strategies and Take-home Message

- Introduction of a sheath wire must be performed carefully. If any resistance is felt during wire advancement, the position of the puncture needle should be corrected until free backflow is visible and easy movement of the wire is possible.
- In the case of uncertain needle location, contrast injections should be performed to rule out a subintimal position.
- Use ultrasound for needle guidance for difficult femoral access.

Further Reading

Kalish J, Eslami M, Gillespie D, et al; Vascular Study Group of New England. Routine use of ultrasound guidance in femoral arterial access for peripheral vascular intervention decreases groin hematoma rates. J Vasc Surg 2015;61(5):1231–1238.

Lo RC, Fokkema MT, Curran T, et al. Routine use of ultrasound-guided access reduces access site-related complications after lower extremity percutaneous revascularization. J Vasc Surg 2015;61(2):405–412

Stone PA, Campbell JE. Complications related to femoral artery access for transcatheter procedures. Vasc Endovasc Surg 2012;46(8):617–623

Tsetis D. Endovascular treatment of complications of femoral arterial access. Cardiovasc Interv Radiol 2010;33(3):457–468

Retrograde groin access complicated by external iliac artery dissection (case 2)

Patient History

A 72-year-old man with a long history of peripheral vascular disease presented with worsening claudication in his left leg. A high-grade stenosis of the left common femoral artery (CFA) was detected by ultrasound. The vascular surgeon requested diagnostic angiography (DA) before reconstructive surgery.

Initial Treatment Received

Status post right femoropopliteal bypass graft.

Problems Encountered during Treatment

Following local anesthesia in the right groin, retrograde puncture of the CFA was performed. Insertion of an introducer wire and placement of the 5F sheath were uneventful; however, angiography revealed extensive dissection of the right external iliac artery (EIA). During the procedure the patient developed rest pain in his right leg.

Imaging Plan

Angiography.

Resulting Complication

Extensive dissection of the right EIA (**Fig. 4.55**).

Possible Strategies for Complication Management

- Crossover recanalization of the true lumen from a retrograde left groin approach; angioplasty and consecutive stent placement (not preferred because of high-grade stenosis in the left CFA).
- Recanalization from a transbrachial approach; angioplasty and consecutive stent placement.
- Abort procedure. Removal of the sheath and manual compression of the groin (not preferred

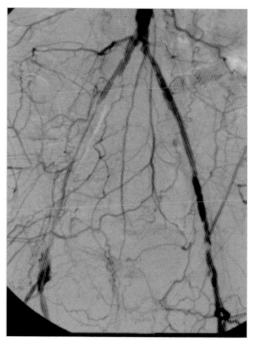

Fig. 4.55 Digital subtraction angiography (DSA) showing extensive dissection of the right EIA. Note the calcified plaque in the left EIA with high-grade stenosis.

because patient showed signs of acute limb ischemia).
- Surgery (if an endovascular approach fails).

Final Complication Management

Following retrograde puncture of the left brachial artery a 90-cm-long 6F sheath was positioned into the infrarenal aorta. The right iliac artery was recanalized with a diagnostic catheter and a 0.035-inch guidewire. Two self-expanding stents were implanted and postdilatated. Postinterventional angiography showed no residual stenosis or dissection (**Fig. 4.56**).

Complication Analysis

Despite uneventful puncture and sheath insertion, iatrogenic dissection of the right iliac access occurred. This complication is more common in patients with heavily diseased peripheral arteries. It can be treated endovascularly from the contralateral groin or a transbrachial approach as shown in this case.

Prevention Strategies and Take-home Message

- Iliac artery dissection from arterial groin access is rare, but potentially limb threatening.

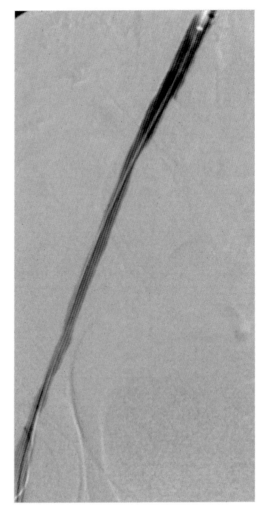

Fig. 4.56 DSA of the right groin following transbrachial stent placement showing successfully reconstituted lumen of the EIA.

- Introduction of the sheath must be performed carefully. If any resistance is felt during wire placement the position of the puncture needle should be corrected until free advancement is possible.
- If femoral access is difficult use ultrasound for needle guidance.
- Hemodynamically relevant iatrogenic dissection should be treated.

Further Reading

Kalish J, Eslami M, Gillespie D, et al; Vascular Study Group of New England. Routine use of ultrasound guidance in femoral arterial access for peripheral vascular intervention decreases groin hematoma rates. J Vasc Surg 2015;61(5):1231–1238

Lo RC, Fokkema MT, Curran T, et al. Routine use of ultrasound-guided access reduces access site-related complications after lower extremity percutaneous revascularization. J Vasc Surg 2015;61(2):405–412

Stone PA, Campbell JE. Complications related to femoral artery access for transcatheter procedures. Vasc Endovasc Surg 2012;46(8):617–623

Tsetis D. Endovascular treatment of complications of femoral arterial access. Cardiovasc Interv Radiol 2010;33(3):457–468

Superficial femoral artery wire perforation during access creation

Patient History

A 55-year-old man with claudication in his right leg presented for endovascular therapy. Noninvasive imaging showed a short-segment distal superficial femoral artery (SFA) occlusion.

Initial Treatment Received

Planned SFA intervention using antegrade puncture technique.

Problems Encountered during Treatment

For unknown reasons a distal direct puncture of the SFA was performed. Following arterial backflow from the puncture needle a sheath guidewire was advanced. Despite resistance during wire advancement a 6F 45-cm-long sheath was inserted. Immediately after access, the patient complained of tenderness and pain in his right groin.

Imaging Plan

Angiography via the sheath.

Resulting Complication

Angiography showed the direct SFA puncture and acute rupture of the artery approximately 2 cm distally to the sheath entry point (**Fig. 4.57**). Note the very low entry point of the sheath (*arrow*) in relation to the femoral head (**Fig. 4.58**). The ostium of the sheath was close to the site of the rupture (**Fig. 4.59**).

Possible Strategies for Complication Management

- Removal of the sheath and manual compression of the groin (not preferred because of distal sheath entry point and active bleeding).
- Antegrade access to the right common femoral artery (CFA) from a left contralateral retrograde groin approach.

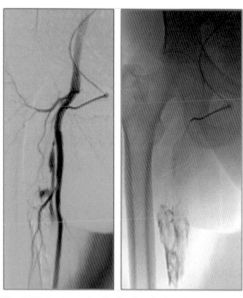

Fig. 4.57 Angiography via the sheath showing rupture of the SFA.

- Further endovascular treatment (stent graft, embolization).
- Surgery (if an endovascular approach fails).

Final Complication Management

Endovascular treatment was performed from a left retrograde femoral approach. Following a crossover maneuver with a curved diagnostic

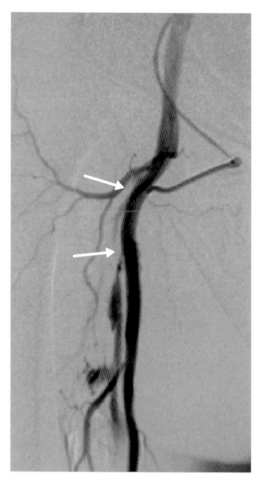

Fig. 4.59 Digital subtraction angiography (DSA) of the right femoral artery showing contrast extravasation and sheath entry point (*arrows*).

catheter and a hydrophilic 0.035-inch guidewire, a 6F 45-cm-long sheath was positioned with its tip in the external iliac artery. The guidewire was advanced distally to the malplaced sheath. To stop the bleeding, a 6 × 60-mm balloon catheter was inflated covering both the sheath entry point and the vessel rupture (images not shown). The sheath was then removed. After 10 minutes there was still bleeding from the ruptured SFA; thus, stent graft placement was indicated. A 6 × 60-mm stent graft (Fluency, Bard PV) was implanted successfully stopping the bleeding (**Fig. 4.60**).

Complication Analysis

In this case two problems were encountered. First, the distal direct puncture of the right SFA was already a risk factor for the development of a pseudoaneurysm because the location cannot

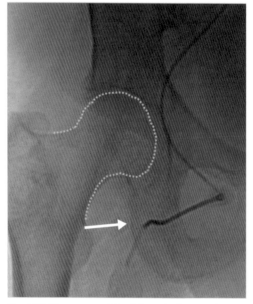

Fig. 4.58 Fluoroscopy of the right groin showing the distal entry point of the vascular sheath (*arrow*) in relation to the femoral head (*dotted line*).

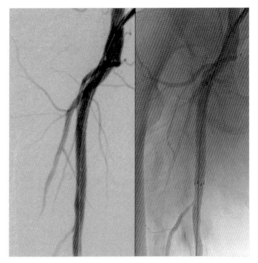

Fig. 4.60 Femoral DSA and diagnostic angiography after stent graft placement showing successful hemostasis.

easily be controlled with manual compression. In addition—due to uncontrolled wire advancement—there was rupture of the proximal SFA with active bleeding that was not managed by internal tamponade. A stent graft long enough to cover both openings in the artery was used successfully to close the vessel injuries without further clinical sequelae for the patient.

Prevention Strategies and Take-home Message

- In the case of challenging groin anatomy, ultrasound guidance should be used to ensure safe access to the CFA.
- Femoral arterial puncture should aim at the mid-third of the femoral head at least 1 cm below the origin of the inferior epigastric artery. In this segment the artery can be compressed against the femoral head to achieve hemostasis.
- The inguinal crease is an unreliable landmark when aiming at the CFA, especially in obese patients.
- Direct SFA puncture should be avoided because it is not easily managed by manual compression.
- Guidewires should not be advanced against resistance.
- Always be prepared to access the contralateral groin to be able to detect and treat vessel injury from failed inguinal puncture.

Further Reading

Gutzeit A, Graf N Schoch E, Sautter T, Jenelten R, Binkert CA. Ultrasound guided antegrade femoral access: comparison between the common femoral artery and the superficial femoral artery. Eur Radiol 2011;21(6):1323–1328

Kalish J, Eslami M, Gillespie D, et al; Vascular Study Group of New England. Routine use of ultrasound guidance in femoral arterial access for peripheral vascular intervention decreases groin hematoma rates. J Vasc Surg 2015;61(5):1231–1238

Lechner G, Jantsch H, Waneck R, Kretschmer G. The relationship between the common femoral artery, the inguinal crease, and the inguinal ligament: a guide to accurate angiographic puncture. Cardiovasc Interv Radiol 1988;11(3):165–169

Lee MS, Applegate B, Rao SV, Kirtane AJ, Seto A, Stone GW. Minimizing femoral artery access complications during percutaneous coronary intervention: a comprehensive review. Catheter Cardiovasc Interv 2014;84(1):62–69

Lo RC, Fokkema MT, Curran T, et al. Routine use of ultrasound-guided access reduces access site-related complications after lower extremity percutaneous revascularization. J Vasc Surg 2015;61(2):405–412

Merriweather N, Sulzbach-Hoke LM. Managing risk of complications at femoral vascular access sites in percutaneous coronary intervention. Crit Care Nurs 2012;32(5):16–29

Stone PA, Campbell JE. Complications related to femoral artery access for transcatheter procedures. Vasc Endovasc Surg 2012;46(8):617–623

Stone PA, Campbell JE, AbuRahma AF. Femoral pseudoaneurysms after percutaneous access. J Vasc Surg 2014;60(5):1359–1366

Tsetis D. Endovascular treatment of complications of femoral arterial access. Cardiovasc Interv Radiol 2010;33(3):457–468

4.2.2 Access Closure

Stent elongation during vascular closure

Patient History

A 62-year-old woman had undergone surgery (patch) of the common femoral artery (CFA) 6 weeks earlier. Upon presentation she still suffered from a limited walking distance (200 m) due to a moderate stenosis of the external iliac artery (EIA) above the inguinal ligament, which had been left untreated for unknown reasons during surgery. The patient was scheduled for endovascular treatment. Treatment plan included retrograde CFA puncture at the level of the patch, direct placement of a self-expanding stent, and closure of the puncture site using a vascular closure device.

Initial Treatment Received

CFA patch; in secondary endovascular procedure direct placement of a self-expanding stent (SES) (8 × 60 mm) followed by percutaneous transluminal angioplasty (PTA) (7 × 60 mm) through a 6F sheath (**Fig. 4.61**). Closure of the puncture site was performed with a StarClose Vascular Closure System (Abbott Vascular).

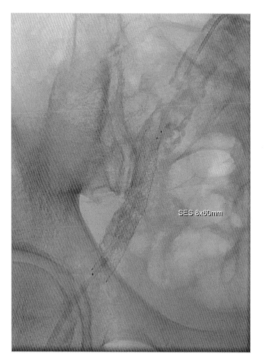

Fig. 4.61 Fluoroscopy of the deployed SES initially showed adequate stent integrity. A 4F diagnostic catheter and a 6F sheath are still in place. Note the distal end of the stent is located 1 cm distally to the innominate line and only a few millimeters proximal to the sheath ostium.

Problems Encountered during Treatment

Removal of the activated closure device after step 1 (unfolding of the nitinol anchor) was a little bit rugged. However, the subsequent procedural steps were unremarkable. The device was successfully removed and hemostasis achieved.

Imaging Plan

Fluoroscopy of the right groin including the EIA.

Resulting Complication

Distraction, elongation, and dislocation of the distal part of the stent towards the entry level of the sheath/closure device (**Fig. 4.62**).

Possible Strategies for Complication Management

- Endovascular management via contralateral groin access with placement of an additional stent using crossover technique. This is only possible if the disintegrated stent is located fully inside the vessel.
- Surgical repair (if an endovascular approach fails).

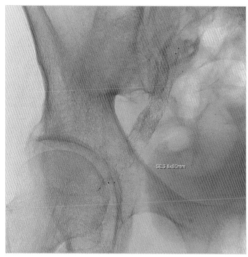

Fig. 4.62 Fluoroscopy of the distracted stent. The struts above and below the innominate line are distracted down towards the entry-level site at the anterior wall of the CFA patch. The distal stent markers are at different levels, indicating the complete disintegration of the distal stent struts.

Final Complication Management

The complication was managed surgically because it was unclear whether parts of the stent had left the vessel through the puncture site. The vessel was visually inspected and the disrupted stent struts were fixed to the vessel wall by intraoperative stenting with an additional SES. In retrospect the endovascular approach using a crossover technique might also have been possible.

Complication Analysis

Apparently, the nitinol anchor of the vascular closure device had engaged the distal end of the stent (**Fig. 4.63**). The stent struts probably got caught by the anchor so that removal of the system resulted in disintegration and dislocation of parts of the stent.

Prevention Strategies and Take-home Message

- Carefully evaluate the level of vessel access in order to guarantee suitability for a vascular closure device (nondiseased, non–heavily calcified CFA, no deep femoral or superficial femoral artery puncture).
- If the puncture level of the CFA is uncertain (i.e., obese patients, nonpalpable pulse), diagnostic angiography should be used in order to gather further anatomical information.

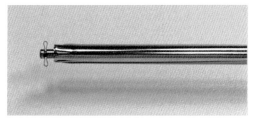

Fig. 4.63 Photograph of the distal part of the StarClose device with the activated nitinol loop anchor. The anchor should help to bring the device into the correct position at the inner side of the anterior arterial vessel wall prior to activating the nitinol clip for vascular closure at the outside of the vascular wall. While bringing down the clip to anterior vessel wall, the anchor is deactivated (infolded into the delivery device).

- Insert and activate vascular closure devices under fluoroscopy to rule out any interaction between devices and stent (struts).
- In the case of a known vascular implant near a puncture site check the correct position of the vascular closure device before activation.
- Use manual compression instead of a closure device if safe application of the device cannot be guaranteed.
- Use contralateral groin or an alternative access routes (radial or brachial approaches) in iliac procedures close inguinal ligament.

Further Reading

Durack JC, Thor Johnson D, Fidelman N, Kerlan RK, LaBerge JM. Entrapment of the StarClose Vascular Closure System after attempted common femoral artery deployment. Cardiovasc Interv Radiol 2012;35(4):942–944

Johnson DT, Durack JC, Fidelman N, Kerlan RK, LaBerge JM. Distribution of reported StarClose SE vascular closure device complications in the manufacturer and user facility device experience database. J Vasc Interv Radiol 2013;24(7):1051–1056

Varghese R, Chess D, Lasorda D. Re-access complication with a Star-Close device. Catheter Cardiovasc Interv 2009;73(7):899–901

Insufficient common femoral artery access close after antegrade Angio-Seal application

Patient History

A 61-year-old man with limited walking distance of 100 m was treated successfully by angioplasty and stent placement in the distal superficial femoral artery (SFA). The patient had typical comorbidities (heavy smoker, hypertension, hyperlipidemia).

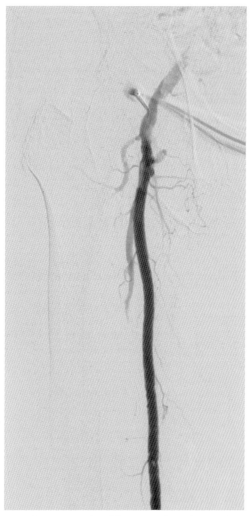

Fig. 4.64 Angiography of the proximal SFA showing the entrance level of the 6F sheath at the mid-part of the CFA.

Initial Treatment Received

Access route was via the ipsilateral common femoral artery (CFA) through a regular 6F sheath (**Fig. 4.64**). Groin puncture and treatment of index lesion was uneventful. Angioplasty (5 × 100 mm) was performed after passing the high-grade stenosis with an 0.018-inch hydrophilic-tip wire. Due to flow-limiting dissection with severe recoil, placement of a self-expanding stent (5 × 100 mm) was performed. Closure of the puncture site was managed with a vascular closure device (Angio-Seal, St. Jude Medical).

Problems Encountered during Treatment

Angio-Seal application was according to the instructions for use; however, during the pulling maneuver the suture tore apart. Because hemostasis was insufficient the procedure was completed by manual compression for 10 minutes. The next day the patient presented with intermittent pain at rest and a limited walking capacity of less than 10 m.

Imaging Plan

Color duplex ultrasound for further evaluation.

Resulting Complication

Dislocation of the entire Angio-Seal anchor with the collagen plug and parts of the suture into the mid-part of the SFA (**Fig. 4.65**).

Possible Strategies for Complication Management

- Retrograde puncture of the contralateral groin. Placement of a long 6F sheath into the ipsilateral SFA using crossover technique. Try to perform a snaring maneuver of the dislodged Angio-Seal using a small snare or a stent retriever (originally intended for thromboembolism removal during acute stroke management).
- Stenting of the iatrogenic stenosis using crossover technique.
- Surgical removal of the dislodged Angio-Seal (if endovascular approach fails).

Final Complication Management

Surgical cut-down of the ipsilateral groin and removal of the dislodged material using Fogarty maneuver.

Complication Analysis

Closure devices with intraluminal anchor and collagen plug need a considerable amount of pulling force to fixate the anchor at the anterior vessel wall. This maneuver gives enough stability for pressing the collagen plug onto the vessel. In most cases successful sealing of the puncture site is achieved. In this case the Angio-Seal suture ruptured and parts of the closure device embolized into the SFA. This is more likely to happen with calcified plaque burden, which might be sharp enough to damage the suture, resulting in rupture. In this particular case the anchor may have been caught intraluminally by plaque material, leading to delivery of collagen material into the vessel.

Prevention Strategies and Take-home Message

- Handle instruments with care. Pull the suture carefully but with enough force to completely

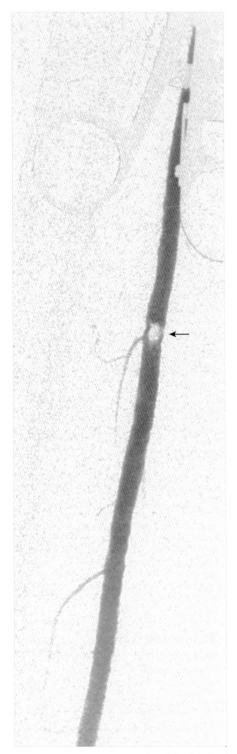

Fig. 4.65 Intraoperative angiography of the dislodged Angio-Seal anchor and plug in the proximal part of the SFA (*arrow*), which resulted in a severe, symptomatic high-grade stenosis.

seal by pushing the collagen down towards the outer anterior vessel wall while holding the suture tight.

- When vascular closure devices do not result in hemostasis and manual compression is to be performed the patient must be clinically observed to rule out complications. Before discharge, the puncture sites should be evaluated by ultrasound to check for local groin complications.

Further Reading

Applegate RJ, Sacrinty M, Kutcher MA, et al. Vascular complications with newer generations of Angio-Seal vascular closure devices. J Interv Cardiol 2006;19(1):67–74

Azmoon S, Pucillo AL, Aronow WS, et al. Vascular complications after percutaneous coronary intervention following hemostasis with the Mynx vascular closure device versus the Angio-Seal vascular closure device. J Invasive Cardiol 2010;22(4):175–178

Carey D, Martin JR, Moore CA, Valentine MC, Nygaard TW. Complications of femoral artery closure devices. Catheter Cardiovasc Interv 2001;52(1):3–7

Corley JA, Kasliwal MK, Tan LA, Lopes DK. Delayed vascular claudication following diagnostic cerebral angiography: a rare complication of the Angio-Seal arteriotomy closure device. J Cerebrovasc Endovasc Neurosurg 2014;16(3):275–280

Eggebrecht H, Von Birgelen C, Naber C, et al. Impact of gender on femoral access complications secondary to application of a collagen-based vascular closure device. J Invasive Cardiol 2004;16(5):247–250

Fargen KM, Velat GJ, Lawson MF, et al. Occurrence of angiographic femoral artery complications after vascular closure with Mynx and Angio-Seal. J Neurointerv Surg 2013;5(2):161–164

Klocker J, Gratl A, Chemelli A, Moes N, Goebel G, Fraedrich G. Influence of use of a vascular closure device on incidence and surgical management of access site complications after percutaneous interventions. Eur J Vasc Endovasc Surg 2011;42(2):230–235

Mukhopadhyay K, Puckett MA, Roobottom CA. Efficacy and complications of Angio-Seal in antegrade puncture. Eur J Radiol 2005;56(3):409–412

Prabhudesai A, Khan MZ. An unusual cause of femoral embolism: angioseal. Ann R Coll Surg Engl 2000;82(5):355–356

Suri S, Nagarsheth KH, Goraya S, Singh K. A novel technique to retrieve a maldeployed vascular closure device. J Endovasc Ther 2015;22(1):71–73

Thalhammer C, Joerg GR, Roffi M, Husmann M, Pfammatter T, Amann-Vesti BR. Endovascular treatment of Angio-Seal-related limb ischemia—primary results and long-term follow-up. Catheter Cardiovasc Interv 2010;75(6):823–827

Wille J, Vos JA, Overtoom TT, Suttorp MJ, Van de Pavoordt ED, De Vries JP. Acute leg ischemia: the dark side of a percutaneous femoral artery closure device. Ann Vasc Surg 2006;20(2):278–281

Impairment of walking capacity after retrograde Angio-Seal access closure

Patient History

A 39-year-old woman was scheduled for percutaneous coronary intervention (PCI). PCI was suc-

cessful and uneventful; a vascular closure device was used for management of vascular access.

Initial Treatment Received

Retrograde 6F access at the level of the common femoral artery (CFA) was used for percutaneous transluminal angioplasty (PTA). The right groin access was closed with an Angio-Seal 6F (St. Jude Medical). Closure of the puncture site was successful and hemostasis initially achieved.

Problems Encountered during Treatment

Angio-Seal application was according to the instructions for use. No adverse events were noted. The next day prior to discharge, the patient reported a limited walking capacity of less than 50 m (ipsilateral, right-side lower limb).

Imaging Plan

Color duplex ultrasound for further evaluation. Additional computed tomography angiography (CTA) was performed.

Resulting Complication

Severe short-segment stenosis was depicted at the puncture site level of the CFA (**Figs. 4.66–4.68**). The Angio-Seal anchor, probably including the

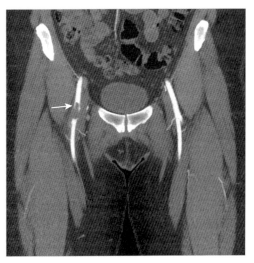

Fig. 4.66 CTA at the level of the CFA (coronal reconstruction). The right CFA is not significantly filled with contrast media (*arrow*), whereas the contralateral side is visible (also a main deep femoral artery branch).

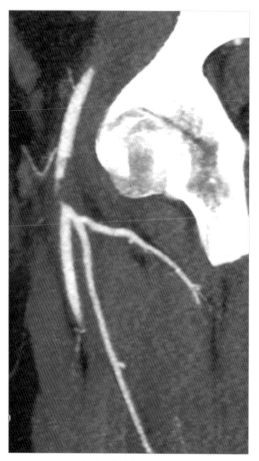

Fig. 4.67 CTA at the level of the CFA (sagittal reconstruction). The right CFA is not significantly filled with contrast media and shows severe stenosis, whereas a main deep femoral artery branch and the origin of the superficial femoral artery (SFA) are not compromised.

plug and parts of the suture, caused a severe stenosis.

Possible Strategies for Complication Management

- Endovascular management with stent placement (con: flexion zone, near femoral bifurcation).
- Open surgical groin access with removal of foreign body and reconstruction of the CFA.

Final Complication Management

Surgical cut-down of the ipsilateral groin and re-moval of the Angio-Seal material and finalizing open repair with patch plasty (**Fig. 4.69**).

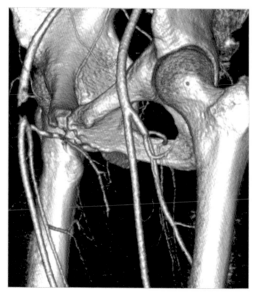

Fig. 4.68 CTA (volume-rendering technique) at the level of the CFA. The right CFA is not significantly filled with contrast media, whereas the contralateral side appears uncompromised.

Complication Analysis

Closure devices with intraluminal anchor and col-lagen plug need a considerable amount of pulling force to fixate the anchor to the anterior vessel wall. This maneuver is necessary to stabilize the anchor before pressing the collagen plug onto the vessel. In the current case the anchor and parts of the collagen plug were found inside the vessel lumen. This complication is possible when the anchor is caught by plaque material inside the vessel so that delivery of the collagen material can end up in the vessel lumen. In the present case no plaque or underlying CFA stenosis was visible. The initial pulling maneuver of the suture was probably insufficient so that collagen mate-rial was delivered to the anchor still located inside the vessel and away from the puncture site.

Prevention Strategies and Take-home Message

- Handle instruments with care. Pull the suture carefully, but with enough force to achieve complete sealing when pushing the collagen down towards the outer anterior vessel wall.
- When a vascular closure device is used patients should be evaluated clinically and/or by Doppler ultrasound before they are discharged to rule out complications.

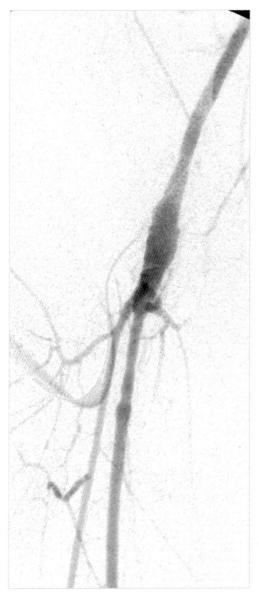

Fig. 4.69 Intraoperative angiography after Angio-Seal removal and groin repair by patch plasty at the CFA level.

Further Reading

Applegate RJ, Sacrinty M, Kutcher MA, et al. Vascular complications with newer generations of Angio-Seal vascular closure devices. J Interv Cardiol 2006;19(1):67–74

Azmoon S, Pucillo AL, Aronow WS, et al. Vascular complications after percutaneous coronary intervention following hemostasis with the Mynx vascular closure device versus the Angio-Seal vascular closure device. J Invasive Cardiol 2010;22(4):175–178

Carey D, Martin JR, Moore CA, Valentine MC, Nygaard TW. Complications of femoral artery closure devices. Catheter Cardiovasc Interv 2001;52(1):3–7

Corley JA, Kasliwal MK, Tan LA, Lopes DK. Delayed vascular claudication following diagnostic cerebral angiography: a rare complication of the Angio-Seal arteriotomy closure device. J Cerebrovasc Endovasc Neurosurg 2014;16(3):275–280

Eggebrecht H, Von Birgelen C, Naber C, et al. Impact of gender on femoral access complications secondary to application of a collagen-based vascular closure device. J Invasive Cardiol 2004;16(5):247–250

Fargen KM, Velat GJ, Lawson MF, et al. Occurrence of angiographic femoral artery complications after vascular closure with Mynx and Angio-Seal. J Neurointerv Surg 2013;5(2):161–164

Klocker J, Gratl A, Chemelli A, Moes N, Goebel G, Fraedrich G. Influence of use of a vascular closure device on incidence and surgical management of access site complications after percutaneous interventions. Eur J Vasc Endovasc Surg 2011;42(2):230–235

Mukhopadhyay K, Puckett MA, Roobottom CA. Efficacy and complications of Angio-Seal in antegrade puncture. Eur J Radiol 2005;56(3):409–412

Prabhudesai A, Khan MZ. An unusual cause of femoral embolism: angioseal. Ann R Coll Surg Engl 2000;82(5):355–356

Thalhammer C, Joerg GR, Roffi M, Husmann M, Pfammatter T, Amann-Vesti BR. Endovascular treatment of Angio-Seal-related limb ischemia—primary results and long-term follow-up. Catheter Cardiovasc Interv 2010;75(6):823–827

Wille J, Vos JA, Overtoom TT, Suttorp MJ, Van de Pavoordt ED, De Vries JP. Acute leg ischemia: the dark side of a percutaneous femoral artery closure device. Ann Vasc Surg 2006;20(2):278–281

Lack of clinical improvement after successful stent placement in the ipsilateral external iliac artery and retrograde Angio-Seal access closure

Patient History

A 78-year-old woman with peripheral vascular disease was treated with stenting of the external iliac artery (EIA) for moderate calcified stenosis. The intervention was performed via retrograde access through the common femoral artery (CFA). Closure of the puncture site was done with a 6F Angio-Seal (St. Jude Medical) and hemostasis was achieved immediately.

Because there was lack of clinical improvement with an unchanged walking distance of 200 m, the patient was scheduled for additional percutaneous transluminal angioplasty (PTA) of a moderate tandem stenosis located in the mid-part and distal part of the ipsilateral superficial femoral artery (SFA) 2 weeks after the index procedure.

Initial Treatment Received

Retrograde 6F access at the level of the CFA for EIA stenosis. Closure of the puncture site was performed with Angio-Seal 6F.

Problems Encountered during Treatment

Angio-Seal application was according to instructions for use. No adverse events were noted. Hemostasis was achieved.

Imaging Plan

Antegrade puncture of the CFA was done under local anesthesia, and a 6F sheath was placed into the mid-part of the CFA. For digital subtraction angiography (DSA), contrast medium was hand injected through the sheath.

Resulting Complication

High-grade CFA stenosis due to intravascular location of the retrograde Angio-Seal closure (**Fig. 4.70**). The Angio-Seal anchor, probably including the plug and parts of the suture, caused a severe stenosis, which was even more pronounced by added obstruction from the sheath.

Possible Strategies for Complication Management

- Endovascular management with crossover stent placement (con: flexion zone, near femoral bifurcation).
- Open surgical groin access with removal of foreign body and reconstruction of the CFA.

Final Complication Management

Surgical cut-down of the ipsilateral groin and removal of the Angio-Seal material.

Complication Analysis

Closure devices with intraluminal anchor and collagen plug need a considerable amount of pulling force to fixate the anchor to the anterior vessel wall. This maneuver is necessary to stabilize the anchor before pressing the collagen plug onto the vessel. In the current case the anchor and parts of the collagen plug were found inside the vessel lumen. This complication is possible when the anchor is caught by plaque material inside the vessel so that delivery of the collagen material can end up in the vessel lumen. In this case no plaque or underlying CFA stenosis were visible. The initial pulling maneuver of the suture was probably insufficient so that collagen material was delivered

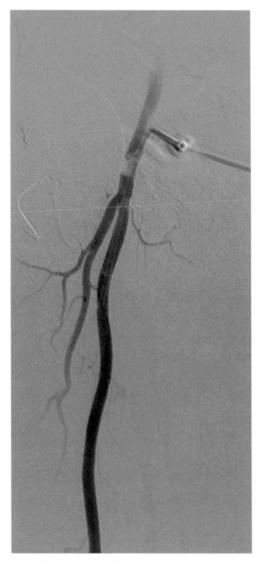

Fig. 4.70 Angiography of the CFA and the SFA showing a high-grade stenosis resulting from the retrograde Angio-Seal closure.

to the anchor still located inside the vessel and away from the puncture site.

Prevention Strategies and Take-home Message

- Handle instruments with care. Pull the suture carefully, but with enough force to achieve complete sealing when pushing the collagen down towards the outer anterior vessel wall.

• When a vascular closure device is used, patients should be evaluated clinically and/or by Doppler ultrasound before they are discharged to rule out complications.

Further Reading

Applegate RJ, Sacrinty M, Kutcher MA, et al. Vascular complications with newer generations of Angio-Seal vascular closure devices. J Interv Cardiol 2006;19(1):67–74

Azmoon S, Pucillo AL, Aronow WS, et al. Vascular complications after percutaneous coronary intervention following hemostasis with the Mynx vascular closure device versus the Angio-Seal vascular closure device. J Invasive Cardiol 2010;22(4):175–178

Carey D, Martin JR, Moore CA, Valentine MC, Nygaard TW. Complications of femoral artery closure devices. Catheter Cardiovasc Interv 2001;52(1):3–7

Corley JA, Kasliwal MK, Tan LA, Lopes DK. Delayed vascular claudication following diagnostic cerebral angiography: a rare complication of the Angio-Seal arteriotomy closure device. J Cerebrovasc Endovasc Neurosurg 2014;16(3):275–280

Eggebrecht H, Von Birgelen C, Naber C, et al. Impact of gender on femoral access complications secondary to application of a collagen-based vascular closure device. J Invasive Cardiol 2004;16(5):247–250

Fargen KM, Velat GJ, Lawson MF, et al. Occurrence of angiographic femoral artery complications after vascular closure with Mynx and Angio-Seal. J Neurointerv Surg 2013;5(2):161–164

Klocker J, Gratl A, Chemelli A, Moes N, Goebel G, Fraedrich G. Influence of use of a vascular closure device on incidence and surgical management of access site complications after percutaneous interventions. Eur J Vasc Endovasc Surg 2011;42(2):230–235

Mukhopadhyay K, Puckett MA, Roobottom CA. Efficacy and complications of Angio-Seal in antegrade puncture. Eur J Radiol 2005;56(3):409–412

Prabhudesai A, Khan MZ. An unusual cause of femoral embolism: Angio-Seal. Ann R Coll Surg Engl 2000;82(5):355–356

Thalhammer C, Joerg GR, Roffi M, Husmann M, Pfammatter T, Amann-Vesti BR. Endovascular treatment of Angio-Seal-related limb ischemia—primary results and long-term follow-up. Catheter Cardiovasc Interv 2010;75(6):823–827

Wille J, Vos JA, Overtoom TT, Suttorp MJ, Van de Pavoordt ED, De Vries JP. Acute leg ischemia: the dark side of a percutaneous femoral artery closure device. Ann Vasc Surg 2006;20(2):278–281

Embolization of ExoSeal plug into the common femoral artery during antegrade groin closure

Patient History

A 67-year-old woman underwent percutaneous transluminal angioplasty (PTA) and superficial femoral artery (SFA) stent placement via antegrade access to the common femoral artery (CFA). After successful treatment, a vascular closure device was used to achieve immediate hemostasis of the puncture site.

Initial Treatment Received

Uneventful PTA and SFA stent placement with application of a 6F ExoSeal vascular closure device (Cordis/Johnson & Johnson).

Problems Encountered during Treatment

The closure device was used according to instructions for use. However, loading of the device, gradual removal of the standard 6F sheath, and activation of the ExoSeal plug seemed a little difficult with a lot of friction. After activation and sheath/ExoSeal removal no hemostasis was achieved, even after 5 minutes of additional manual compression. Manual compression was needed for another 10 minutes until complete hemostasis was achieved.

Imaging Plan

Color duplex ultrasound of the groin.

Resulting Complication

Embolization of the collagen plug into the common femoral arterial lumen, resulting in severe obstruction (**Fig. 4.71**).

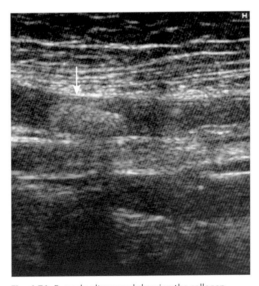

Fig. 4.71 B-mode ultrasound showing the collagen plaque (*arrow*) inside the vessel lumen instead of outside of the anterior vessel wall.

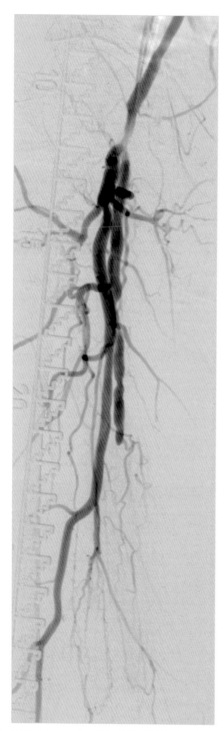

Fig. 4.72 Angiography of the right-side infrainguinal arteries prior to SFA recanalization, which was followed by PTA and stent placement, and final vascular closure using an ExoSeal system. Note the entrance level of the antegrade-placed sheath. The sheath crosses a severely narrowed area of the distal CFA.

Possible Strategies for Complication Management

- Endovascular management with crossover stent placement (con: high material burden, femoral flexion zone, near femoral bifurcation).
- Open surgical groin access with removal of foreign body and reconstruction of the CFA.

Final Complication Management

This complication was resolved by surgically inspecting the vessel and removal of the collagen plug. An endovascular approach using crossover technique with snaring of the plug or stenting might have been possible, but bore the risk of downstream embolization or other complications. The surgical approach for resolving this complication was deemed more appropriate.

Complication Analysis

A severely stenosed CFA at the entrance level of the sheath (**Fig. 4.72**) probably contributed to this complication. Due to the resulting friction forces during ExoSeal placement and activation, there was misplacement of the plaque into the vessel lumen.

Prevention Strategies and Take-home Message

- Evaluate vessel access carefully in order to guarantee suitability for a vascular closure device (nondiseased, non–heavily calcified CFA, no deep femoral or SFA puncture).
- When experiencing unexpected friction or other irregularities while applying a closure device, consider aborting the procedure and do manual compression instead.

Further Reading

Kara K, Mahabadi AA, Rothe H, et al. Safety and effectiveness of a novel vascular closure device: a prospective study of the ExoSeal compared to the Angio-Seal and ProGlide. J Endovasc Ther 2014;21(6):822–828

High-grade superficial femoral artery stenosis following cardiac catheterization

Patient History

A 75-year-old woman presented with new onset of claudication in her right leg following diagnostic cardiac catheterization 2 weeks earlier. Color Doppler ultrasound showed a short-segment high-grade stenosis of the right superficial femoral artery (SFA). Significant comorbidities were arterial hypertension, coronary heart disease, and diabetes.

Initial Treatment Received

Status post diagnostic cardiac catheterization via retrograde 7F access in the right groin. Closure of the puncture site was performed with Angio-Seal 6F (St. Jude Medical).

Problems Encountered during Treatment

The procedure report did not note any problems during the procedure or after puncture site closure. Hemostasis had been reached using the vascular closure device; no bleeding complications in the groin were documented.

Imaging Plan

Retrograde puncture of the contralateral common femoral artery (CFA) using the crossover maneuver and placement of a 45-cm-long 6F sheath into the right external iliac artery (EIA). Digital subtraction angiography with contrast medium injections through the sheath.

Resulting Complication

There was dissection and high-grade SFA stenosis, most likely due to intravascular location of parts of the Angio-Seal applied 2 weeks earlier (**Fig. 4.73**). The angiogram also revealed that the initial puncture was not in the CFA, but located directly in the SFA.

Possible Strategies for Complication Management

- Endovascular management with recanalization and crossover stent placement.
- Endovascular management with primary atherectomy.
- Open surgical groin access with removal of foreign body and reconstruction of the femoral artery.

Final Complication Management

Endovascular management with recanalization and crossover stent placement (**Figs. 4.74** and **4.75**).

Complication Analysis

Percutaneous vascular closure devices, especially when designed with an intraluminal component,

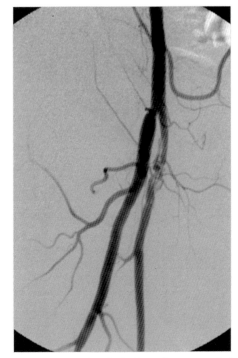

Fig. 4.73 Angiography of right femoral artery revealed a dissection and high-grade stenosis in the proximal aspect of the SFA, most likely resulting from the Angio-Seal device placed 2 weeks earlier.

may lead to iatrogenic vessel stenosis. Direct puncture of the SFA—as had been done here—is also associated with a greater likelihood of complications. Due to the relatively small vessel lumen of the SFA and the distance between skin level and the puncture site, malfunctioning of a vascular closure device is not uncommon in this situation. In this case, because of the distal location of the resulting stenosis, percutaneous endovascular management with stent placement solved the problem.

Prevention Strategies and Take-home Message

- When a vascular closure device is used, patients should be evaluated clinically and/or by Doppler ultrasound before they are discharged to rule out complications.
- In case of challenging groin anatomy, ultrasound guidance should be used to establish safe access to the CFA.
- The puncture should always be aimed at the mid-level of the CFA over the femoral head.
- Do not use vascular closure devices in small access vessels.

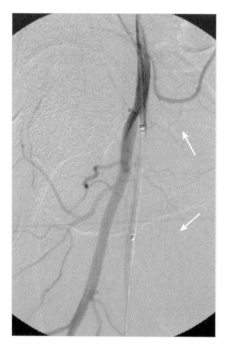

Fig. 4.74 Angiogram before deployment of a 6 × 40-mm self-expanding nitinol stent (*arrows*).

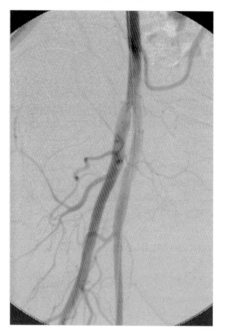

Fig. 4.75 Following stent implantation and mild balloon angioplasty no residual stenosis was detected.

Further Reading

Applegate RJ, Sacrinty M, Kutcher MA, et al. Vascular complications with newer generations of Angio-Seal vascular closure devices. J Interv Cardiol 2006;19(1):67–74

Azmoon S, Pucillo AL, Aronow WS, et al. Vascular complications after percutaneous coronary intervention following hemostasis with the Mynx vascular closure device versus the Angio-Seal vascular closure device. J Invasive Cardiol 2010;22(4):175–178

Carey D, Martin JR, Moore CA, Valentine MC, Nygaard TW. Complications of femoral artery closure devices. Catheter Cardiovasc Interv 2001;52(1):3–7

Corley JA, Kasliwal MK, Tan LA, Lopes DK. Delayed vascular claudication following diagnostic cerebral angiography: a rare complication of the Angio-Seal arteriotomy closure device. J Cerebrovasc Endovasc Neurosurg 2014;16(3):275–280

Eggebrecht H, Von Birgelen C, Naber C, et al. Impact of gender on femoral access complications secondary to application of a collagen-based vascular closure device. J Invasive Cardiol 2004;16(5):247–250

Fargen KM, Velat GJ, Lawson MF, et al. Occurrence of angiographic femoral artery complications after vascular closure with Mynx and Angio-Seal. J Neurointerv Surg 2013;5(2):161–164

Klocker J, Gratl A, Chemelli A, Moes N, Goebel G, Fraedrich G. Influence of use of a vascular closure device on incidence and surgical management of access site complications after percutaneous interventions. Eur J Vasc Endovasc Surg 2011;42(2):230–235

Mukhopadhyay K, Puckett MA, Roobottom CA. Efficacy and complications of Angio-Seal in antegrade puncture. Eur J Radiol 2005;56(3):409–412

Prabhudesai A, Khan MZ. An unusual cause of femoral embolism: Angio-Seal. Ann R Coll Surg Engl 2000;82(5):355–356

Thalhammer C, Joerg GR, Roffi M, Husmann M, Pfammatter T, Amann-Vesti BR. Endovascular treatment of Angio-Seal-related limb ischemia—primary results and long-term follow-up. Catheter Cardiovasc Interv 2010;75(6):823–827

Wille J, Vos JA, Overtoom TT, Suttorp MJ, Van de Pavoordt ED, De Vries JP. Acute leg ischemia: the dark side of a percutaneous femoral artery closure device. Ann Vasc Surg 2006;20(2):278–281

Diffuse pelvic bleeding from expanding retroperitoneal hematoma

Patient History

A 74-year-old woman following diagnostic cardiac catheterization was referred to the vascular surgery department for open repair of a pseudoaneurysm of the common femoral artery (CFA) (**Fig. 4.76**). Hours before the scheduled operation the patient developed signs of peripheral circulatory failure and needed fluid resuscitation.

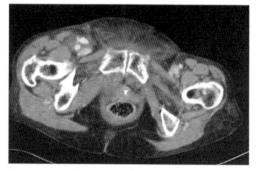

Fig. 4.76 Pseudoaneurysm of the groin after cardiac catheterization.

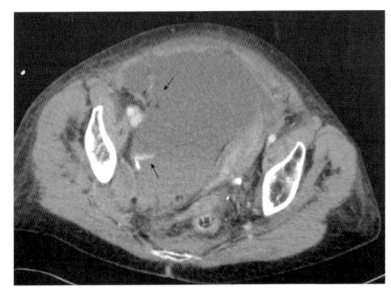

Fig. 4.77 Huge expanding retroperitoneal hematoma of the pelvis with multiple small active bleeding sites.

Initial Treatment Received

Diagnostic cardiac catheterization had been performed. Access closure was with manual compression.

Problems Encountered during Treatment

Postprocedure development of a pseudoaneurysm of the right femoral artery.

Imaging Plan

Computed tomography angiography (CTA) to evaluate extent of groin aneurysm and identification of active bleeding.

Resulting Complication

CTA confirmed diagnosis of a pseudoaneurysm in the right groin. However, in addition there was a huge expanding retroperitoneal hematoma of the pelvis with multiple small diffuse active bleeding sites (**Fig. 4.77**).

Possible Strategies for Complication Management

- Endovascular management (embolization with coils, glue or collagen sponge).
- Medical treatment with transfusion of blood cells and/or replacement of clotting factors.
- Surgical repair (if endovascular management fails).

Final Complication Management

The patient was transferred to the Angio Suite. The left CFA was punctured and a 45-cm-long 6F sheath was placed into the right common iliac artery (CIA). The right internal iliac artery (IIA) was cannulated using a 4F diagnostic catheter. Selective angiography revealed multiple small bleeding spots in the distal collateral network of the IIA (**Figs. 4.78a, b** and **4.79**). For embolization, a gelfoam sponge slurry with contrast medium was prepared and injected into the IIA until complete stasis was achieved (**Fig. 4.80**).

Complication Analysis

In this case a pseudoaneurysm of the CFA apparently progressed to a retroperitoneal hematoma. Because no single bleeding source was identified, the active bleeding was likely due to expansion of the groin hematoma with consecutive rupture

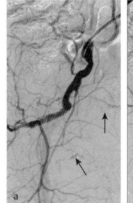
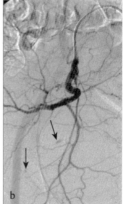

Fig. 4.78 (a,b) Selective angiogram of the right IIA. No major bleeding arteries are identified, unless small side branch bleeding is identified (*arrows*).

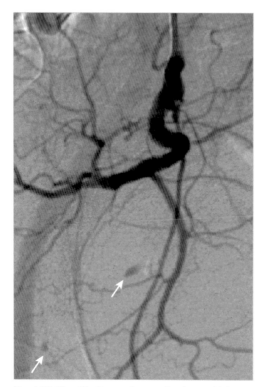

Fig. 4.79 Magnification angiogram showing multiple small peripheral branches with extravasation (*arrows*).

of multiple smaller arteries. With ongoing hemorrhage, disseminated intravascular coagulation (DIC) developed, preventing hematoma from compressing the arterial feeders. In this situation temporary nonselective embolization of the IIA with gelfoam sponge stopped the active bleeding and worsening of hemodynamic compromise. Two days after successful embolization and consolidation of coagulation parameters the hematoma was removed and the pseudoaneurysm closed surgically. The patient fully recovered.

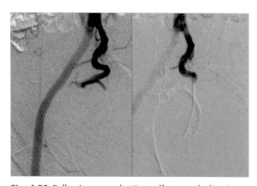

Fig. 4.80 Following nonselective gelfoam embolization, total stasis within the IIA was achieved.

Prevention Strategies and Take-home Message

- Be aware of potentially fatal retroperitoneal progression of a pseudoaneurysm previously contained in the groin.
- Be familiar with endovascular embolization techniques.
- In a patient with a compromised coagulation system, primary operative management of diffuse pelvic bleeding should be avoided.

Further Reading

Cale L, Constantino R. Strategies for decreasing vascular complications in diagnostic cardiac catheterization patients. Dimens Crit Care Nurs 2012;31(1):13–17

Görich J, Brambs HJ, Allmenröder C, et al. The role of embolization treatment of acute hemorrhage. Rofo 1993;159(4):379–387. [In German]

Merriweather N, Sulzbach-Hoke LM. Managing risk of complications at femoral vascular access sites in percutaneous coronary intervention. Crit Care Nurs 2012;32(5):16–29

Stone PA, Campbell JE. Complications related to femoral artery access for transcatheter procedures. Vasc Endovasc Surg 2012; 46(8):617–623

Stone PA, Campbell JE, AbuRahma AF. Femoral pseudoaneurysms after percutaneous access. J Vasc Surg 2014;60(5):1359–1366

Tavris DR, Wang Y, Jacobs S, et al. Bleeding and vascular complications at the femoral access site following percutaneous coronary intervention (PCI): an evaluation of hemostasis strategies. J Invasive Cardiol 2012;24(7):328–334

Velmahos GC, Chahwan S, Hanks SE, et al. Angiographic embolization of bilateral internal iliac arteries to control life-threatening hemorrhage after blunt trauma to the pelvis. Am Surg 2000;66(9):858–862

Wiley JM, White CJ, Uretsky BF. Noncoronary complications of coronary intervention. Catheter Cardiovasc Interv 2002;57(2):257–265

Xu JQ. Effectiveness of embolization of the internal iliac or uterine arteries in the treatment of massive obstetrical and gynecological hemorrhages. Eur Rev Med Pharmacol Sci 2015;19(3):372–374

Intravascular application of an Angio-Seal collagen plug

Patient History

A 68-year-old man underwent coronary angiography via retrograde access to the right common femoral artery (CFA). A vascular closure device was used to achieve hemostasis of the puncture site. A few days after the procedure, the patient was readmitted with new onset of claudication in his right leg. Clinical examination was unremarkable.

Initial Treatment Received

Uneventful coronary angiography with application of a 6F Angio-Seal vascular closure device (St. Jude Medical).

Problems Encountered during Treatment

The closure device was used according to the instructions for use. Hemostasis was achieved immediately.

Imaging Plan

Color duplex ultrasound of the groin; computed tomography angiography (CTA).

Resulting Complication

There was high-grade stenosis of the CFA allegedly due to an intravascular position of the collagen plug and anchor complex (**Fig. 4.81**).

Possible Strategies for Complication Management

- Endovascular management with stent placement (con: high material burden, flexion zone).
- Open surgical groin access with removal of foreign body and patch reconstruction.

Final Complication Management

This complication was solved surgically. Intraoperative angiography (**Fig. 4.82**) confirmed high-grade stenosis from the foreign body. Surgery revealed that the collagen plug on the intravascular anchor had been placed partly inside the lumen. The foreign body was removed

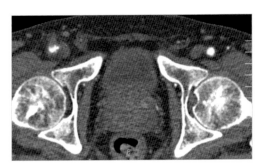

Fig. 4.81 Axial image from CTA at the level of the puncture. Note high-grade stenosis in the right CFA.

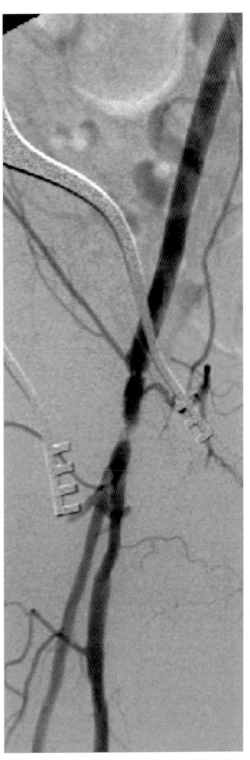

Fig. 4.82 Intraoperative angiography of the high-grade stenosis in the right CFA after Angio-Seal application.

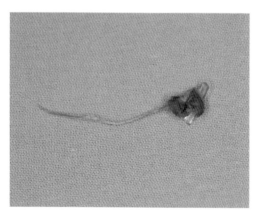

Fig. 4.83 Removed suture, collagen plug, and anchor.

(**Fig. 4.83**) and the vessel reconstructed by patch plasty.

Complication Analysis

The reason for this complication remains unclear. During Angio-Seal placement the anchor probably became attached to a plaque in the CFA. When pushing the collagen plug down, the material must have entered the vessel lumen, leading to an intravascular position of the device.

Prevention Strategies and Take-home Message

- Evaluate vessel access carefully in order to guarantee suitability for a vascular closure device (nondiseased, non–heavily calcified CFA, no deep femoral or superficial femoral artery puncture).
- When experiencing unexpected friction or other irregularities while applying a closure device consider aborting the procedure and doing manual compression instead.
- Carefully follow the instructions for use and do not hesitate to ask a colleague if something is unclear.

Further Reading

Carey D, Martin JR, Moore CA, Valentine MC, Nygaard TW. Complications of femoral artery closure devices. Catheter Cardiovasc Interv 2001;52(1):3–7
Corley JA, Kasliwal MK, Tan LA, Lopes DK. Delayed vascular claudication following diagnostic cerebral angiography: a rare complication of the Angio-Seal arteriotomy closure device. J Cerebrovasc Endovasc Neurosurg 2014;16(3):275–280

Klocker J, Gratl A, Chemelli A, Moes N, Goebel G, Fraedrich G. Influence of use of a vascular closure device on incidence and surgical management of access site complications after percutaneous interventions. Eur J Vasc Endovasc Surg 2011;42(2):230–235
Wille J, Vos JA, Overtoom TT, Suttorp MJ, Van de Pavoordt ED, De Vries JP. Acute leg ischemia: the dark side of a percutaneous femoral artery closure device. Ann Vasc Surg 2006;20(2):278–281

Embolization of ExoSeal plug into the distal superficial femoral artery during antegrade groin closure

Patient History

A 70-year-old woman underwent coronary angiography via retrograde access to the common femoral artery (CFA). After successful treatment, a vascular closure device was used to achieve immediate hemostasis of the puncture site. One week later, the patient was admitted to the hospital with claudication (limited walking capacity 20 m). Before coronary angiography, no history of claudication was reported. Clinical examination at rest showed a pale ispsilateral forefoot (**Fig. 4.84**).

Initial Treatment Received

Uneventful coronary angiography with application of a 6F ExoSeal vascular closure device (Cordis/Johnson & Johnson).

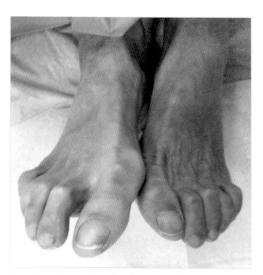

Fig. 4.84 Pale ispsilateral, pale forefoot. Note the adequately colored left foot.

Problems Encountered during Treatment

The closure device was used according to instructions for use. However, after activation and sheath/ ExoSeal removal, no hemostasis was achieved. Manual compression was needed for 5 minutes until complete hemostasis was achieved.

Imaging Plan

Color duplex ultrasound of the groin and femoropopliteal artery.

Resulting Complication

Embolization of the collagen plug into the distal femoral arterial lumen, resulting in severe obstruction (**Fig. 4.85**).

Possible Strategies for Complication Management

- Endovascular management with stent placement (con: high material burden, femoral and popliteal flexion zone, near knee joint).
- Ipsilateral antegrade puncture in order to extract the dislodged collagen by endovascular means such as snaring or aspiration.
- Open surgical groin access with removal of foreign body and reconstruction of the CFA.

Final Complication Management

This complication was solved by endovascular means and stent fixation of the collagen plug. An attempt to snare or aspirate the plug was unsuccessful. Only small amounts of the collagen ma-

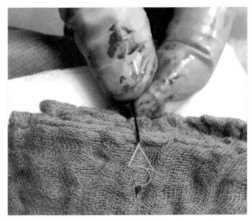

Fig. 4.86 Small amounts of the collagen material removed with a snare.

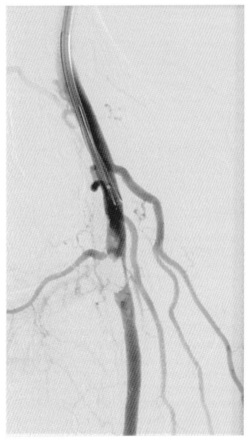

Fig. 4.87 Control angiography after several snaring attempts still shows a high-grade stenosis due to underling atherosclerotic plaque and dislodged collagen.

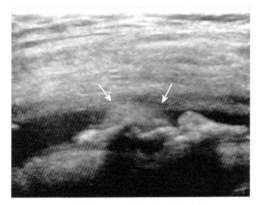

Fig. 4.85 B-mode ultrasound showing the collagen plug (*arrows*) inside the vessel lumen adherent to an intravascular plaque.

terial were removed with a snare (**Figs. 4.86** and **4.87**). An attempt at engaging the material with a stent retriever, originally intended for throm-

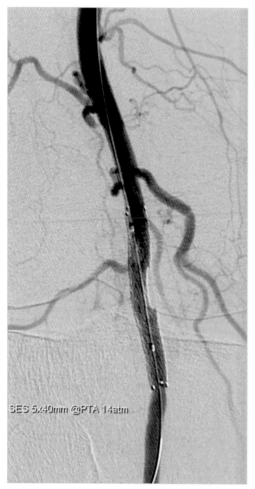

SES 5×40mm @PTA 14atm

Fig. 4.88 Angiography after collagen fixation by stenting (SES 5 × 40 mm) and final PTA (4 × 30 mm at 14 atmospheres [atm] inflated). Note the slight narrowing due to the compressed collagen.

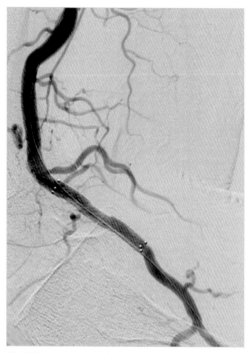

Fig. 4.89 Angiography during 90° knee bending shows an uncompromised femoropopliteal artery segment.

Complication Analysis

The reason for this complication remains unclear. During ExoSeal placement and activation it is probable that there was misplacement of the plug into the vessel lumen.

Prevention Strategies and Take-home Message

- Evaluate the level of vessel access carefully in order to guarantee suitability for a vascular closure device (nondiseased, non–heavily calcified CFA, no deep femoral or superficial femoral artery puncture).
- When experiencing unexpected friction or other irregularities while applying a closure device consider aborting the procedure and doing manual compression instead.
- Follow the instructions for use carefully and do not hesitate to ask a colleague if something is unclear.

bus removal during acute stroke management, failed. The procedure was therefore completed by fixation of the collagen to the vessel wall using a self-expanding stent (SES) (5 × 40 mm) and final percutaneous transluminal angioplasty (PTA) (4 × 30 mm; **Figs. 4.88** and **4.89**). Finally, no signs of distal embolization at the origin of the below the knee arteries were visible (**Fig. 4.90**) and the foot arteries are patent. The main feeding vessels are the posterior and anterior tibial arteries (**Fig. 4.91**).

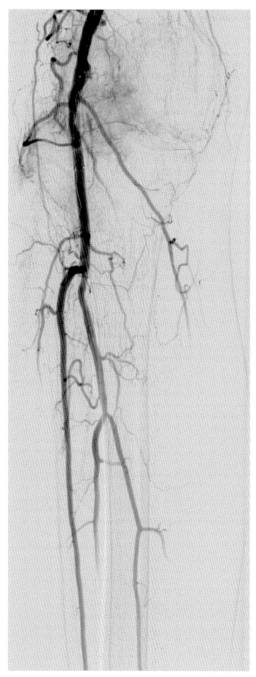

Fig. 4.90 No signs of distal embolization at the origin of the below the knee arteries.

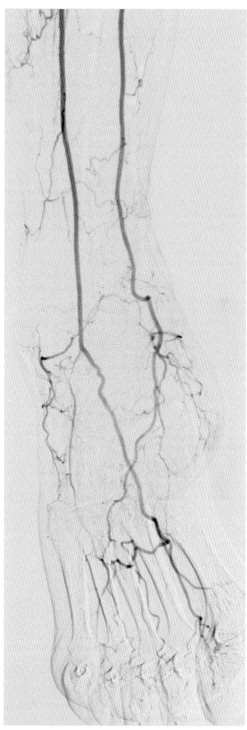

Fig. 4.91 Even the foot arteries are patent. The main feeder vessels are the posterior and anterior tibial artery.

Further Reading

Boersma D, Van Strijen MJ, Kloppenburg GT, Van den Heuvel DA, De Vries JP. Endovascular retrieval of a dislodged femoral arterial closure device with alligator forceps. J Vasc Surg 2012;55(4):1150–1152

Cahill TJ, Choji K, Kardos A. Fluoroscopy-guided snare retrieval of the celt ACD® metallic vascular closure device following failed deployment. Catheter Cardiovasc Interv 2014;83(4):556–559

Cikirikcioglu M, Cherian S, Keil V, et al. Surgical treatment of complications associated with the Angio-Seal vascular closure device. Ann Vasc Surg 2011;25(4):557.e1–e4

Kara K, Mahabadi AA, Rothe H, et al. Safety and effectiveness of a novel vascular closure device: a prospective study of the ExoSeal compared to the Angio-Seal and ProGlide. J Endovasc Ther 2014;21(6):822–828

Maxien D, Behrends B, Eberhardt KM, et al. Endovascular treatment of acute limb ischemia caused by an intravascularly deployed bioabsorbable plug of a vascular closure device. Vasa 2013;42(2):144–148

Schiele TM, Rademacher A, Meissner O, Klauss V, Hoffmann U. Acute limb ischemia after femoral arterial closure with a vascular sealing device: successful endovascular treatment. Vasa 2004;33(4):252–256

Suri S, Nagarsheth KH, Goraya S, Singh K. A novel technique to retrieve a maldeployed vascular closure device. J Endovasc Ther 2015;22(1):71–73

4.2.3 Intravenous Access

Port line dislocation into the right heart

Patient History

A 73-year-old woman suffering from breast cancer had received a port line 4 weeks previously. During routine lung X-ray, dislocation of the distal intravenous line into the right atrium was noticed; parts of the line protruded into the right ventricle. She had no clinical symptoms from this catheter dislodgement.

Initial Treatment Received

A port line from the left subclavian vein (LSV) was placed 4 weeks ago.

Problems Encountered during Treatment

Placements of port line and port chamber were uneventful. During routine X-ray of the chest, a dislocation of the port catheter was noticed.

Imaging Plan

Fluoroscopy of the chest.

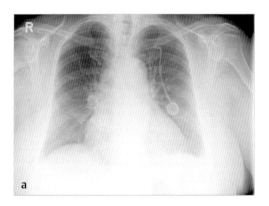

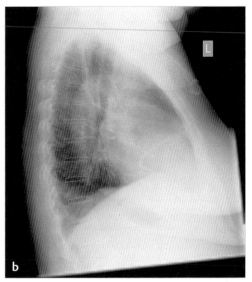

Fig. 4.92 Chest X-ray presenting a dislocation of the entire intravenous part of the port catheter into the right heart (atrium and partially ventricle). Port chamber and extravascular part of the port line are still in place. Posterior-anterior projection (a) and lateral projection (b).

Resulting Complication

Port line dislocation into the right heart (Fig. 4.92a, b).

Possible Strategies for Complication Management

- Foreign body removal under fluoroscopy. Snaring techniques from retrograde venous groin approach via a 12F sheath. A brachial or jugular approach should be avoided due to large sheath size.

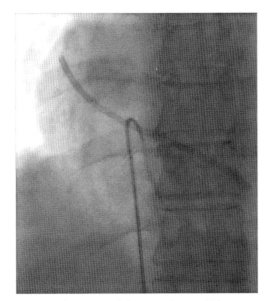

Fig. 4.93 Fluoroscopy of the port catheter, which was already hooked with a Simmons catheter, ready for pulling down into the IVC.

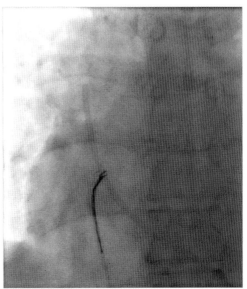

Fig. 4.94 Already snared port catheter from the distal end, which protruded into the IVC. The snare fixed the catheter in the mid-section.

Final Complication Management

Puncture of the right common femoral vein (CFV) under local anesthesia and insertion of a 12F sheath. Advancement of a snare (different manufacturers available) and engagement of the port catheter. In this case, prior to the successful snaring maneuver, the port line was retracted and removed into the inferior vena cava (IVC) using a 5F Simmons catheter (**Fig. 4.93**). In the smaller IVC, snaring was successful and both snare and catheter were removed via the sheath (**Figs. 4.94–4.96**). After sheath removal, the procedure was completed by manual compression. Control fluoroscopy of the chest showed the extravenous part of the port line (**Fig. 4.97**).

Complication Analysis

Disruption of the port line at the entrance level of the LSV. Decreased fatigue resistance of the catheter material resulted in catheter rupture and dislodgement into the right heart.

Prevention Strategies and Take-home Message

- Inspect the port line for any material damage or fatigue prior to implantation.

- Avoid any kinking or sharp manipulation of the port line.
- Rule out any narrowing of the port line at the entrance level of the vessel.
- Be careful with any sutures affecting the port line.

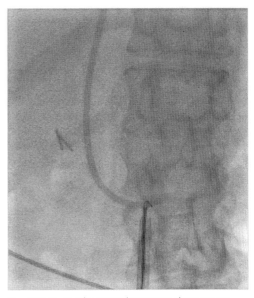

Fig. 4.95 During the retrieval maneuver, the snare was repositioned carefully onto one of the port catheter ends in order to retrieve an unkinked catheter into the large sheath.

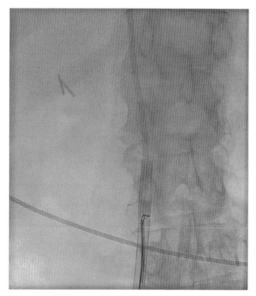

Fig. 4.96 The end of the port catheter was withdrawn into the sheath and fixed with the snare during the entire foreign body retrieval.

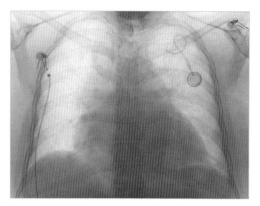

Fig. 4.97 Final fluoroscopic control in order to rule out any further port catheter dislocation or disintegration after retrieval. The extravascular part of the port line was still in place.

Further Reading

Bostan M, Durakoğlugil ME, Satiroğlu O, Erdivanli B, Tufan G. Retrieval of embolized tip of port catheter from branch of right pulmonary artery using a macro snare catheter. Interv Med Appl Sci 2014;6(2):93–95

Choksy P, Zaidi SS, Kapoor D. Removal of intracardiac fractured port-A catheter utilizing an existing forearm peripheral intravenous access site in the cath lab. J Invasive Cardiol 2014;26(2):75–76

Chuang MT, Wu DK, Chang CA, et al. Concurrent use of pigtail and loop snare catheters for percutaneous retrieval of dislodged central venous port catheter. Kaohsiung J Med Sci 2011;27(11):514–519

Colón-Casasnovas NE, Lugo-Vicente H. Distal fragmented port catheter: case report and review of literature. Bol Asoc Med P R 2008;100(1):70–75

Elkhoury MI, Boeckx WD, Chahine EG, Feghali MA. Retrieval of port-A catheter fragment from the main and right pulmonary arteries 3 years after dislodgement. J Vasc Access 2008;9(4):296–298

Hara M, Takayama S, Imafuji H, Sato M, Funahashi H, Takeyama H. Single-port retrieval of peritoneal foreign body using SILS port: report of a case. Surg Laparosc Endosc Percutan Tech 2011;21(3):e126–e129

Kawata M, Ozawa K, Matsuura T, et al. Percutaneous interventional techniques to remove embolized silicone port catheters from heart and great vessels. Cardiovasc Interv Ther 2012;27(3):196–200

Motta Leal Filho JM, Carnevale FC, Nasser F, et al. Endovascular techniques and procedures, methods for removal of intravascular foreign bodies. Rev Bras Cir Cardiovasc 2010;25(2):202–208

Sowinski H, Kobayashi D, Turner DR. Transcutaneous removal of an intravenous catheter fragment using a spider FX™ Embolic Protection device. Catheter Cardiovasc Interv 2015;86(3):467–471

Wang PC, Liang HL, Wu TH, et al. Percutaneous retrieval of dislodged central venous port catheter: experience of 25 patients in a single institute. Acta Radiol 2009;50(1):15–20

Wang SC, Tsai CH, Hou CP, et al. Dislodgement of port-A catheters in pediatric oncology patients: 11 years of experience. World J Surg Oncol 2013;11:191

Port line dislocation into the right pulmonary artery

Patient History

A 74-year-old woman suffering from malignant lymphoma was scheduled for a port implantation before initiation of chemotherapy. During implantation, dislocation of entire port line occurred. Initial attempts to remove the catheter failed. Immediate chest X-ray showed the port catheter projecting into the right pulmonary artery trunk.

Initial Treatment Received

Port line insertion from the left subclavian vein.

Problems Encountered during Treatment

During placement of the port line in the operating room, the entire catheter dislodged. Postoperative X-ray of the chest showed dislocation of the port catheter into the right pulmonary artery.

Imaging Plan

Fluoroscopy of the chest.

Resulting Complication

Port line dislocation into the right pulmonary artery (**Fig. 4.98**).

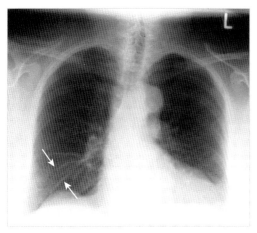

Fig. 4.98 Chest X-ray posterior-anterior projection showing the dislocated port catheter (*arrow*) in the right pulmonary artery (and the lower lobe artery).

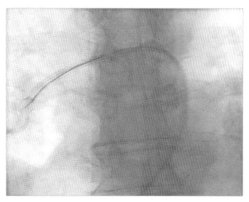

Fig. 4.99 Fluoroscopy of the port catheter that has been snared and is ready for retraction into the IVC.

Possible Strategies for Complication Management

• Foreign body removal under fluoroscopy. Snaring techniques from retrograde venous groin approach via a 12F sheath. A brachial or jugular approach should be avoided due to large sheath size.

Final Complication Management

Puncture of the right common femoral vein (CFV) under local anesthesia and insertion of a 12F sheath. After placement of a 5F pigtail catheter into the right pulmonary artery a rotating maneuver was performed to engage the port catheter; however, it was unsuccessful. A 7F 90-cm-long sheath (Terumo) was therefore positioned into the right lower lobe artery. A 0.035-inch Teflon-coated wire was formed into a snare and advanced through the 7F sheath. Using the distal loop of the wire as a snare the port catheter was pulled back and fixed to the distal end of the sheath.

During retrieval towards the main pulmonary artery, the port catheter was close to becoming dislodged again so it was held in that position. Then a regular 0.035-inch snare was advanced through the 7F sheath inside the 12F sheath. Passing the distal end of the long 7F sheath, the snare was used to grab the port catheter and finally remove it through the right heart into the inferior vena cava (IVC) (**Figs. 4.99** and **4.100**). Close to the groin, at the entrance level to the vein, both the snared catheter and the 12F sheath were fixed with a clamp because it was not possible to remove the entangled port catheter percutaneously (**Fig. 4.101**).

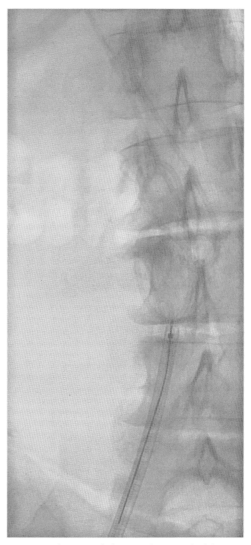

Fig. 4.100 The entangled port catheter reached the distal part of the 12F sheath. Nevertheless, removal through the sheath failed.

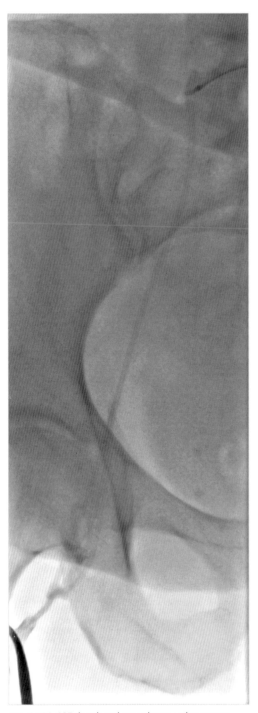

Fig. 4.101 12F sheath and snared port catheter were fixed at the entrance level of the CFV. In order to avoid fragmentation during forceful removal, it was decided to perform veinotomy for safe and complete removal of the port catheter.

All material was removed surgically through veinotomy. Control fluoroscopy of the chest showed no remaining parts of the port line.

Complication Analysis

During surgery the entire port line was lost through the entrance level of the left subclavian vein. Foreign body removal was begun endovascularly, but had to be completed surgically.

Prevention Strategies and Take-home Message

- Be very aware of the port line at all times during implantation.
- When preparing the port chamber, fixate the proximal end of the port line.

Further Reading

Bostan M, Durakoğlugil ME, Satiroğlu O, Erdivanli B, Tufan G. Retrieval of embolized tip of port catheter from branch of right pulmonary artery using a macro snare catheter. Interv Med Appl Sci 2014;6(2):93–95

Choksy P, Zaidi SS, Kapoor D. Removal of intracardiac fractured port-A catheter utilizing an existing forearm peripheral intravenous access site in the cath lab. J Invasive Cardiol 2014;26(2):75–76

Chuang MT, Wu DK, Chang CA, et al. Concurrent use of pigtail and loop snare catheters for percutaneous retrieval of dislodged central venous port catheter. Kaohsiung J Med Sci 2011;27(11):514–519

Colón-Casasnovas NE, Lugo-Vicente H. Distal fragmented port catheter: case report and review of literature. Bol Asoc Med P R 2008;100(1):70–75

Elkhoury MI, Boeckx WD, Chahine EG, Feghali MA. Retrieval of port-A catheter fragment from the main and right pulmonary arteries 3 years after dislodgement. J Vasc Access 2008;9(4):296–298

Hara M, Takayama S, Imafuji H, Sato M, Funahashi H, Takeyama H. Single-port retrieval of peritoneal foreign body using SILS port: report of a case. Surg Laparosc Endosc Percutan Tech 2011;21(3):e126–3129.

Kawata M, Ozawa K, Matsuura T, et al. Percutaneous interventional techniques to remove embolized silicone port catheters from heart and great vessels. Cardiovasc Interv Ther 2012;27(3):196–200

Motta Leal Filho JM, Carnevale FC, Nasser F, et al. Endovascular techniques and procedures, methods for removal of intravascular foreign bodies. Rev Bras Cir Cardiovasc 2010;25(2):202–208

Sowinski H, Kobayashi D, Turner DR. Transcutaneous removal of an intravenous catheter fragment using a spider FX™ Embolic Protection device. Catheter Cardiovasc Interv 2015;86(3):467–471

Wang PC, Liang HL, Wu TH, et al. Percutaneous retrieval of dislodged central venous port catheter: experience of 25 patients in a single institute. Acta Radiol 2009;50(1):15–20

Wang SC, Tsai CH, Hou CP, et al. Dislodgement of port-A catheters in pediatric oncology patients: 11 years of experience. World J Surg Oncol 2013;11:191

Hemoptysis after subclavian vein catheterization in a patient with low platelets

Patient History

A 49-year-old woman with a history of acute lymphoblastic leukemia relapse was referred for central venous catheter placement. The patient had a platelet count of less than 15,000 and normal clotting parameters.

Initial Treatment Received

A 6F double lumen peripherally inserted central catheter (PICC) was chosen for insertion through a standard arm approach. After repeatedly failed attempts to push the microintroducer's guidewire into a suitable arm vein, due to thrombotic occlusion, the peripheral access sites were abandoned. It was decided to place the line through a right subclavian vein (SCV) access.

Problems Encountered during Treatment

A sonographically guided puncture of the right SCV was made via an out-of-plane approach (transversal plane). The needle punctured the vein through-and-through with the first attempt, but after withdrawing the needle the guidewire could easily pass intraluminally and the line placement was completed as usual. Immediately after the puncture the patient experienced a paroxysmal cough and gross hemoptysis. Due to con-

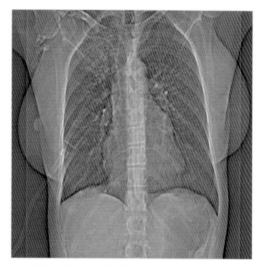

Fig. 4.102 CT 'scout' film showing central line placement through the right SCV. Note the steep angle of approach, due to out-of-plane ultrasound guidance, and also the right upper lobe density, immediately below the access site.

tinuing hemoptysis on the ward she received a platelet transfusion, with no improvement.

Imaging Plan

The patient was referred for emergency chest computed tomography (CT) with an indication of life-threatening massive hemoptysis (**Fig. 4.102**). CT revealed a small peripheral pleural collection with contrast extravasation on the right upper lobe, just below the right SCV access site (**Fig. 4.103**). Lung window CT showed a large dif-

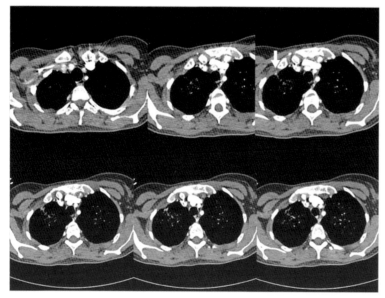

Fig. 4.103 Chest CT images showing a small contrast extravasation and pleural collection, bellow the SCV access site in the right upper lobe periphery (*arrow*).

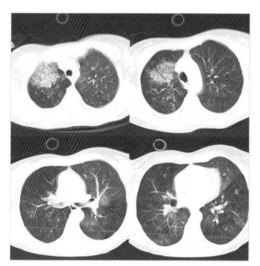

Fig. 4.104 Lung window CT images showing diffuse densities, especially in the right upper lung field, but also in the middle and lower fields bilaterally, consistent with diffuse pulmonary hemorrhage.

fuse density in the right upper lobe, along with multiple focal densities in the middle and lower lung fields—findings consistent with diffuse pulmonary hemorrhage (**Fig. 4.104**). Due to continuing hemoptysis the patient developed dyspnea and tachypnea with resultant O_2 saturation drop to around 60% and she was intubated. Based on contrast extravasation seen on CT scan the patient was referred for bronchial artery angiography and embolization. The angiography of subclavian artery, thyrocervical trunk, and bronchial arteries on the right was unremarkable (**Fig. 4.105**) and the

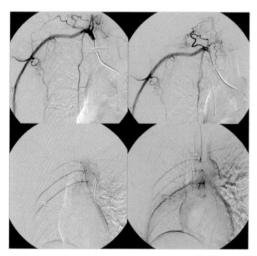

Fig. 4.105 Digital subtraction angiography of right thyrocervical trunk, subclavian artery, and bronchial arteries showing no contrast extravasation.

patient was admitted to the Intensive Care Unit (ICU), transferred after 48 hours to the hematology ward, and discharged home a few days later.

Resulting Complication

Inadvertent through-and-through SCV puncture caused a small pleural and lung injury from the needle, initiating a paroxysmal cough reflex, which in turn, due to a low platelet count, caused massive pulmonary hemorrhage.

Possible Strategies for Complication Management

- Ultrasound-guided SCV puncture via the out-of-plane approach (transversal plane) increases the risk of inadvertently puncturing the underlying pleura or lung, causing hemorrhage or pneumothorax. The sonographically guided in-plane approach (supra- or infraclavicular) is considered safer, because it allows for a better view of the needle tip. Additionally, an in-plane approach with a conventional linear probe forces the operator to use a more lateral access site, close to the axillary–subclavian vein junction where there is less risk of lung puncture.
- A right internal jugular vein (IJV) approach would be a safer option, despite the inconvenience to the patient and possible increased infection rate.

Final Complication Management

The patient was treated with intubation, platelet transfusion, and supportive therapy in the ICU. A small peripheral pleural lung extravasation on chest CT was not confirmed during angiography and no embolization was performed.

Complication Analysis

Inadvertent pleura or lung puncture during right SCV catheterization in a patient with low platelets, causing paroxysmal cough and massive hemoptysis due to pulmonary hemorrhage in both lungs.

Prevention Strategies and Take-home Message

- Patients with coagulation disorders are best treated by peripherally inserted lines, such as PICCs, but their prone-to-bleeding veins do not allow for multiple catheterization attempts. Adequate experience is essential.

- A sonographically guided in-plane approach is a safer option for supra- or infraclavicular puncture of the SCV.
- IJV is also a justified approach, despite inconvenience to the patient and possible increased infection rate.
- Paroxysmal coughing can lead to serious complications in patients with severe coagulation disorders.

Further Reading

Lennon M, Zaw NN, Pöpping DM, Wenk M. Procedural complications of central venous catheter insertion. Minerva Anestesiol 2012;78(11):1234–1240

Ruesch S, Walder B, Tramèr MR. Complications of central venous catheters: internal jugular versus subclavian access—a systematic review. Crit Care Med 2002; 30(2):454–460

Puncture of the common femoral vein with external pudendal artery injury

Patient History

A 46-year-old woman on hemodialysis (HD) presented with thrombosis of her arm HD fistula. It was decided to temporarily place a percutaneous dialysis catheter through the left common femoral vein (CFV).

Initial Treatment Received

Percutaneous insertion of the temporary dialysis catheter into the left CFV using the traditional "blind" landmark method.

Problems Encountered during Treatment

During attempts to gain percutaneous access to the left CFV the patient developed a rapidly expanding upper thigh and labial hematoma (**Fig. 4.106**) and quickly became hemodynamically unstable.

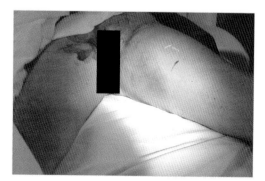

Fig. 4.106 Expanding left upper thigh and labial hematoma developed during attempts to gain percutaneous CFV access.

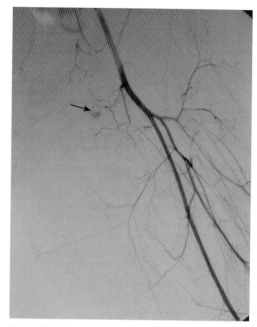

Fig. 4.107 DSA through contralateral femoral approach demonstrates active contrast extravasation from left SEPA.

Imaging Plan

Digital subtraction angiography (DSA) through percutaneous contralateral retrograde access to the right common femoral artery (CFA).

Resulting Complication

Left superficial external pudendal artery (SEPA) injury with active bleeding (**Figs. 4.107** and **4.108**).

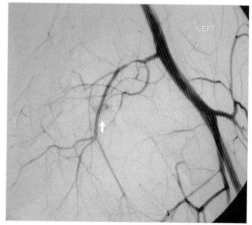

Fig. 4.108 Selective left common femoral angiogram shows active contrast extravasation from a branch of SEPA (*arrow*) in more detail.

Possible Strategies for Complication Management

- Catheterization of the feeder vessel and selective coil embolization.
- Alternative agents for embolization: glue, large particles, gelfoam.
- Stent graft implantation in the CFA in the unlikely occasion of failure to catheterize the SEPA.
- Surgery (if endovascular approach fails).

Final Complication Management

Endovascular treatment via contralateral retrograde CFA access was decided upon. The left SEPA was selectively catheterized with a 4F cobra catheter and successfully embolized in its proximal part with 4-mm platinum coils (**Fig. 4.109**). No attempt was made for a more distal superselective embolization due to the patient's hemodynamic instability.

Complication Analysis

Perforation of left SEPA branch during percutaneous CFV access attempts using the traditional "blind" landmark method. In general this complication is very rare during this type of procedure. This complication was managed by endovascular means.

Prevention Strategies and Take-home Message

- Using ultrasound guidance instead of the traditional "blind" landmark technique for

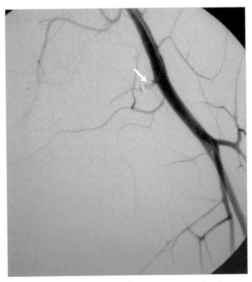

Fig. 4.109 Final angiogram demonstrating no further active extravasation due to successful coiling of the left proximal SEPA (*arrow*).

percutaneous femoral venous access is strongly advised.
- The use of ultrasound guidance is associated with significantly less risk of arterial puncture and hematomas and less time to insert venous catheters or sheaths, as well as a higher success rate for inserting the catheter or sheath on the first attempt.
- Inadvertent arterial puncture during percutaneous femoral venous access can be life threatening, requiring immediate endovascular repair.
- Interventionists performing CFV punctures should be familiar with the anatomy of the superficial and deep external pudendal arteries and be aware that these arteries could potentially be injured during the procedure.

Further Reading

Baum PA, Matsumoto AH, Teitelbaum GP, Zuurbier RA, Barth KH. Anatomical relationship between the common femoral artery and vein: CT evaluation and clinical significance. Radiology 1989;173(3):775–777

Port line migration during surgical explant

Patient History

A 77-year-old woman with a totally implantable vascular access device (TIVAD) for chemotherapy was referred to the surgeon who had initially performed the implantation for TIVAD removal.

Initial Treatment Received

After the surgeon exposed the implanted port using the initial incision he noticed that the device was detached from its catheter. In an effort to secure the catheter in the subcutaneous tunnel a fairly large chest incision was made, but eventually the catheter was lost into the venous system.

Problems Encountered during Treatment

The patient was referred to the Interventional Radiology Unit (IRU) for percutaneous removal of the migrated TIVAD catheter.

Imaging Plan

The catheter appeared in one piece on the chest X-ray (**Fig. 4.110**) with its central tip resting in the right ventricle and the peripheral tip in the right internal jugular vein (IJV).

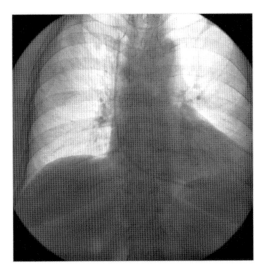

Fig. 4.110 Initial chest radiograph showing the catheter fragment's initial position.

Resulting Complication

The TIVAD catheter was presumably cut during port exposure and during the attempt to grasp it the surgeon pushed it even further into the subcutaneous tissues and then into the venous system.

Possible Strategies for Complication Management

- Accessing the venous system using a large sheath from the jugular or femoral approach, or both, in difficult cases, to create support.
- Using a commercially available snare or making an improvised snare using a guide catheter or long sheath and a folded guidewire.
- Refer the patient to a vascular surgeon to expose the peripheral tip of the catheter in the right IJV.

Final Complication Management

The right common femoral vein (CFV) was accessed under local anesthesia and a short 10F vascular sheath was placed. A commercially available snare (SeQure 20-mm, Lifetech Scientific) was used to securely grasp the peripheral tip of the catheter, and the snare–catheter assembly was dragged into the 10F sheath and out of the body (**Fig. 4.111a, b**). The sheath was then removed and compression hemostasis applied.

The patient was anticoagulated using a prophylactic dose of low molecular weight heparin (LMWH) to prevent pericatheter thrombosis and in the unlikely event of pulmonary embolism. During the immediate postoperative follow-up the

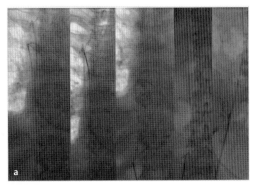

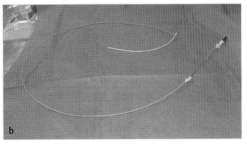

Fig. 4.111 **(a)** Catheter fragment, step-by-step snaring, and removal through the right CFV sheath. **(b)** The snared catheter after removal.

patient complained of an enlarging painful hematoma around her chest incision. Visual inspection confirmed the increased swelling and she was referred for an emergency chest computed tomography (CT), which confirmed a subcutaneous hematoma presenting acute contrast extravasation from venous collaterals (**Fig. 4.112**). A vascular surgeon surgically drained the hematoma.

Complication Analysis

Accidental catheter cut during TIVAD removal is a common complication. Another possible cause

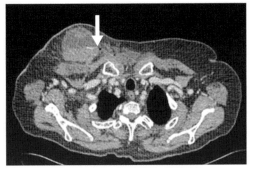

Fig. 4.112 Contrast-enhanced chest CT, showing a large subcutaneous hematoma formation (*arrow*) with acute contrast extravasation, caused by surgical exploration in an attempt to find the migrated catheter.

may be the "pinch-off" phenomenon, where the catheter is chronically compressed and ruptured between the clavicle and the first rib. Pinch-off is rare nowadays due to the wide use of the IJV for central venous access.

Prevention Strategies and Take-home Message

- Some surgeons, for fear of catheter disconnection, prefer to use a separate incision from below to expose and remove a TIVAD. This leaves the patient with an extra scar and is rarely, if ever, necessary if some simple rules are followed.
- Familiarity with the TIVAD that needs removal is crucial. To assess the type of device implanted, study the patient's files and if no information can be found perform a preoperative chest radiograph. Most devices have a unique appearance on X-rays.
- A chest radiograph is obviously indicated when looking for a detached catheter, to determine its location and whether it is in one piece—factors that can affect the removal plan.
- When exposing a TIVAD, blunt dissection using scissors or a simple mosquito forceps is preferable because catheters are notoriously easy to cut! Moreover, some devices have a small plastic safety sleeve to connect the port to the catheter, which can be easily removed if force is applied.
- To implant TIVADs, sonographically guided IJV punctures are preferable, which, among other benefits, will prevent "pinch-off" syndrome. Moreover, in the case of accidental catheter dislodgement during removal, the catheter tip is almost always lost in subcutaneous tissues and every attempt to grasp it pushes it even deeper. It is hopeless to chase a migrated catheter tip with forceps. Instead, the catheter may be easily exposed and removed from the IJV puncture.

Further Reading

Bostan M, Durakoğlugil ME, Satiroğlu O, Erdivanli B, Tufan G. Retrieval of embolized tip of port catheter from branch of right pulmonary artery using a macro snare catheter. Interv Med Appl Sci 2014;6(2):93–95

Choksy P, Zaidi SS, Kapoor D. Removal of intracardiac fractured port-A catheter utilizing an existing forearm peripheral intravenous access site in the cath lab. J Invasive Cardiol 2014;26(2):75–76

Chuang MT, Wu DK, Chang CA, et al. Concurrent use of pigtail and loop snare catheters for percutaneous retrieval of dislodged central venous port catheter. Kaohsiung J Med Sci 2011;27(11):514–519

Colón-Casasnovas NE, Lugo-Vicente H. Distal fragmented port catheter: case report and review of literature. Bol Asoc Med P R 2008;100(1):70–75

Elkhoury MI, Boeckx WD, Chahine EG, Feghali MA. Retrieval of port-A catheter fragment from the main and right pulmonary arteries 3 years after dislodgement. J Vasc Access 2008;9(4):296–298

Hara M, Takayama S, Imafuji H, Sato M, Funahashi H, Takeyama H. Single-port retrieval of peritoneal foreign body using SILS port: report of a case. Surg Laparosc Endosc Percutan Tech 2011;21(3):e126–e129

Kawata M, Ozawa K, Matsuura T, et al. Percutaneous interventional techniques to remove embolized silicone port catheters from heart and great vessels. Cardiovasc Interv Ther 2012;27(3):196–200

Motta Leal Filho JM, Carnevale FC, Nasser F, et al. Endovascular techniques and procedures, methods for removal of intravascular foreign bodies. Rev Bras Cir Cardiovasc 2010;25(2):202–208

Sowinski H, Kobayashi D, Turner DR. Transcutaneous removal of an intravenous catheter fragment using a spider FX™ Embolic Protection device. Catheter Cardiovasc Interv 2015;86(3):467–471

Wang PC, Liang HL, Wu TH, et al. Percutaneous retrieval of dislodged central venous port catheter: experience of 25 patients in a single institute. Acta Radiol 2009;50(1):15–20

Wang SC, Tsai CH, Hou CP, et al. Dislodgement of port-A catheters in pediatric oncology patients: 11 years of experience. World J Surg Oncol 2013;11:191

Incidental insertion of a venous central line into the subclavian artery

Patient History

A 78-year-old woman was scheduled for central venous line placement to facilitate hemofiltration therapy on the Intensive Care Unit (ICU) after surgery.

Initial Treatment Received

Right-side subclavian catheter placement (10F).

Problems Encountered during Treatment

Pulsatile arterial backflow during incidental placement of the venous line into the subclavian artery.

Imaging Plan

Angiography via the catheter in order to verify the intra-arterial position and to determine the arterial puncture level.

Resulting Complication

Inadvertent subclavian arterial puncture and large lumen catheter placement (**Figs. 4.113** and **4.114**).

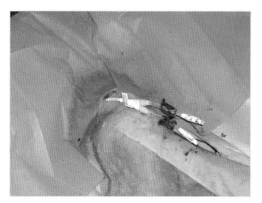

Fig. 4.113 Photograph showing the right-side subclavian puncture site.

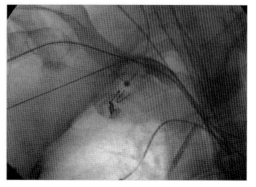

Fig. 4.115 Catheterization of the right-side subclavian artery and positioning of an 8 × 40-mm balloon for short-term inflation during catheter retrieval and sheath insertion for the Angio-Seal closure device.

Possible Strategies for Complication Management

- Insertion of a 0.035-inch guidewire and vascular closure with an 8F Angio-Seal (e.g., St. Jude Medical).
- Insertion of a 0.035-inch guidewire and vascular closure with one or two suture-mediated closure devices (e.g., Abbott Vascular 6F ProGlide or 10F Prostar).
- Transarterial balloon tamponade.
- Implantation of a stent graft after removal of the arterial "central line."
- Manual compression of the subclavian puncture site (unlikely to be successful).
- Surgery (if an endovascular approach fails).

Final Complication Management

Retrograde puncture of the right groin and 7F sheath insertion. Diagnostic angiography for anatomical evaluation of the aortic arch. Catheterization of the right subclavian artery and

prophylactic positioning of an 8 × 40-mm balloon for short-term inflation during the catheter retrieval.

After placement of a 0.035-inch guidewire through the central line, and removal of the catheter, an Angio-Seal closure device was introduced (**Figs. 4.115** and **4.116**). "Off-label" application of the 8F Angio-Seal device. Unfor-

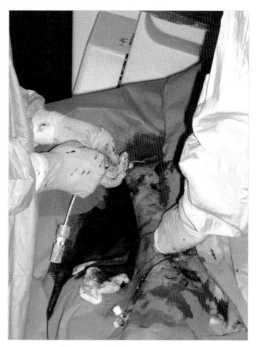

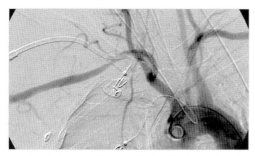

Fig. 4.114 Angiography via a 4F pigtail catheter placed in the aortic arch. Note the correct position of the contralateral left-side central line ending in the proximal superior vena cava.

Fig. 4.116 Placement of an 8F Angio-Seal closure device, while the balloon catheter is inflated in order to avoid any bleeding during device exchange and positioning.

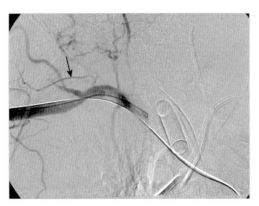

Fig. 4.117 Control angiography still showing some contrast extravasation (*arrow*) after final Angio-Seal placement.

tunately, control angiography of the left subclavian artery (LSA) showed contrast extravasation at the puncture site level (**Fig. 4.117**). The decision was made to implant a covered stent from the groin (Viabahn 8 × 50 mm). After stent graft placement, the subclavian artery was sealed (**Fig. 4.118**).

Complication Analysis

Puncture of the subclavian vein without ultrasound guidance resulted in inadvertent subclavian artery puncture and large-bore arterial central line insertion.

Prevention Strategies and Take-home Message

- When subclavian vein puncture for central line placement is difficult, a B-mode ultrasound should be used in order to gather further anatomical information.

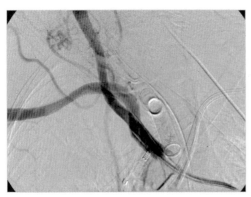

Fig. 4.118 Final angiography after placement of a covered stent from the groin.

- Once a subclavian vessel has been punctured, the venous position should be verified before a large-bore catheter is inserted.
- If there is arterial backflow from the needle it should be removed and manual compression performed. An increase of the access diameter by inserting the catheter should be avoided.
- Perform every vessel puncture with great care even if the procedure seems simple!
- Use B-mode ultrasound, whenever possible.

Further Reading

Chan CC, Lee V, Chu W, Tam YH, Li CK, Shing MM. Carotid jugular arteriovenous fistula: an unusual complication of internal jugular vein catheterization in children. Pediatr Blood Cancer 2012;59(7):1302–1304

Lennon M, Zaw NN, Pöpping DM, Wenk M. Procedural complications of central venous catheter insertion. Minerva Anestesiol 2012;78(11):1234–1240

Ruesch S, Walder B, Tramèr MR. Complications of central venous catheters: internal jugular versus subclavian access—a systematic review. Crit Care Med 2002;30(2):454–460

Schütz N, Doll S, Bonvini RF. Erroneous placement of central venous catheter in the subclavian artery: retrieval and successful hemostasis with a femoral closure device. Catheter Cardiovasc Interv 2011;77(1):154–157

Central venous port line separation

Patient History

A 54-year-old woman came to the outpatient oncology clinic for a chemotherapy follow-up appointment for breast cancer. Attempts to flush the Port-A-Cath device were unsuccessful. A chest X-ray was performed.

Initial Treatment Received

Four years previously the patient had been diagnosed with breast cancer. As part of the treatment regimen a Port-A-Cath device was inserted for central venous access for chemotherapy.

Problems Encountered during Treatment

There were no problems encountered during the initial insertion of the Port-A-Cath device based on a review of the procedure notes and postprocedure imaging from 4 years prior.

Imaging Plan

Usually, no dedicated additional imaging is required, because the dislocated catheter is already visualized by chest X-ray. If this was not yet done, a chest X-ray is indicated for exact catheter location.

Resulting Complication

Chest X-ray performed at time of current presentation demonstrated separation of the catheter from the central venous port hub (**Fig. 4.119**).

Possible Strategies for Complication Management

- Endovascular treatment via right internal jugular vein to snare catheter fragment.
- Endovascular treatment via right common femoral vein (CFV) to snare catheter fragment.

Final Complication Management

Endovascular access was obtained via the right CFV under ultrasound guidance using a micropuncture kit. An 8F vascular sheath was inserted. Using a 0.035-inch 145-cm-long Rosen wire and an 80-cm-long angled 5F MPA (multipurpose A) catheter, cannulation into the inferior vena cava (IVC) was performed. Fluoroscopy showed the catheter fragment overlying the upper chest. The angled MPA catheter and wire were advanced into the superior vena cava (SVC).

Contrast was injected through the MPA catheter and a central venogram was done (**Fig. 4.120**). Venogram showed the proximal tip of the catheter located in the right brachiocephalic vein

and the distal tip in the right ventricle based on catheter position. Neither the proximal nor the distal tip could be grabbed with a loop snare as the proximal tip was embedded in the vein wall and the distal tip appeared to be located near the tricuspid valve. Using a reverse curve VS-1 catheter, the middle of the catheter was hooked. The reverse-curve catheter was twisted and the catheter fragment brought down into the suprarenal IVC. At this point a 20-mm loop snare was used to engage the proximal edge of the catheter. The snare was brought to the middle of

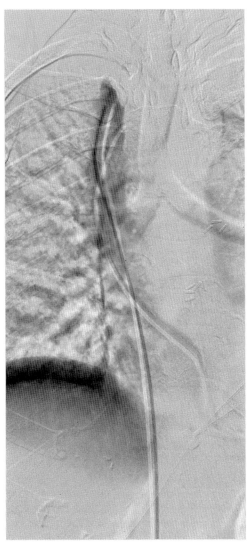

Fig. 4.120 Venogram showing the proximal tip of the catheter located in the right brachiocephalic vein and the distal tip in the right ventricle based on catheter position.

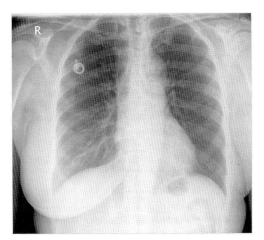

Fig. 4.119 Separated catheter from the central venous port hub.

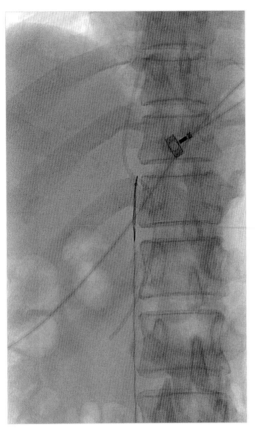

Fig. 4.121 The snare was brought to the middle of the catheter fragment, tightened, and the catheter was cinched down.

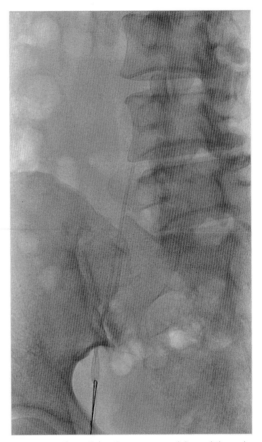

Fig. 4.122 The catheter fragment was delivered through an 8F sheath from the right CFV access.

the catheter fragment, tightened, and the catheter was cinched down (**Fig. 4.121**). The catheter fragment was then infolded and delivered through an 8F sheath from the right CFV access (**Fig. 4.122**).

Fluoroscopy of the chest and abdomen demonstrated no evidence of any retained catheter fragments (**Fig. 4.123**). Using local anesthetic and blunt dissection, the port device was removed from the right anterior chest.

Complication Analysis

Fracture, dehiscence, and separation of central venous access devices are not uncommon. Removing endovascular foreign bodies is one of the key skills of an interventional radiologist. In this case neither the proximal nor the distal tip of the catheter could be snared in the chest, which is not uncommon. "Hooking" the catheter fragment using a reverse-curve catheter is a useful technique to expose the edges of the catheter for a snaring maneuver in the IVC in a "lower risk environment."

Prevention Strategies and Take-home Message

- Intravascular foreign bodies are a common occurrence. Having multiple techniques and access points for retrieval is critical.
- Carefully delineating the anatomy with endovascular contrast is critical prior to any intervention.
- Always have the equipment and a plan in place if your initial access site or equipment is unsuccessful in retrieving the intravascular foreign body.

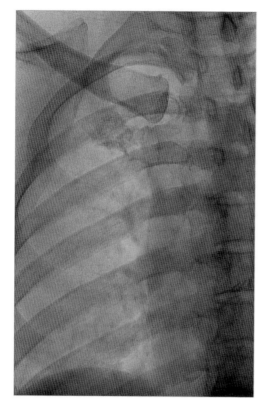

Fig. 4.123 Fluoroscopy of the chest and abdomen showing no evidence of any retained catheter fragments.

Further Reading

Bostan M, Durakoğlugil ME, Satiroğlu O, Erdivanli B, Tufan G. Retrieval of embolized tip of port catheter from branch of right pulmonary artery using a macro snare catheter. Interv Med Appl Sci 2014;6(2):93–95

Choksy P, Zaidi SS, Kapoor D. Removal of intracardiac fractured port-A catheter utilizing an existing forearm peripheral intravenous access site in the cath lab. J Invasive Cardiol 2014;26(2):75–76

Chuang MT, Wu DK, Chang CA, et al. Concurrent use of pigtail and loop snare catheters for percutaneous retrieval of dislodged central venous port catheter. Kaohsiung J Med Sci 2011;27(11):514–519

Colón-Casasnovas NE, Lugo-Vicente H. Distal fragmented port catheter: case report and review of literature. Bol Asoc Med P R 2008;100(1):70–75

Elkhoury MI, Boeckx WD, Chahine EG, Feghali MA. Retrieval of port-A catheter fragment from the main and right pulmonary arteries 3 years after dislodgement. J Vasc Access 2008;9(4):296–298

Hara M, Takayama S, Imafuji H, Sato M, Funahashi H, Takeyama H. Single-port retrieval of peritoneal foreign body using SILS port: report of a case. Surg Laparosc Endosc Percutan Tech 2011;21(3):e126–e129

Kawata M, Ozawa K, Matsuura T, et al. Percutaneous interventional techniques to remove embolized silicone port catheters from heart and great vessels. Cardiovasc Interv Ther 2012;27(3):196–200

Motta Leal Filho JM, Carnevale FC, Nasser F, et al. Endovascular techniques and procedures, methods for removal of intravascular foreign bodies. Rev Bras Cir Cardiovasc 2010;25(2):202–208

Sowinski H, Kobayashi D, Turner DR. Transcutaneous removal of an intravenous catheter fragment using a spider FX™ Embolic Protection device. Catheter Cardiovasc Interv 2015;86(3):467–471

Wang PC, Liang HL, Wu TH, et al. Percutaneous retrieval of dislodged central venous port catheter: experience of 25 patients in a single institute. Acta Radiol 2009;50(1):15–20

Wang SC, Tsai CH, Hou CP, et al. Dislodgement of port-A catheters in pediatric oncology patients: 11 years of experience. World J Surg Oncol 2013;11:191

Venous access complication—fibrin sheath and adherent thrombus—and how to avoid embolic complications

Patient History

An obese, elderly woman presented with problems with her permacath. Dialysis nurses reported that injection inflow was possible but aspiration was limited. Thrombosis of one of the catheter channels was suspected.

Initial Treatment Received

A standard in the dialysis practice of one of the contributing authors is to inject 10 mg of recombinant tissue plasminogen activator (rtPA) in 1.9 mL normal saline (the dead space volume of the catheter) into each lumen. This avoids any systemic thrombolysis.

When this failed to improve blood flow the patient was referred to angiography. Angiography revealed an extensive fibrin sheath with a large thrombus at the distal end of the permacath projecting into the right atrium (**Fig. 4.124**). Anticoagulation was begun with low molecular weight heparin (LMWH) (enoxaparin).

Problems Encountered during Treatment

During flushing of the permacath for angiography, the catheter began to extrude until the fibrin cuff, previously in a subcutaneous tunnel, appeared at the skin surface.

Imaging Plan

Computed tomography (CT) venogram and further angiography.

Resulting Complication

Imaging revealed a large atrial thrombus and extensive fibrin sheath with partial occlusion of the

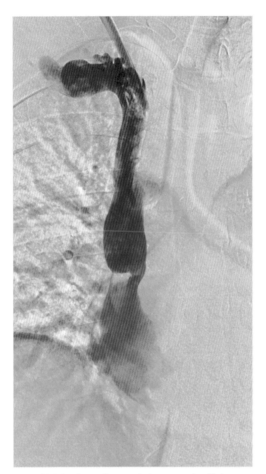

Fig. 4.124 Angiography revealed an extensive fibrin sheath with a large thrombus at the distal end of the permacath projecting into the right atrium.

superior vena cava (SVC). The permacath had extruded further almost to the junction of the subclavian and jugular veins. The patient had been off dialysis for 3 days.

Possible Strategies for Complication Management

- Insertion of alternative venous access:
  - Patient refused as she had had two prior failed permacaths via the left internal jugular vein.
  - Femoral vein access was considered risky because of obesity and infection risk.
- Removal of the permacath and hope the thrombus does not detach from the catheter.
- Insertion of a new permacath from higher in the right internal jugular vein or subclavian vein.

- Open thoracotomy and thrombectomy.
- Replacement of permacath with protection against pulmonary embolus.

Final Complication Management

Via an ultrasound guided femoral vein puncture in the thigh, a long 12F venous sheath was inserted into the hepatic portion of the inferior vena cava (IVC). A 24-mm-diameter self-expanding sinus-XL nitinol stent (OptiMed) was partially deployed immediately below the atrial thrombus to act as a trap for any loose thrombus (**Fig. 4.125**). A 5F

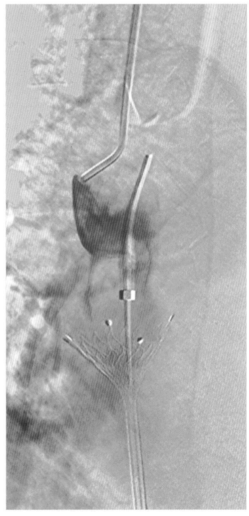

Fig. 4.125 Angiography via diagnostic catheter showing a 24-mm diameter self-expanding Optimed Sinus XL nitinol stent, partially deployed immediately below the atrial thrombus to act as a trap for any loose thrombus.

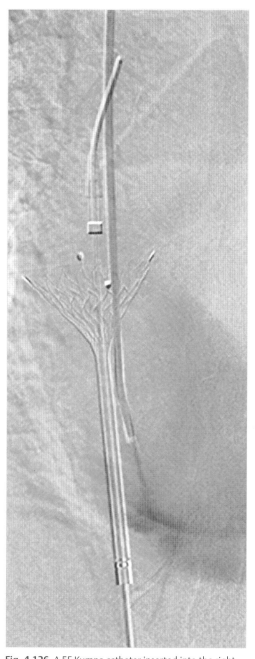

Fig. 4.126 A 5F Kumpe catheter inserted into the right internal jugular vein and a wire guide passed beyond the thrombus. The thrombus deflected the wire guide either into the right atrium or into the open stent.

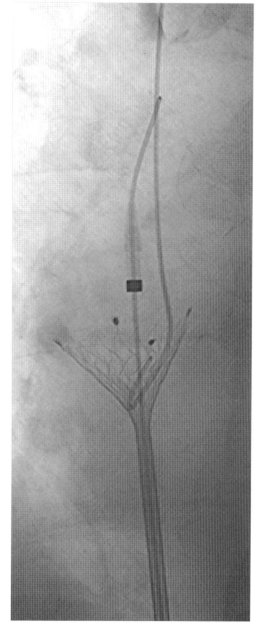

Fig. 4.127 The stent was closed around the wire guide and withdrawn until the guidewire could be released in the inferior vena cava.

Kumpe catheter was then inserted into the right internal jugular vein and a wire guide passed beyond the thrombus. Since the thrombus deflected the wire guide either into the right atrium (**Fig. 4.126**) or into the open stent (**Fig. 4.127**) the stent was closed around the wire guide and withdrawn until the guidewire could be released in the IVC (**Fig. 4.128**). The nitinol stent was then repositioned partly opened below the thrombus and the permacath removed.

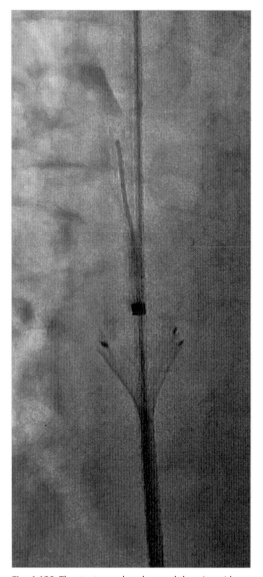

Fig. 4.128 The stent was closed around the wireguide and withdrawn until the guidewire could be released in the inferior vena cava.

A new long permacath was inserted from the high right internal jugular puncture down to the IVC, flushed and heparin locked (**Fig. 4.129**).

Once it was apparent the thrombus was not mobile, the nitinol stent was sheathed and removed.

Anticoagulation has been continued with the expectation that the thrombus will resolve completely.

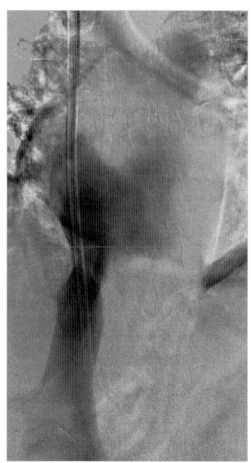

Fig. 4.129 A new long permacath inserted from the high right internal jugular puncture down to the IVC, flushed and heparin locked.

Complication Analysis

Inadequate flushing and failure to recognize a fibrin sheath early resulted in a potentially life-threatening thrombus formation.

Prevention Strategies and Take-Home Message

- Permacath withdrawal is more common in obese patients especially if the tunneled portion is long and in a pendulant portion of the chest.
- Early management of fibrin sheaths is preferred.
- Think outside the box for solutions.
- Know how far a stent can be deployed before it cannot be recaptured.

Further Reading

Gabriel J. Preventing and managing complications of CVADs. Nurs Times 2013;109(40):20–23

Gaddh M, Antun A, Yamada K, et al. Venous access catheter-related thrombosis in patients with cancer. Leuk Lymphoma 2014;55(3):501–508

Latham GJ, Thompson DR. Thrombotic complications in children from short-term percutaneous central venous catheters: what can we do? Paediatr Anaesth 2014;24(9):902–911

Mino JS, Gutnick JR, Monteiro R, Anzlovar N, Siperstein AE. Line-associated thrombosis as the major cause of hospital-acquired deep vein thromboses: an analysis from National Surgical Quality Improvement Program data and a call to re-assess prophylaxis strategies. Am J Surg 2014;208(1):45–49

Nayeemuddin M, Pherwani AD, Asquith JR. Imaging and management of complications of central venous catheters. Clin Radiol 2013;68(5):529–544

Zochios V, Umar I, Simpson N, Jones N. Peripherally inserted central catheter (PICC)-related thrombosis in critically ill patients. J Vasc Access 2014;15(5):329–337

4.3 Lesion Treatment–Related Complications

4.3.1 Catheter Guidance and Navigation

Wire Advancement

Uncontrolled advancement of a hydrophylic 0.035-inch guidewire

Patient History

A 69-year-old patient suffered from acute abdominal and right flank pain, developing several hours following diagnostic coronary angiography via retrograde access to the right common femoral artery (CFA). Apart from his coronary heart disease no further comorbidities were reported. During coronary angiography a vascular closure device was used successfully and immediate hemostasis of the puncture site was achieved. The patient now presented with clinical signs of hypovolemia, controllable by means of fluid resuscitation. Clinical inspection of the right groin did not show significant hematoma or active bleeding.

Initial Treatment Received

Diagnostic coronary angiography.

Problems Encountered during Treatment

Unremarkable procedure, no complications reported!

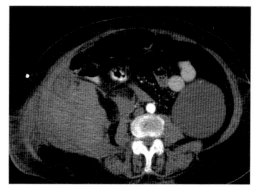

Fig. 4.130 Contrast-enhanced axial CT scan showing a huge retroperitoneal hematoma.

Imaging Plan

Computed tomography angiography (CTA).

Resulting Complication

There is active retroperitoneal bleeding with a huge right retroperitoneal hematoma proven by contrast-enhanced CTA (**Figs. 4.130** and **4.131**).

Possible Strategies for Complication Management

- Endovascular treatment via ipsilateral or contralateral retrograde access to the CFA.

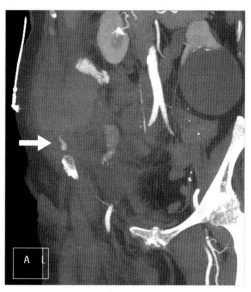

Fig. 4.131 Coronal maximum intensity projection (MIP) reconstructions show the feeder vessel (deep circumflex iliac artery) and the location of active bleeding (*arrow*).

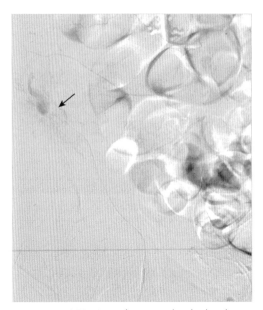

Fig. 4.132 A 2.7F microcatheter was already placed at the target lesion via a retrograde access to the CFA (4F sheath). The source of bleeding was verified by contrast media injection (*arrow*).

- Catheterization of the feeder vessel, for example using a microcatheter and followed by selective microcoil embolization.
- Alternative agents for embolization: glue, large particles, gelfoam.
- Surgery (if an endovascular approach fails).

Final Complication Management

Endovascular treatment via ipsilateral retrograde access to the CFA (4F sheath). Catheterization of the feeder vessel with a microcatheter (2.7F) followed by selective microcoil embolization (**Figs. 4.132** and **4.133**).

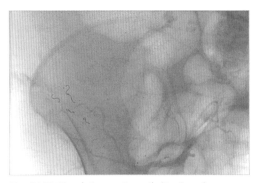

Fig. 4.133 Five platinum microcoils (2 × 5 mm) were placed at the bleeding site.

Complication Analysis

Suspected uncontrolled advancement of a hydrophylic guidewire during the initial procedure (after further interviewing the operating cardiologist), resulted in side-branch perforation.

Prevention Strategies and Take-home Message

- Guidewire advancement should be constantly controlled under fluoroscopy, especially when using hydrophilic-coated wires!
- Wires should never be pushed against resistance without fluoroscopic guidance!

Further Reading

Axelrod DJ, Freeman H, Pukin L, Guller J, Mitty HA. Guidewire perforation leading to fatal perirenal hemorrhage from transcortical collaterals after renal artery stent placement. J Vasc Interv Radiol 2004;15(9):985–987

Blake PG, Uldall R. Cardiac perforation by a guidewire during subclavian catheter insertion. Int J Artif Organs 1989;12(2):111–113

Durão C, Barros A, Guerreiro R, Pedrosa F. "Death by a thread"—peritonitis due to visceral perforation by a guidewire, during proximal femur osteosynthesis with DHS: a fatal case and legal implications. Forensic Sci Int 2015;249:e12–e14

Hiroshima Y, Tajima K, Shiono Y, et al. Soft J-tipped guidewire-induced cardiac perforation in a patient with right ventricular lipomatosis and wall thinning. Intern Med 2012;51(18):2609–2612

Hong YM, Lee SR. A case of guidewire fracture with remnant filaments in the left anterior descending coronary artery and aorta. Korean Circ J 2010;40(9):475–477

Lee SY, Kim SM, Bae JW, et al. Renal artery perforation related with hydrophilic guidewire during coronary intervention: successful treatment with polyvinyl alcohol injection. Can J Cardiol 2012;28(5):612.e5–e7

Tanaka S, Nishigaki K, Ojio S, et al. Transcatheter embolization by autologous blood clot is useful management for small side-branch perforation due to percutaneous coronary intervention guidewire. J Cardiol 2008;52(3):285–289

Störger H, Ruef J. Closure of guidewire-induced coronary artery perforation with a two-component fibrin glue. Catheter Cardiovasc Interv 2007;70(2):237–240

Hydrophylic guidewires and side-branch perforation (case 1)

Patient History

A 61-year-old male patient suffering from peripheral artery occlusive disease (PAOD) presented a 10-cm occlusion of the superficial femoral artery (SFA) during magnetic resonance angiography (MRA). The patient was scheduled for SFA recanalization. After antegrade groin access and administration of 5,000 IU of heparin and 1,000 mg ASA (aspirin) intravenously, the lesion was recanalized successfully using a hydrophilic-coated 0.018-inch wire. The procedure was completed by placement of a self-expanding stent.

During the procedure, the patient complained of a short, self-limiting, heavy pain localized in the ipsilateral calf. The operator instantly retracted the guidewire for 4–5 cm, with its tip being left distally from the treated lesion. Control angiography for run-off evaluation showed contrast extravasation of the proximal and distal *inferior* medial genicular artery.

Initial Treatment Received

SFA recanalization via antegrade approach followed by plain old balloon angioplasty (POBA) and stent placement (self-expanding stent [SES]).

Problems Encountered during Treatment

Apart from the patient complaining of a short episode of heavy sharp pain in the calf during POBA and stent placement, the intervention was uneventful. However, bleeding from an infragenual side branch was noticed during control angiography (**Fig. 4.134**).

Imaging Plan

Selective/superselective angiography in order to visualize the exact source of bleeding (**Fig. 4.135**).

Resulting Complication

Side-branch perforation.

Possible Strategies for Complication Management

- Manual compression of the calf at the level of the detected bleeding source for 3 minutes. Repetition of manual compression procedure until bleeding stops.
- Placement of a pressure cuff, which is applied for 3 minutes between systolic and diastolic pressure; pedal pulses should be palpable; repetition for another 3 minutes if warranted; inflation for 1–3 minutes to 20 mm Hg suprasystolic pressure might be

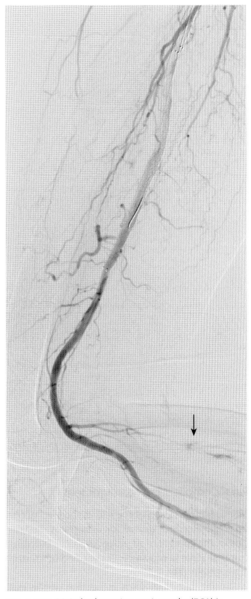

Fig. 4.134 Digital subtraction angiography (DSA) in a lateral projection and 90° knee bending after stent placement in the mid-part SFA. A moderate contrast blush (*arrow*) was noticed at the level of the inferior medial genicular artery.

helpful in dedicated situations resistant to mild compression (adapted from the instructions for use for FemoStop [St. Jude Medical] compression clamp).
- Selective catheterization of the feeder vessel using a microcatheter with embolization (coil, glue, collagen sponge).

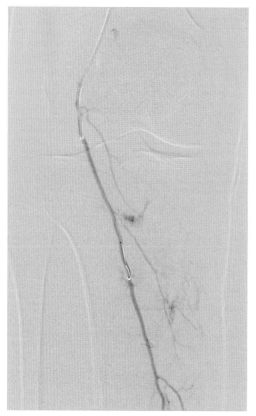

Fig. 4.135 Angiography via 4F angle-tip diagnostic catheter and 0.018-inch guidewire in place. Contrast extravasation was verified at the proximal and distal part of the inferior medial genicular artery.

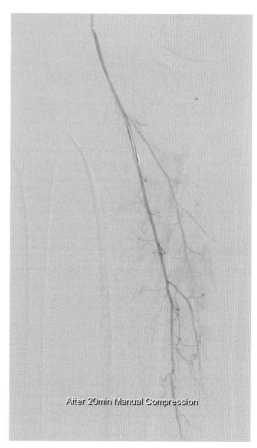

Fig. 4.136 Final angiographic control after 20 minutes of manual compression. No signs of residual bleeding were visible.

Final Complication Management

Manual compression of the calf at the level of the detected bleeding source for 3 minutes. Repetition of the compression procedure until bleeding stopped. Final hemostasis was verified by control angiography (**Fig. 4.136**).

Clinical follow-up with inspection of the calf and Doppler assessment to rule out development of compartment syndrome.

Complication Analysis

Uncontrolled hydrophilic guidewire advancement resulted in perforation of a calf vessel side branch.

Prevention Strategies and Take-home Message

• Always be aware of the position of the distal end of hydrophilic guidewires.

• Secure wires carefully during catheter or device exchange (advancement and removal).
• Whenever possible, keep visual control over the hydrophilic tip of the guidewire.
• Take patients' complaints seriously and check what could be responsible for the onset of new symptoms during the intervention.

Further Reading

Axelrod DJ, Freeman H, Pukin L, Guller J, Mitty HA. Guidewire perforation leading to fatal perirenal hemorrhage from transcortical collaterals after renal artery stent placement. J Vasc Interv Radiol 2004;15(9):985–987

Blake PG, Uldall R. Cardiac perforation by a guidewire during subclavian catheter insertion. Int J Artif Organs 1989;12(2):111–113

Durão C, Barros A, Guerreiro R, Pedrosa F. "Death by a thread"—peritonitis due to visceral perforation by a guidewire, during proximal femur osteosynthesis with DHS: a fatal case and legal implications. Forensic Sci Int 2015;249:e12–e14

Hiroshima Y, Tajima K, Shiono Y, et al. Soft J-tipped guide-wire-induced cardiac perforation in a patient with right ventricular lipomatosis and wall thinning. Intern Med 2012;51(18):2609–2612

Hong YM, Lee SR. A case of guidewire fracture with remnant filaments in the left anterior descending coronary artery and aorta. Korean Circ J 2010;40(9):475–477

Lee SY, Kim SM, Bae JW, et al. Renal artery perforation related with hydrophilic guidewire during coronary intervention: successful treatment with polyvinyl alcohol injection. Can J Cardiol 2012;28(5):612.e5–e7

Störger H, Ruef J. Closure of guidewire-induced coronary artery perforation with a two-component fibrin glue. Catheter Cardiovasc Interv 2007;70(2):237–240

Tanaka S, Nishigaki K, Ojio S, et al. Transcatheter embolization by autologous blood clot is useful management for small side-branch perforation due to percutaneous coronary intervention guidewire. J Cardiol 2008;52(3):285–289

Hydrophylic guidewires and side-branch perforation (case 2)

Patient History

A 68-year-old man suffering from peripheral artery occlusive disease (PAOD) presented with multiple high-grade stenoses of the superficial femoral artery (SFA) during diagnostic magnetic resonance angiography (MRA). The patient was scheduled for SFA percutaneous transluminal angioplasty (PTA) and optional stenting. After antegrade groin access and administration of 5,000 IU of heparin and 1000 mg ASA (aspirin) intravenously, the lesions were passed successfully using a hydrophilic-coated 0.018-inch wire. The procedure was completed by placement of multiple self-expanding stents (SESs) due to multi-level flow-limiting dissections and elastic recoil despite repeated long-term plain old balloon angioplasty (POBA). Several devices (PTA catheters and stent delivery catheters) had been advanced, removed, and exchanged; a 0.018-inch guidewire was left in place during the entire procedure.

During the procedure (probably during device removal or advancement), the patient complained of a short, self-limiting, heavy pain attack in the ipsilateral calf. The guidewire was retracted immediately for a few centimeters and positioned in the popliteal artery (PIII), still distal from the treated lesion. During control angiography, extravasation of contrast media in two different infragenual side branches was depicted (**Fig. 4.137**).

Initial Treatment Received

SFA multilevel lesion treatment via an antegrade approach followed by POBA and stent placement (SESs).

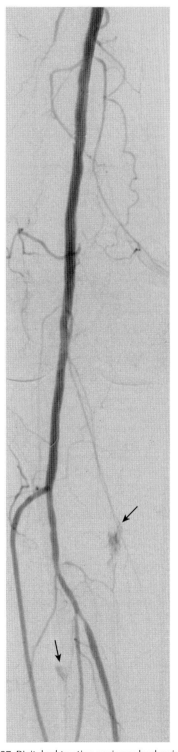

Fig. 4.137 Digital subtraction angiography showing a moderate contrast blush (*arrows*) at the level of the inferior medial genicular artery and more distally from a peroneal artery side branch.

Problems Encountered during Treatment

Apart from the patient complaining of a self-limiting severe sharp pain during POBA and stent placement, the intervention was uneventful. However, bleeding from infragenual side branches was noticed during control angiography.

Imaging Plan

Selective angiography in order to visualize the exact source of bleeding.

Resulting Complication

Side-branch perforation.

Possible Strategies for Complication Management

- Manual compression of the calf at the level of detected bleeding source for 3 minutes. Repetition of compression procedure until bleeding stops.
- Placement of a pressure cuff, which is applied for 3 minutes between systolic and diastolic pressure; pedal pulses should be palpable; repetition for another 3 minutes if warranted; short-term inflation for 1–3 minutes to 20 mm Hg suprasystolic pressure might be helpful in dedicated situations resistant to mild compression (adapted from the instructions for use for FemoStop [St. Jude Medical] compression clamp).
- Selective catheterization of the feeder vessel by microcatheter and embolization (coil, glue, collagen sponge).

Final Complication Management

Inflation of a pressure cuff placed below the knee at the level of detected bleeding source for 3 minutes at diastolic pressure. Repetition of compression procedure by carefully inflating the cuff until bleeding stopped as proven in the final angiographic control (**Fig. 4.138**). Proof of hemostasis by control angiography. Clinical follow-up with inspection of the calf and Doppler assessment to rule out development of compartment syndrome.

Complication Analysis

Uncontrolled hydrophilic guidewire advancement resulted in perforation of calf vessel side branches.

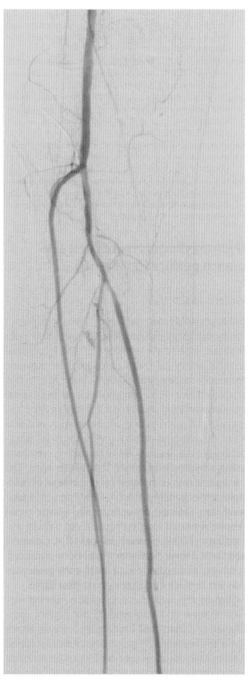

Fig. 4.138 Angiography via 4F angle-tip diagnostic catheter and 0.018-inch guidewire in place. Significant contrast extravasation was no longer visible.

Prevention Strategies and Take-home Message

- Always be aware of the position of the distal end of hydrophilic guidewires.

- Secure wires carefully during catheter or device exchange (advancement and removal).
- Whenever possible, keep visual control over the hydrophilic tip of the guidewire.
- Take patients' complaints seriously and check what could be responsible for the onset of new symptoms during the intervention.

Further Reading

Axelrod DJ, Freeman H, Pukin L, Guller J, Mitty HA. Guidewire perforation leading to fatal perirenal hemorrhage from transcortical collaterals after renal artery stent placement. J Vasc Interv Radiol 2004;15(9):985–987

Blake PG, Uldall R. Cardiac perforation by a guidewire during subclavian catheter insertion. Int J Artif Organs 1989;12(2):111–113

Durão C, Barros A, Guerreiro R, Pedrosa F. "Death by a thread"—peritonitis due to visceral perforation by a guidewire, during proximal femur osteosynthesis with DHS: a fatal case and legal implications. Forensic Sci Int 2015;249:e12–e14

Hiroshima Y, Tajima K, Shiono Y, et al. Soft J-tipped guidewire-induced cardiac perforation in a patient with right ventricular lipomatosis and wall thinning. Intern Med 2012;51(18):2609–2612

Hong YM, Lee SR. A case of guidewire fracture with remnant filaments in the left anterior descending coronary artery and aorta. Korean Circ J 2010;40(9):475–477

Lee MS, Applegate B, Rao SV, Kirtane AJ, Seto A, Stone GW. Minimizing femoral artery access complications during percutaneous coronary intervention: a comprehensive review. Catheter Cardiovasc Interv 2014;84(1):62–69

Störger H, Ruef J. Closure of guidewire-induced coronary artery perforation with a two-component fibrin glue. Catheter Cardiovasc Interv 2007;70(2):237–240

Tanaka S, Nishigaki K, Ojio S, et al. Transcatheter embolization by autologous blood clot is useful management for small side-branch perforation due to percutaneous coronary intervention guidewire. J Cardiol 2008;52(3):285–289

Flow-limiting axillary artery dissection after failed transbrachial approach for percutaneous coronary intervention

Patient History

A 62-year-old patient suffered from a pulseless right brachial artery 4 weeks after percutaneous coronary intervention (PCI; drug-eluting stent [DES] left anterior descending [LAD]) via a transradial approach. Comorbidities were hypertension and smoking history for 10 years. Since discharge after PCI, the patient was on ASA (aspirin), statins, and antihypertensive triple therapy. Two weeks after PCI, the patient reported arm pain during stress and motoric weakness. A symptomatic distal subclavian or axillary artery stenosis was suspected based on clinical and Doppler ultrasound examination.

Initial Treatment Received

PCI was planned using a right-side transradial approach. A guide catheter of unknown size (6F or 7F) failed to catheterize the left coronary artery. Attempts to exchange the catheter via a guidewire failed. A snaring maneuver from the groin, after completing PCI from an inguinal approach, was successful for catheter removal. Final angiography of the brachiocephalic trunk and the subclavian artery showed no damage of the vessels, where the catheter kinked (angiogram not available). Patient's discharge was uneventful.

Doppler ultrasound 3 days after PCI depicted triphasic flow signals for all peripheral right arm arteries (axillary, brachial, radial, and ulnar).

Two weeks later the patient presented with symptoms, as described above.

Problems Encountered during Treatment

Failed placement of a guiding catheter via a transradial approach in order to perform PCI. Manipulation with the guiding catheter resulted in catheter kinking. Catheter removal via a radial approach failed. In order to avoid any vessel damage, the distal and kinked catheter was snared from a groin approach and successfully removed (no images available). Attempts made to overcome this problem using a hydrophilic-coated guidewire resulted in scaling of the coating.

Imaging Plan

Angiography of the right upper extremity from the groin.

Resulting Complication

Short-distance circumscriptive flow-limiting dissection of the right axillary artery (**Fig. 4.139**).

Possible Strategies for Complication Management

- Endovascular treatment via retrograde groin access from a common femoral artery (CFA) or retrograde radial/brachial ipsilateral access.

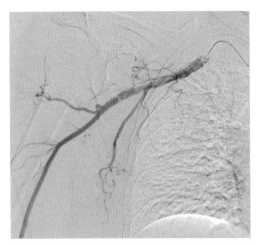

Fig. 4.139 Diagnostic, selective angiography of the right subclavian artery shows a short-distance, circumscriptive flow-limiting dissection of the right axillary artery.

- Crossing the lesion and performing long-term percutaneous transluminal angioplasty (PTA) or cutting-balloon angioplasty (CBA), if PTA is not sufficient.
- Surgery (if an endovascular approach fails).

Final Complication Management

Endovascular treatment via retrograde groin access from the right CFA (6F sheath, 90 cm long). The sheath was placed in the subclavian artery. A 4F JB catheter (125 cm) was placed in front of the lesion. Wire (0.018-inch Terumo) crossing failed (**Fig. 4.140**). The reverse side of an 0.018-inch wire could pass the dissection membrane. After verified successful lesion crossing with the catheter, the reverse-side flexible wire tip was placed beyond the lesion and long-term PTA with a 7 × 40-mm balloon was performed (**Fig. 4.141**).

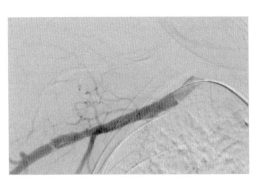

Fig. 4.140 Failed Terumo wire (0.018-inch) crossing.

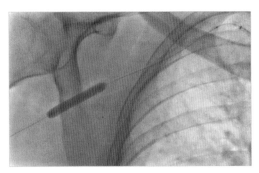

Fig. 4.141 After successful lesion crossing (with reverse side of the Terumo wire), long-term PTA with a 7 × 40-mm balloon was performed.

Final angiography in neutral (**Fig. 4.142**) and elevated (**Fig. 4.143**) arm position showed an immediate contrast run-off; peripheral pulses were palpable.

Complication Analysis

A manipulation of a guide catheter placed for transradial PCI led to catheter kinking in the axillary artery, resulting in a flow-limiting dissection.

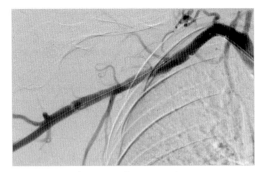

Fig. 4.142 Final angiography in neutral arm position showing an immediate contrast run-off.

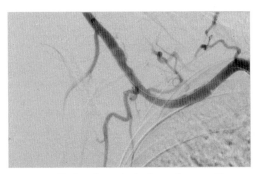

Fig. 4.143 Final angiography in elevated arm position showing an immediate contrast run-off.

Prevention Strategies and Take-home Message

- Careful manipulation of endovascular instruments.
- If a severe resistance is noticed or unknown forces are acting during guidewire or (guide) catheter placement and manipulation, all further manipulations should be carried out with great care.
- All wire and catheter advancements should be done under fluoroscopic control.

Further Reading

Axelrod DJ, Freeman H, Pukin L, Guller J, Mitty HA. Guidewire perforation leading to fatal perirenal hemorrhage from transcortical collaterals after renal artery stent placement. J Vasc Interv Radiol 2004;15(9):985–987

Blake PG, Uldall R. Cardiac perforation by a guidewire during subclavian catheter insertion. Int J Artif Organs 1989;12(2):111–113

Durão C, Barros A, Guerreiro R, Pedrosa F. "Death by a thread"—peritonitis due to visceral perforation by a guidewire, during proximal femur osteosynthesis with DHS: a fatal case and legal implications. Forensic Sci Int 2015;249:e12–e14

Hiroshima Y, Tajima K, Shiono Y, et al. Soft J-tipped guidewire-induced cardiac perforation in a patient with right ventricular lipomatosis and wall thinning. Intern Med 2012;51(18):2609–2612

Hong YM, Lee SR. A case of guidewire fracture with remnant filaments in the left anterior descending coronary artery and aorta. Korean Circ J 2010;40(9):475–477

Lee SY, Kim SM, Bae JW, et al. Renal artery perforation related with hydrophilic guidewire during coronary intervention: successful treatment with polyvinyl alcohol injection. Can J Cardiol 2012;28(5):612.e5–e7

Störger H, Ruef J. Closure of guidewire-induced coronary artery perforation with a two-component fibrin glue. Catheter Cardiovasc Interv 2007;70(2):237–240

Tanaka S, Nishigaki K, Ojio S, et al. Transcatheter embolization by autologous blood clot is useful management for small side-branch perforation due to percutaneous coronary intervention guidewire. J Cardiol 2008;52(3):285–289

Potentially fatal complication from superior vena cava angioplasty to facilitate permanent dialysis access

Patient History

A 55-year-old woman on chronic dialysis had a failed internal jugular vein (IJV) catheter due to superior vena cava (SVC) obstruction and subsequently a temporary femoral catheter for dialysis was placed. She was referred for SVC angioplasty to facilitate permanent dialysis access placement from the right IJV.

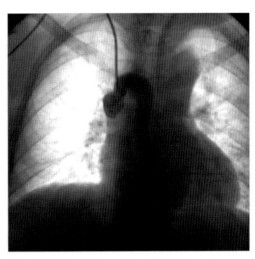

Fig. 4.144 Complete "cup-shaped" SVC obstruction below azygos vein confluence with resultant azygos vein collateral circulation.

Initial Treatment Received

The right IJV was accessed using ultrasound and a 6F vascular sheath was placed. The initial angiography showed complete SVC obstruction at a level just centrally to the azygos vein confluence, which resulted in remarkable dilatation and flow reversal of the azygos, making it the main collateral to the inferior vena cava (IVC) (**Fig. 4.144**).

Problems Encountered during Treatment

During attempted catheterization of the obstruction a straight-tipped stiff hydrophylic guidewire was advanced beyond the level of the obstruction (**Fig. 4.145**) but after catheter advancement and a brief hand injection it was discovered that the catheter was indeed in the pericardial cavity. The catheter was pulled back and a new angiography from the sheath proved there was apparent SVC dissection contrast media extravasation from the SVC into the pericardial cavity (**Fig. 4.146**). The patient stated she had difficulty breathing and chest pain, had a fall in blood pressure, and nonpalpable radial pulses. She also presented with distended neck veins. Low blood pressure and distended neck veins are recognized as the first two signs of the Beck's triad for cardiac tamponade (the third being muffled heart sounds).

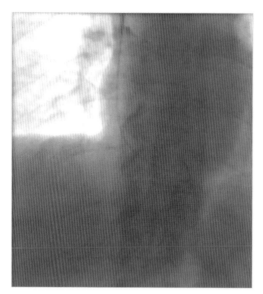

Fig. 4.145 Passage of straight-tipped stiff guidewire through the level of the obstruction as visualized on fluoroscopy.

Imaging Plan

An upper abdominal ultrasound verified the presence of a large pericardial collection of blood about 4 cm in anterior thickness, presumably hemopericardium. Using a subxiphoid transhepatic approach, a 15-cm 18G needle was used to enter the pericardium. In the mean time an emergency anesthesiology team started resuscitating the patient. Blood aspiration from the pericardium using the 18G needle and 20-mL syringe suction proved to be inefficiently slow, so a standard J-type Teflon-coated guidewire was used (**Fig. 4.147**) to insert a 5F pigtail catheter. After removing about 200 mL of blood, again, due to insufficient drainage, the 5F pigtail was exchanged over the wire for a standard 8F pericardiocentesis set using a set of dilators. A total of approximately 500 mL of blood was drained from the pericardial cavity, with remarkable improvement in the patient. A completion angiography with the drainage tube in place showed no extravasation (**Fig. 4.148**). The drainage tube remained for 24 hours but with no additional drainage and was removed. A peritoneal dialysis catheter was then

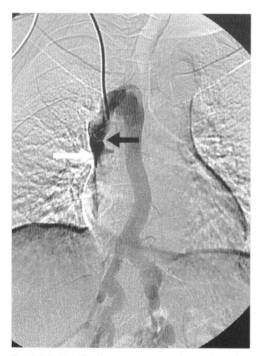

Fig. 4.146 Digital subtraction angiography run from the sheath confirms SVC wall dissection beyond the level of the obstruction (*black arrow*) and site of wall rupture with extravasation into the pericardial cavity (*white arrow*).

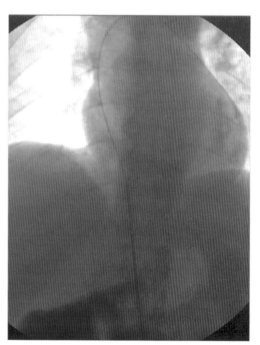

Fig. 4.147 Sonographically guided needle puncture and guidewire insertion into the pericardial cavity.

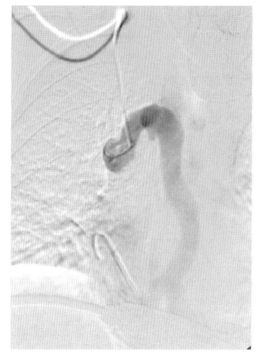

Fig. 4.148 Final angiography, showing no extravasation and final position of the 8F drainage tube.

inserted, the femoral catheter removed, and the patient was discharged from the hospital.

Resulting Complication

Active bleeding from SVC catheter dissection and perforation to the pericardial cavity, creating acute pericardial tamponade.

Possible Strategies for Complication Management

- Supporting the guidewire used to cross the obstruction with an inflated 16-mm balloon to center the crossing effort in the middle of the obstruction, could have prevented SVC dissection and perforation. The balloon could be also used as a safeguard, to inflate it in case SVC perforation occurs. It probably would have helped in this case to have an assistant inflate a balloon in the SVC while the primary operator tried to access the pericardium, but the presence of the resuscitation anesthesiology team allowed little room for sterile work around the patient's IJV.

Final Complication Management

Percutaneous sonographically guided placement of an 8F drainage tube in the pericardial cavity.

Complication Analysis

Dissection across an SVC obstruction by the guidewire and catheter along with perforation of SVC into the pericardial cavity, resulting in acute hemopericardium causing acute cardiac tamponade.

Prevention Strategies and Take-home Message

- Be prepared and always have an appropriately sized balloon to inflate across a perforation.
- Patients on dialysis are usually in a volume-depleted state, making them more prone to developing severe cardiac tamponade as a result of hemopericardium. Patients' intravascular volume expansion and emergency team activation should be established immediately.
- Plain needle aspiration in acute cardiac tamponade is insecure because it can cause loss of position, myocardial or coronary vessel injury, and is slow and cumbersome. It should be exchanged for a drain catheter as soon as possible.

Further Reading

O'Horo SK, Soares GM, Dubel GJ. Acute pericardial effusion during endovascular intervention for superior vena cava syndrome: case series and review. Semin Interv Radiol 2007;24(1):82–86

Oshima K, Takahashi T, Ishikawa S, Nagashima T, Hirai K, Morishita Y. Superior vena cava rupture caused during balloon dilatation for treatment of SVC syndrome due to repetitive catheter ablation—a case report. Angiology 2006;57(2):247–249

Tempelhof M, Campbell J, Ilkhanoff L. Sinus arrest following angioplasty and stenting for superior vena cava syndrome. J Invasive Cardiol 2014;26(2):E21–E23

Swelling of the supraclavicular area after unsuccessful recanalization of an occluded axillofemoral bypass graft

Patient History

A 68-year-old patient suffered from critical ischemia of both legs. The patient had a previous aortobifemoral graft placed surgically 3 years ago, followed by surgical repair of a distal anastomotic pseudoaneurysm 4 weeks ago. The patient presented with acute critical leg ischemia of the right leg. Duplex ultrasound demonstrated an occluded right limb of the aortobifemoral graft. The patient underwent an emergent right axillary artery to right common femoral artery (CFA) surgical graft placement. The patient returned 3 weeks later with critical right leg ischemia and an occluded right axillary artery to CFA graft.

Initial Treatment Received

The patient underwent a percutaneous endovascular attempt at recanalization of the axillary artery to CFA graft, which was unsuccessful.

Problems Encountered during Treatment

The procedure notes indicate an inability to cannulate the axillary artery to femoral artery graft from a right subclavian artery approach (**Fig. 4.149**). The patient subsequently developed swelling in the supraclavicular area on the right and presented to the Emergency Department 48 hours later.

Imaging Plan

Computed tomography angiography (CTA).

Resulting Complication

A large pseudoaneurysm arising from the right subclavian artery (**Figs. 4.150** and **4.151**).

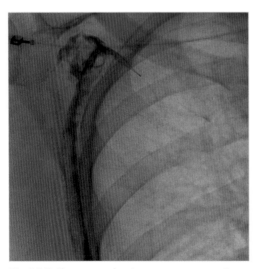

Fig. 4.149 Fluoroscopy showing contrast extravasation in the surrounding tissue; a guidewire and a catheter are still in place.

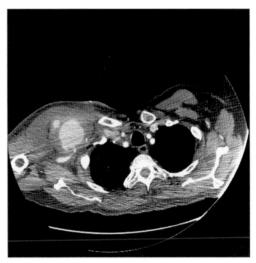

Fig. 4.150 Contrast-enhanced computed tomography (CT) depicts a large pseudoaneurysm arising from the right subclavian artery.

Possible Strategies for Complication Management

- Endovascular treatment via ipsilateral or contralateral retrograde access to the CFA with catheterization of the feeder vessel and placement of covered stent.
- Embolization of pseudoaneurysm.
- Thrombin injection into pseudoaneurysm.
- Surgery (if an endovascular approach fails).

Final Complication Management

Endovascular treatment via a right retrograde access to the CFA followed by insertion of a 90-cm-

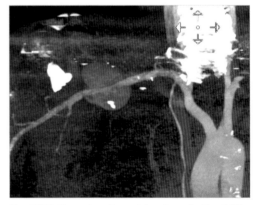

Fig. 4.151 Coronal maximum intensity projection (MIP) reconstruction shows the large pseudoaneurysm arising from the mid-part of the right subclavian artery, located at suspected anastomosis site.

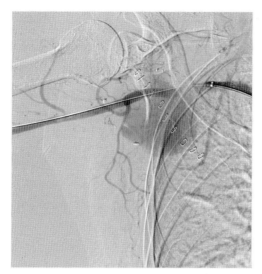

Fig. 4.152 Diagnostic angiogram via retrograde groin access demonstrates a large pseudoaneurysm arising from the mid-right subclavian artery.

long 7F vascular sheath. Selective catheterization of right brachiocephalic artery using a 5F, 90°-angled catheter. Diagnostic angiogram demonstrated a large pseudoaneurysm arising from the mid-right subclavian artery (**Fig. 4.152**). The subclavian artery was crossed with an angled catheter and 0.035-inch, 260-cm-long Teflon-coated steel wire. A 7 × 40-mm covered stent was placed with complete exclusion of the pseudoaneurysm. There was no evidence of an endoleak (**Fig. 4.153**). Groin closure was performed using a "preclose technique" with use of two suture-mediated closure devices.

Complication Analysis

Suspected uncontrolled advancement of a hydrophilic guidewire during the initial proce-

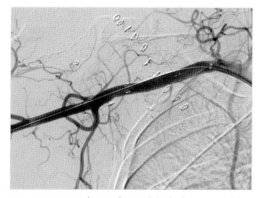

Fig. 4.153 No evidence of an endoleak after successful placement of a 7 × 40-mm covered stent.

dure resulted in perforation of right subclavian artery.

Prevention Strategies and Take-home Message

- Guidewire advancement should be controlled under fluoroscopy, especially when using hydrophilic-coated wires!
- Wires should never be pushed against resistance without fluoroscopic guidance.
- Nonhydrophilic wires, if possible, when trying to cannulate or cross a vessel.

Further Reading

Thompson CS, Rodriguez JA, Ramaiah VG, Olsen D, Diethrich EB. Pseudoaneurysm of the aortic arch after aortosubclavian bypass treated with endoluminal stent grafting—a case report. Vasc Endovasc Surg 2003;37(5):375–379

Uncontrolled advancement of a hydrophilic 0.018-inch guidewire

Patient History

An 87-year-old woman with peripheral vascular disease presented with rest pain in her right leg. She was scheduled for recanalization of a distal superficial femoral artery (SFA)/popliteal artery occlusion (**Fig. 4.154**).

Initial Treatment Received

Following antegrade access to the right common femoral artery (CFA) and insertion of a 6F sheath, the lesion was recanalized using a diagnostic catheter and a straight 0.018-inch hydrophylic guidewire V18 (Boston Scientific). The lesion was passed intraluminally and balloon angioplasty was performed (**Fig. 4.155**).

Problems Encountered during Treatment

During recanalization of the lesion the guidewire slipped into a collateral and the patient suddenly complained of sharp pain in her distal thigh/ knee region.

Imaging Plan

Angiography.

Resulting Complication

There was perforation of a genual side branch from the guidewire, which had been advanced

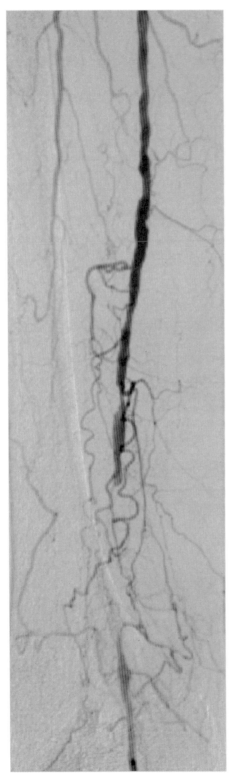

Fig. 4.154 Preinterventional angiography showing distal SFA occlusion.

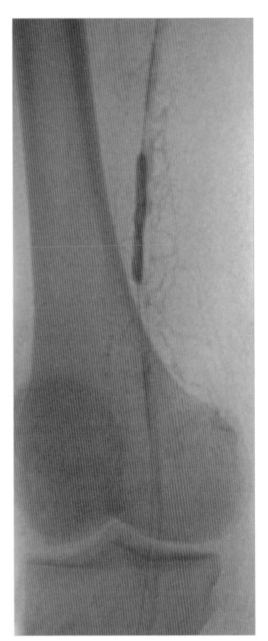

Fig. 4.155 Fluoroscopy image of angioplasty balloon.

too far into the vessel in an uncontrolled fashion (**Fig. 4.156**).

Possible Strategies for Complication Management

• Wait and see.
• Manual compression of the calf at the level of the detected bleeding source.

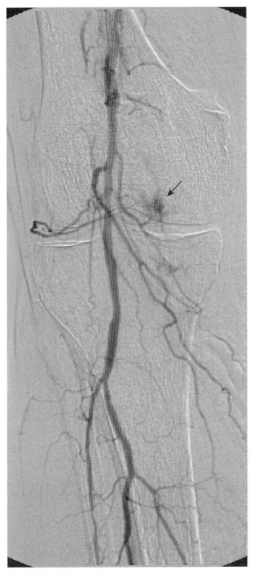

Fig. 4.156 Digital subtraction angiography image showing ruptured genual collateral indicated by contrast media blush (*arrow*).

- Placement of a pressure cuff.
- Selective catheterization of the feeder vessel using a microcatheter for embolization (coil, glue, collagen sponge).

Final Complication Management

Endovascular treatment with catheterization of the feeder vessel using a microcatheter (2.7F) followed by selective microcoil embolization (**Figs. 4.157** and **4.158**).

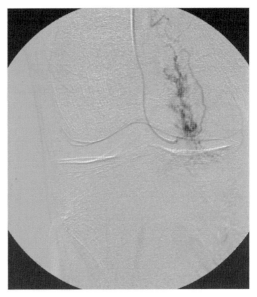

Fig. 4.157 Contrast injection through a microcatheter showing side-branch rupture with active bleeding.

Complication Analysis

Suspected uncontrolled advancement of the hydrophylic guidewire resulted in side-branch perforation. Due to the location of the vessel lac-

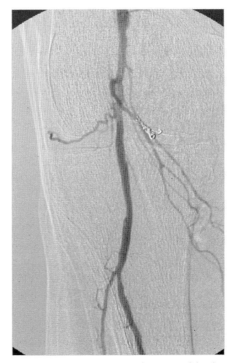

Fig. 4.158 Control angiography after successful coil embolization.

eration, manual compression and/or application of a pressure cuff was not possible.

Prevention Strategies and Take-home Message

- Guidewire advancement should be constantly controlled under fluoroscopy, especially when using hydrophilic-coated wires!
- Wires should never be pushed against resistance without fluoroscopic guidance!

Further Reading

Axelrod DJ, Freeman H, Pukin L, Guller J, Mitty HA. Guidewire perforation leading to fatal perirenal hemorrhage from transcortical collaterals after renal artery stent placement. J Vasc Interv Radiol 2004;15(9):985–987

Hiroshima Y, Tajima K, Shiono Y, et al. Soft J-tipped guidewire-induced cardiac perforation in a patient with right ventricular lipomatosis and wall thinning. Intern Med 2012;51(18):2609–2612

Störger H, Ruef J. Closure of guidewire-induced coronary artery perforation with a two-component fibrin glue. Catheter Cardiovasc Interv 2007;70(2):237–240

Tanaka S, Nishigaki K, Ojio S, et al. Transcatheter embolization by autologous blood clot is useful management for small side-branch perforation due to percutaneous coronary intervention guidewire. J Cardiol 2008;52(3):285–289

Tarar MN, Christakopoulos GE, Brilakis ES. Successful management of a distal vessel perforation through a single 8-F guide catheter: combining balloon inflation for bleeding control with coil embolization. Catheter Cardiovasc Interv 2015

Catheter Placement

Perforation of the left internal thoracic artery

Patient History

A 2-year-old boy had undergone Glenn surgery for pulmonary atresia with intact ventricular septum. Preoperative embolization of extrapulmonary collaterals was additionally planned prior to the Fontan procedure.

Initial Treatment Received

Coil embolization of the extrapulmonary collateral arteries was performed including the left internal thoracic artery from the right femoral approach (**Fig. 4.159**).

Problems Encountered after Treatment

When a 4F Judkins right coronary catheter was inserted into the left internal thoracic artery, test

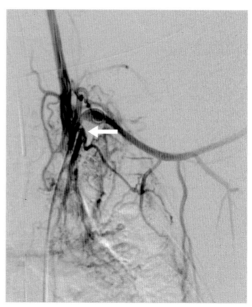

Fig. 4.159 The left subclavian arteriogram showing the angulated origin of the left internal thoracic artery (*arrow*).

contrast injection showed an extravasation indicating vessel perforation at its origin (**Fig. 4.160**). The perforating catheter was not removed in order to avoid active bleeding.

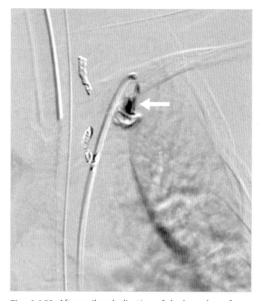

Fig. 4.160 After coil embolization of the branches of thyrocervical trunk, and hooking of a 4F Judkins right catheter into the left internal thoracic artery. Test contrast injection reveals extravasation (*arrow*).

Imaging Plan

Ultrasound to check the bleeding and hematoma.
Left subclavian arteriogram by inserting a new catheter from the left femoral approach.

Resulting Complication

Vital signs remained stable. No hematoma was observed under ultrasound.
No extravasation was seen on the left subclavian arteriogram.

Possible Strategies for Complication Management

- Manual compression after removal of the perforating catheter (unpredictable outcome).
- Embolization of the internal thoracic artery.
- Covered stent in the left subclavian artery (LSA) (cons: too close to the vertebral artery—a small curved vessel in a child).
- Surgical repair (if endovascular approach fails).

Final Complication Management

Through a newly inserted guiding catheter, coil embolization of the left internal thoracic artery was performed under balloon protection of the LSA. Detachable 0.010-inch microcoils were deployed to cover the origin of the left internal thoracic artery (**Figs. 4.161** and **4.162**). Finally, the perforating catheter was removed.

Complication Analysis

Vessel perforation was accidentally induced at the origin of the internal thoracic artery due to the angulation and small vessel size of the child.

Prevention Strategies and Take-home Message

- An angiographic catheter should be gently manipulated in small vessels with angulated origin.
- The perforating catheter should not be removed immediately.
- In coil embolization of the injured vessel, balloon protection technique is helpful to minimize further bleeding and also to prevent coil protrusion into the parent artery.

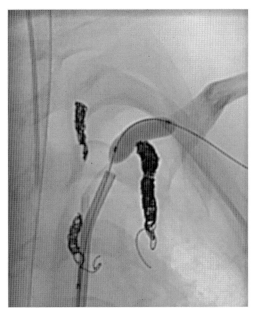

Fig. 4.161 Coil embolization of the left internal thoracic artery using 0.010-inch detachable microcoils under microballoon protection of the LSA.

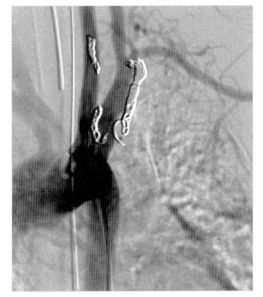

Fig. 4.162 Aortography after coil embolization shows the complete occlusion of the internal thoracic artery without extravasation at its origin.

Further Reading

Agid R, Simons M, Casaubon LK, Sniderman K. Salvage of the carotid artery with covered stent after perforation with dialysis sheath. A case report. Interv Neuroradiol 2012;18(4):386–390

Farooqi F, Alexander J, Sarma A. Rare vascular perforation complicating radial approach to percutaneous coronary angioplasty. BMJ Case Rep 2013;bcr2012007732

Gilchrist IC. Seal it to heal it: potential option for distal wire perforation. Catheter Cardiovasc Interv 2009;73(6):795–796

Maluenda G, Mitulescu L, Ben-Dor I, et al. Transcatheter "thrombin-blood patch" injection: a novel and effective approach to treat catheterization-related arterial perforation. Catheter Cardiovasc Interv 2012;80(6):1025–1032

Masson JB, Al Bugami S, Webb JG. Endovascular balloon occlusion for catheter-induced large artery perforation in the catheterization laboratory. Catheter Cardiovasc Interv 2009;73(4):514–518

Ohira S, Matsushita T, Masuda S, Ishise T. Right ventricular perforation caused by pulmonary artery catheter three days after insertion in a patient with acute pulmonary embolism. Heart Lung Circ 2013;22(12):1040–1042

Roubelakis A, Karangelis D, Kaarne M. Innominate artery perforation during placement of hemodialysis catheter. J Vasc Access 2013;14(4):402

Ziakas A, Economou F, Feloukidis C, Kiratlidis K, Stiliadis I. Left anterior descending artery perforation treated with graft stenting combining dual catheter and side-branch graft stenting techniques. Herz 2012;37(8):913–916

Dissection of the brachiocephalic trunk during diagnostic cerebral angiography

Patient History

A 65-year-old woman was referred for cerebral angiography to assess an intracranial aneurysm.

Initial Procedure

Cerebral angiography was performed via the right brachial approach.

Problems Encountered during Procedure

A 4F modified Simmons reverse-curve catheter was reformed in the ascending aorta. However, it was difficult to advance the reformed catheter from the tortuous brachiocephalic artery to the common carotid artery simply by catheter withdrawal or rotation. After negotiating with a hydrophilic guidewire, test contrast injection revealed stagnation of the contrast material along the right common carotid artery, indicating arterial dissection (**Fig. 4.163**).

Imaging Plan

Brachiocephalic arteriogram to assess extent of pseudolumen.

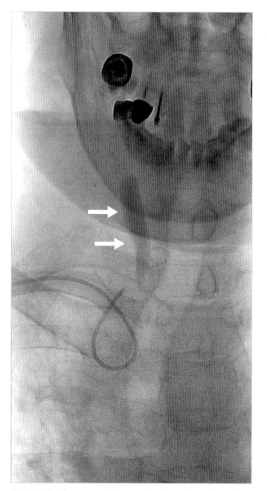

Fig. 4.163 Fluoroscopic image showing stagnation of contrast agent along the right common carotid artery (*arrows*).

Resulting Complication

The angiography revealed an arterial dissection from the brachiocephalic artery to the proximal common carotid artery (**Fig. 4.164**). The patient presented with no symptoms of cerebral ischemia.

Possible Strategies for Complication Management

- Low-pressure compression using a balloon catheter.
- Stent placement.
- Surgical repair (if endovascular approach fails).

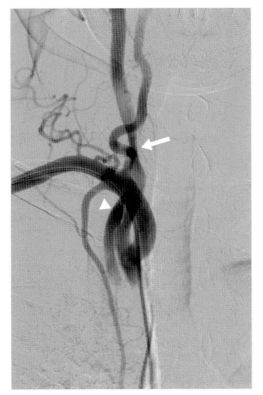

Fig. 4.164 The pseudolumen (*arrowhead*) and stenosis (*arrow*) of the right common carotid artery.

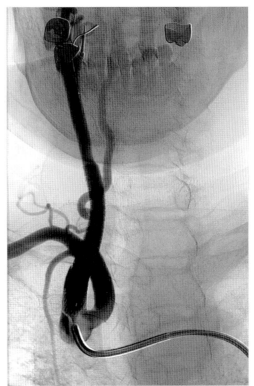

Fig. 4.165 Two carotid stents (10 × 4 cm and 10 × 3 cm) were sequentially placed to repair the arterial dissection.

Final Complication Management

Because of the progressive stenosis in the common carotid artery, carotid stent placement was performed. From the right femoral approach, two self-expanding carotid stents (10 × 4 cm and 10 × 3 cm) were sequentially placed (**Fig. 4.165**).

Complication Analysis

The hydrophilic guidewire accidentally induced the dissection of the right common carotid artery.

Prevention Strategies and Take-home Message

- Guidewire negotiation through a reverse-curve catheter may impair control of the wire tip and lead to vessel injury.
- Different curves of reverse-curve catheters should be available for the tortuous brachiocephalic artery.
- When catheterization is difficult via the brachial or radial artery, consider switching to a femoral artery approach.

Further Reading

Cloft HJ, Jensen ME, Kallmes DF, Dion JE. Arterial dissections complicating cerebral angiography and cerebrovascular interventions. AJNR Am J Neuroradiol 2000;21(3):541–545

Fifi JT, Meyers PM, Lavine SD, Cox V, Silverberg I, Mangla S, Pile-Spellman J. Complications of modern diagnostic cerebral angiography in an academic medical center. J Vasc Interv Radiol 2009;20(4):442–447

Vitek J. In Re: "Arterial dissection complicating cerebral angiography and cerebrovascular interventions." AJNR Am J Neuroradiol 2002;23(4):740–741

Perforation of the fibular artery with a diagnostic catheter

Patient History

A 68-year-old diabetic patient with critical limb ischemia of his right leg presented for selective angiography and possible interventional treatment.

Initial Treatment Received

After antegrade puncture of the right common femoral artery (CFA) a 4F sheath was inserted.

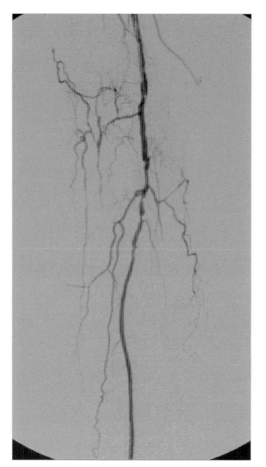

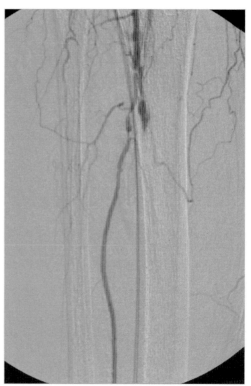

Fig. 4.167 Rupture of the target vessel after a forceful attempt to cross the lesion with a 4F catheter.

Fig. 4.166 Pretreatment angiography of a high-grade stenosis of the fibular artery.

Angiography revealed chronic occlusion of the posterior tibial and anterior tibial artery. The fibular artery was the only vessel reaching the ankle; there was an eccentric short high-grade stenosis in the proximal aspect of this artery (**Fig. 4.166**). Percutaneous transluminal angioplasty (PTA) of the lesion was planned.

Problems Encountered during Treatment

The fibular artery was engaged with a 0.018-inch guidewire through a 4F multipurpose catheter. While the guidewire could be easily positioned in the target vessel, the diagnostic catheter would not follow to verify intraluminal catheter/wire position. Nonetheless, the catheter was advanced further against resistance. When this maneuver failed the catheter was pulled back and primary angioplasty was planned as the next step. How-

ever, angiography showed vessel rupture at the site of the lesion (**Fig. 4.167**).

Imaging Plan

Selective angiography.

Resulting Complication

Iatrogenic perforation of a critical single infragenual artery.

Possible Strategies for Complication Management

- Manual compression of the calf at the level of the detected bleeding source (not possible due to anatomical location of target vessel).
- Placement of a pressure cuff with inflation to suprasystolic level until hemostasis.
- Selective catheterization and embolization (not possible as this was the only vessel supplying the foot).
- Stent graft placement.

Final Complication Management

The stenosis and site of rupture were passed with a low-profile angioplasty balloon (3 × 20 mm) over the 0.018-inch guidewire, which was already in place. Following long-term angioplasty there was still high-grade residual stenosis. The amount of contrast extravasation had worsened, indicating a large defect in the treated artery (**Fig. 4.168**). A 3-mm balloon-expandable stent graft (Graftmaster, Abbott Vascular) was implanted. After this no residual stenosis was seen and the rupture was sealed completely (**Fig. 4.169**).

Complication Analysis

In this patient with critical limb ischemia and a severely stenosed single vessel supplying the foot, recanalization was indicated. Passage of the lesion was difficult due to a high burden of calcified plaque. For recanalization a diagnostic catheter with a 0.035-inch inner lumen was tracked over a 0.018-inch guidewire. Due to the design of the catheter and the wire mismatch at the catheter tip it was not possible to insert the catheter into the target vessel. Undue force applied against resistance led to vessel perforation. With angioplasty alone neither the stenosis nor the vessel rupture could be treated, thus stent graft implantation was performed.

Prevention Strategies and Take-home Message

- Use dedicated low-profile support catheters with suitable guidewires if recanalization of severe stenosis is difficult.
- Never push or pull anything against resistance.
- Have low-profile stent grafts for small lumen arteries available.

Further Reading

Abdool MA, Morrison S, Sullivan H. Iatrogenic perforation of subclavian artery as a complication of coronary angiography

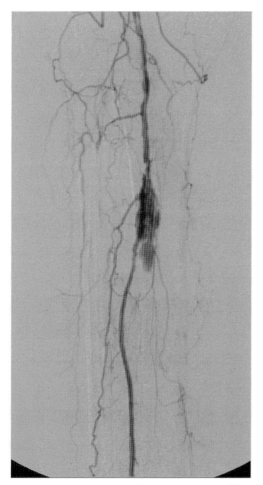

Fig. 4.168 After angioplasty, there was worsening of the hemorrhage and residual stenosis.

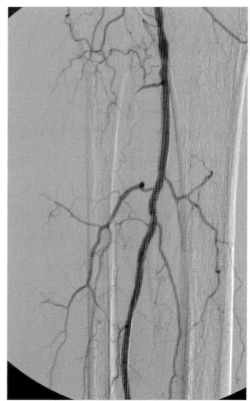

Fig. 4.169 Final result after stent graft implantation.

from the radial route, endovascularly repaired with a covered stent graft. BMJ Case Rep 2013;bcr2012007602

Ekici B, Erkan AF, Kütük U, Töre HF. Successful management of
coronary artery rupture with stent graft: a case report. Case
Rep Med 2014;391843

Meguro K, Ohira H, Nishikido T, et al. Outcome of prolonged balloon inflation for the management of coronary perforation.
J Cardiol 2013;61(3):206–209

Narayan RL, Vaishnava P, Kim M. Radial artery perforation during transradial catheterization managed with a coronary
polytetrafluoroethylene-covered stent graft. J Invasive
Cardiol 2012;24(4):185–187

Yeo KK, Rogers JH, Laird JR. Use of stent grafts and coils in vessel
rupture and perforation. J Interv Cardiol 2008;21(1):86–99

4.3.2 Lesion Crossing

Unexpected stent migration during kissing stent procedure

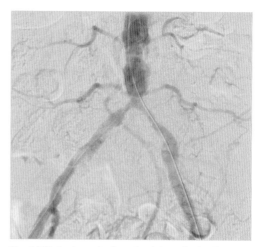

Fig. 4.170 Angiography from the right groin showing a moderate stenosis of the left and right CIA; both lesions involve the aortic bifurcation. A 0.035-inch wire had already been placed from the left groin in the infrarenal aorta.

Patient History

A 70-year-old patient suffered from lifestyle-lim-iting peripheral artery disease. The underlying cause was moderate common iliac artery (CIA) stenosis involving the aortic bifurcation. The pa-tient was scheduled for a kissing stent procedure from bilateral groin access.

Initial Treatment Received

Under local anesthesia, inserting a 6F sheath on each side created retrograde access to the left and right common femoral artery (CFA). Two 0.035-inch guidewires crossed the lesion, one from each side. It was planned to place a 8 × 59-mm stent from the left side and a 9 × 29-mm stent from the right side in a kissing stent configuration in order to treat left and right CIA stenosis (**Fig. 4.170**).

Problems Encountered during Treatment

The stent intended for the left common iliac ar-tery was advanced without any problems to-wards the target lesion, whereas the right-side stent migrated from the balloon still threaded on the guidewire. The operator removed the balloon and the stent was stopped by the sheath opening (**Fig. 4.171**).

Imaging Plan

Fluoroscopy to identify the exact position of the stent and potential damage of the stent, that is, deformation of stent struts.

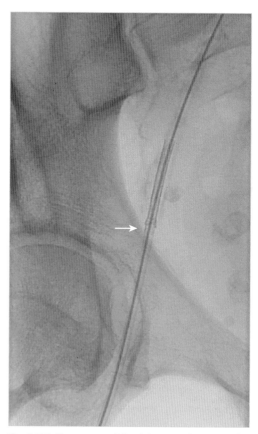

Fig. 4.171 Fluoroscopy of the right groin; the migrated stent still threaded on the guidewire was riding on the sheath. The proximal stent was in a kind of tulip configuration engaging the distal end of the sheath (*arrow*).

Resulting Complication

Stent migration and mild stent deformation.

Possible Strategies for Complication Management

- Endovascular treatment using the ipsilateral retrograde approach via the existing access to the CFA and leaving the guidewire in place in order to balloon the stent in the EIA.
- Endovascular treatment using the ipsilateral retrograde approach with ballooning the stent at the target lesion in order to complete the kissing stent procedure.
- Endovascular treatment with snaring the stent for final removal after upsizing the sheath to at least 9F.
- Surgery (if an endovascular approach fails).

Final Complication Management

Endovascular treatment using the ipsilateral retrograde approach via the existing access to the CFA and leaving the guidewire in place in order to balloon at the target lesion for completion of the kissing stent procedure. To finalize this procedure the following steps were necessary:

A 4 × 80-mm balloon could be inserted through the unexpanded stent. Mild balloon inflation made it possible to bring the stent up towards the target lesion (**Figs. 4.172** and **4.173**). At the intended position the stent was inflated with the 4-mm balloon up to rated burst pressure, achieving a stent diameter of around 4.5 mm. This diameter was sufficient to fix the stent at the aortic bifurcation (**Fig. 4.174**) where the contralateral stent was already deployed. The procedure was completed by an exchange of the balloon for an 8 × 40-mm balloon, which was inflated simultaneously with the contralateral 8 × 60-mm balloon (**Fig. 4.175**).

Complication Analysis

Suspected uncontrolled advancement of a balloon-expandable stent resulted in stent migration.

Prevention Strategies and Take-home Message

- Stent advancement should be controlled under fluoroscopy, especially when using balloon-expandable stents.

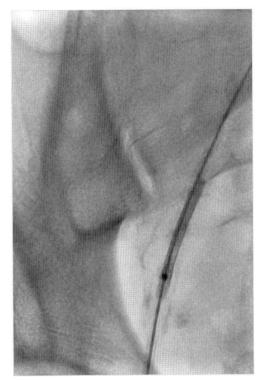

Fig. 4.172 A 4 × 80-mm balloon was already slightly inflated after a successful threading maneuver.

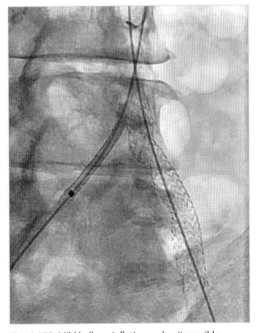

Fig. 4.173 Mild balloon inflation makes it possible to bring the stent up towards the target lesion. The contralateral stent was already inflated.

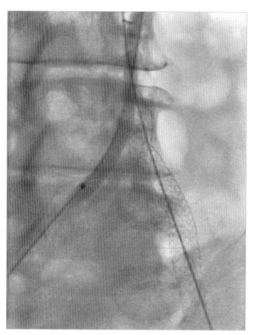

Fig. 4.174 Balloon inflation at rated burst pressure in order to fix the stent at the target lesion.

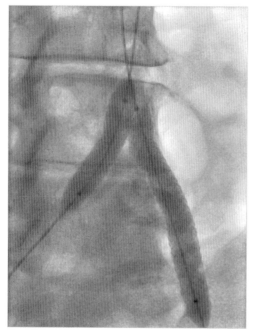

Fig. 4.175 Simultaneous balloon inflation (kissing balloon, left 8 × 60 mm and right 8 × 40 mm) resulting in an adequate stent position.

- If a stent is unable to cross a lesion, careful predilatation is warranted!
- If stent removal is necessary in case of primary placement failure at the target lesion, remove the stent carefully, especially at the entrance of the sheath and the level of the hemostatic valve!
- Never push or pull a stent delivery catheter in an uncontrolled fashion when resistance is encountered.

Further Reading

Broadbent LP, Moran CJ, Cross DT III, Derdeyn CP. Management of neuroform stent dislodgement and misplacement. AJNR Am J Neuroradiol 2003;24(9):1819–1822

Meadows J, Teitel D, Moore P. Anatomical and technical predictors of stent malposition during implantation for vascular obstruction in patients with congenital and acquired heart disease. JACC Cardiovasc Interv 2010;3(10):1080–1086

Taherioun M, Namazi MH, Safi M, et al. Stent underexpansion in angiographic guided percutaneous coronary intervention, despite adjunctive balloon post-dilatation, in drug eluting stent era. ARYA Atheroscler 2014;10(1):13–17

Stent migration during vertebral artery stenting

Patient History

A 69-year-old patient suffered from severe symptoms of vertebrobasilar insufficiency, refractory to optimized medical treatment. Upon interdisciplinary consensus, the decision was made to treat the underlying cause—a high-grade vertebral artery stenosis close to the basilar artery. The contralateral vertebral artery was occluded. The patient was scheduled for a balloon-expandable drug-eluting stent placement from right-side groin access, performed under general anesthesia.

Initial Treatment Received

Under general anesthesia, a 6F, 90-cm-long sheath was placed in the right common femoral artery (CFA). The sheath was advanced using the telescope technique towards the left subclavian artery (LSA), followed by catheterization of the origin of the left vertebral artery with a 2.7F microcatheter in combination with a 0.014-inch guidewire. The guidewire crossed the lesion located at the level of the V4 segment, and the distal end of the wire was placed in the basilar artery (**Fig. 4.176**). A 2.75 × 12-mm paclitaxel-eluting balloon-expand-

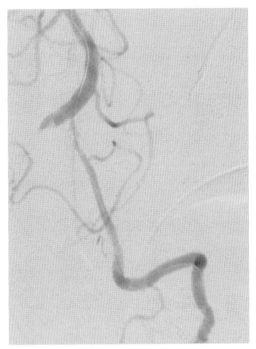

Fig. 4.176 Angiography of the left vertebral artery via the sheath placed in the LSA. The guidewire crossed the lesion located at the level of the V4 segment and the distal end was placed in the basilar artery.

able stent, intended for use in coronary arteries, was planned to be deployed at the target lesion.

Problems Encountered during Treatment

The balloon (mounted stent) was advanced towards the target lesion without any problems. When the proximal and distal markers of the balloon were clearly identified at the target lesion, it was impossible to identify the stent. A magnified image could not visualize the stent. It was supposed that the stent had been lost somewhere on the way up to the lesion. The proximal part of the vertebral artery was a little elongated as is often seen (**Fig. 4.177**). The operator removed the balloon, keeping the guidewire in a stable position. Fluoroscopy identified the stent at the level of the elongated V1 segment, still threaded on the guidewire.

Imaging Plan

Fluoroscopy to identify the exact position of and damage to the stent, that is, deformation of stent struts.

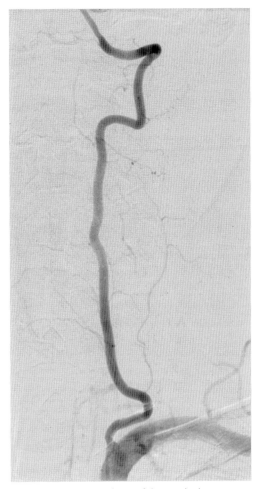

Fig. 4.177 The proximal part of the vertebral artery was a little elongated. Problems were probably encountered at this level.

Resulting Complication

Stent migration at the level of the V1 elongation.

Possible Strategies for Complication Management

- Endovascular treatment using an ipsilateral retrograde approach via the existing access coming from the CFA towards the subclavian artery and leaving the guidewire in place in order to try to balloon the stent at the proximal vertebral artery, that is, by threading the stent with a small balloon diameter.
- Endovascular treatment via the existing access leaving the guidewire in place in order to thread the balloon through the stent and trying

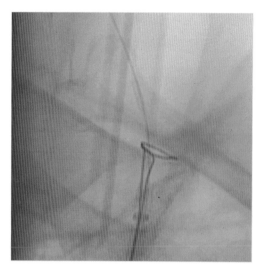

Fig. 4.178 Fluoroscopy of the already opened snare, which was still lodged beyond the stent.

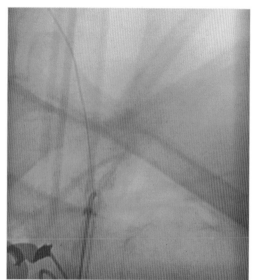

Fig. 4.179 Fluoroscopy of the closed snare at the entrance level of the sheath. The stent was still outside the sheath. At this point the foreign body retrieval maneuver has to be performed very carefully.

to advance both towards the target lesion in order to complete stent procedure.

- Endovascular treatment via the existing access and trying to snare the stent, which is still on the guidewire, for final removal of both.

Final Complication Management

Endovascular treatment via the existing access and snaring both the stent on the guidewire and the guidewire itself for final removal of both. To finalize this procedure the following steps were necessary:

Threading the snare on the wire and advancing it towards the stent while keeping the guidewire in a stable position (**Fig. 4.178**). When the snare caught the stent, it was closed carefully and was retrieved with the wire into the 6F sheath outside the body (**Fig. 4.179**).

Finally, a new guidewire was placed; a new stent was advanced carefully, especially at the level of the elongated V1 segment. At the target lesion, the stent was deployed. Final angiography showed a well-deployed stent without any remaining stenosis (**Fig. 4.180**).

Complication Analysis

Suspected uncontrolled advancement of a balloon-expandable stent resulted in stent migration.

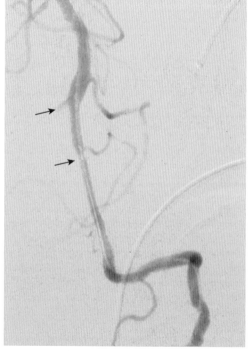

Fig. 4.180 Final angiography showing a well-deployed stent (*arrows*) without any remaining stenosis.

Prevention Strategies and Take-home Message

- Stent advancement should be controlled under fluoroscopy, especially when using balloon-expandable stents.
- If a stent is unable to cross a lesion, careful predilatation is warranted!
- If stent removal is necessary in a case of primary placement failure at the target lesion, remove the stent carefully, especially at the entrance of the sheath and the level of the hemostatic valve.
- Never push or pull a stent delivery catheter in an uncontrolled fashion when resistance is encountered.

Further Reading

Broadbent LP, Moran CJ, Cross DT III, Derdeyn CP. Management of neuroform stent dislodgement and misplacement. AJNR Am J Neuroradiol 2003;24(9):1819–1822

Meadows J, Teitel D, Moore P. Anatomical and technical predictors of stent malposition during implantation for vascular obstruction in patients with congenital and acquired heart disease. JACC Cardiovasc Interv 2010;3(10):1080–1086

Taherioun M, Namazi MH, Safi M, et al. Stent underexpansion in angiographic guided percutaneous coronary intervention, despite adjunctive balloon post-dilatation, in drug eluting stent era. ARYA Atheroscler 2014;10(1):13–17

Irreversible support catheter entrapment during superficial femoral artery chronic total occlusion treatment

Patient History

An 80-year-old woman patient presented with critical limb ischemia and osteomyelitis of the forefoot. The patient had a prior history of operative reduction and internal fixation (ORIF) of the right femur secondary to proximal femoral fracture.

Initial Treatment Received

Femoral angiogram demonstrated a short-segment superficial femoral artery (SFA) occlusion at the site of cerclage wires (**Fig. 4.181**). A hydrophilic wire was advanced through the occlusion. However, the lesion could not be crossed with a standard diagnostic catheter. Instead, a TrailBlazer (Ev3) support catheter was advanced successfully through the lesion (*arrows*, **Fig. 4.181**).

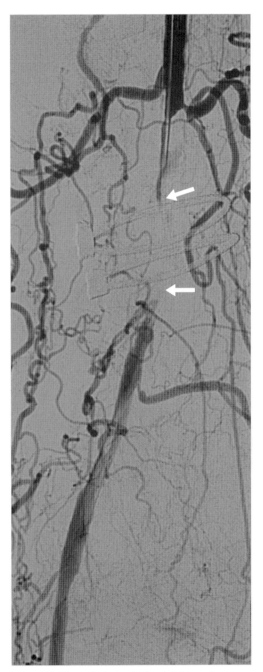

Fig. 4.181 The occlusion at the level of the cerclage wires (*arrows*).

Imaging Plan

Angiogram.

Problems Encountered during Treatment

The TrailBlazer catheter could not be withdrawn to allow for angioplasty.

Resulting Complication

Multiple attempts to remove the catheter failed and with increased traction the catheter snapped with the distal end embedded distal to the stricture (**Fig. 4.182**).

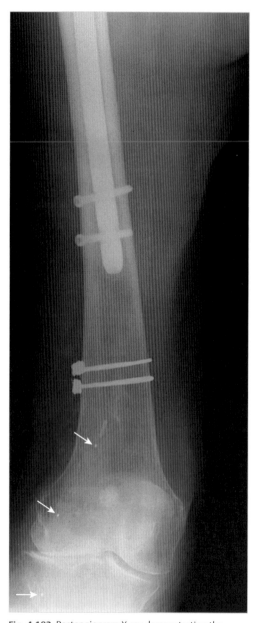

Fig. 4.182 Postangiogram X-ray demonstrating the radiopaque markers (*arrows*) of the TrailBlazer catheter distal to the cerclage wires.

Possible Strategies for Complication Management

- Attempt endovascular snaring.
- Surgical retrieval (if endovascular approach fails).

Final Complication Management

Endovascular retrieval using snare techniques was attempted but because the more proximal end of the catheter was not readily accessible this proved fruitless. The patient ultimately underwent successful surgical removal of the foreign body and surgical bypass.

Complication Analysis

Performing angioplasty in the region of prior surgery can be difficult. It may be more appropriate for a patient to undergo primary surgical revascularization.

Prevention Strategies and Take-home Message

- Arteries within areas of previous surgery may develop resistant fibrotic structures.
- These stenoses may respond poorly to endovascular therapy and primary surgical revascularization should be considered.
- Avoid using excessive tractional force when removing catheters.

Further Reading

Aydin H, Kandemir O, Günaydin S, Zorlutuna Y. A peeled off and entrapped intraaortic balloon catheter in the femoral artery: an unusual complication. Interact Cardiovasc Thorac Surg 2004;3(2):314–316

Conti JB, Geiser E, Curtis AB. Catheter entrapment in the mitral valve apparatus during radiofrequency ablation. Pacing Clin Electrophysiol 1994;17(10):1681–1685

Jahollari A, Sarac A, Ozal E. Intra-aortic balloon pump rupture and entrapment. Case Rep Vasc Med 2014;378672

Lorusso R, De Cicco G, Ettori F, Curello S, Gelsomino S, Fucci C. Emergency surgery after saphenous vein graft perforation complicated by catheter balloon entrapment and hemorrhagic shock. Ann Thorac Surg 2008;86(3):1002–1004

Taniguchi N, Mizuguchi Y, Takahashi A. Longitudinal stent elongation during retraction of entrapped jailed guidewire in a side branch with balloon catheter support: a case report. Cardiovasc Revasc Med 2015;16(1):52–54

Retrograde iliac dissection

Patient History

A 71-year-old man with chronic intermittent claudication in his left leg was scheduled for interventional therapy. Noninvasive imaging had detected a stenosis of the left external iliac artery (EIA). The patient was scheduled for recanalization from a left retrograde approach.

Initial Treatment Received

Following retrograde puncture of the left common femoral artery (CFA) and placement of a 6F sheath, digital subtraction angiography (DSA) was performed through the sheath. Retrograde injection of contrast medium revealed long-segment mild to moderate stenosis of the EIA starting at the iliac bifurcation (**Fig. 4.183**). Recanalization with a multipurpose catheter over a standard hydrophilic guidewire (0.035-inch) was attempted.

Problems Encountered during Treatment

During the recanalization procedure, passage of the guidewire through the EIA into the common iliac artery (CIA) was more difficult than expected. The guidewire primarily took a subintimal course at the level of the iliac bifurcation. Injection of contrast medium through the sheath

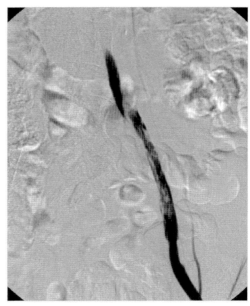

Fig. 4.184 Retrograde contrast injection showing extensive EIA dissection.

now showed extensive dissection of the EIA with allegedly occluded internal iliac artery (IIA) (**Fig. 4.184**).

Imaging Plan

Contralateral retrograde access from the right groin; angiography with a catheter placed into the infrarenal aorta.

Resulting Complication

Iatrogenic dissection of the left EIA, reaching into the CFA (**Fig. 4.185**). The femoral pulse, which was present at the beginning of the intervention, was no longer palpable. The patient did not complain of rest pain at this time.

Possible Strategies for Complication Management

- Abort procedure. Heparinization, second-look angiography after 1–2 days.
- Antegrade recanalization from the already established contralateral approach; percutaneous transluminal angioplasty (PTA) and/or stent placement.
- Surgery (if endovascular measures fail).

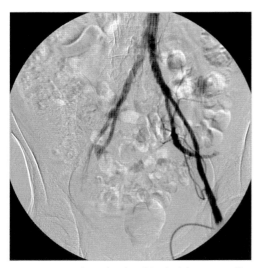

Fig. 4.183 DSA through a sheath in the left common iliac artery showing mild to moderate stenosis of the left EIA.

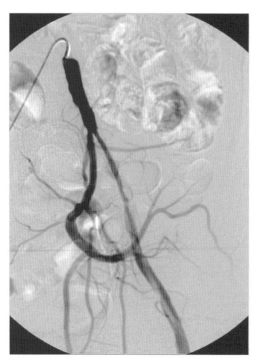

Fig. 4.185 Angiography from a right retrograde contralateral approach with contrast medium injection shows dissection of the left EIA reaching into the CFA. The IIA is still patent.

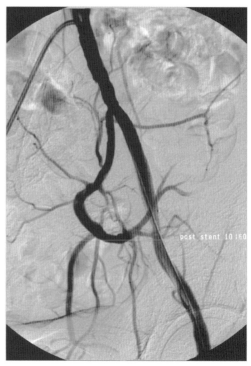

Fig. 4.186 Following crossover stent placement there is still dissection in the distal aspect of the left EIA.

Final Complication Management

The dissection in the left EIA was passed using a 0.035-inch guidewire through a 4F Rösch inferior mesenteric (RIM) catheter (Cordis/Johnson & Johnson). The wire was exchanged for a stiffer Teflon-coated steel wire. A 45-cm-long 6F sheath was positioned into the CIA. A self-expanding stent (SES; 10 × 60 mm) was implanted starting in the distal CFA. After this there was still a dissecting membrane present in the distal EIA (**Fig. 4.186**). Long-term PTA using an 8-mm balloon was now performed (8 atmospheres [atm], 5 minutes). Control angiography showed a good result without dissection or residual stenosis (**Fig. 4.187**)

Complication Analysis

This case of mild to moderate stenosis of an iliac artery seemed like a straightforward intervention, but turned out to be rather complicated. The hydrophilic-coated guidewire initially entered the subintimal space and dissected the diseased artery. Retrograde injections through the sheath possibly aggravated the problem, leading to worsening of the anatomical lesion. Recanalization in an antegrade fashion from a contralateral groin approach was possible and treatment of the lesion was successful.

Prevention Strategies and Take-home Message

- Consider initial antegrade recanalization of isolated lesions of the EIA from a crossover approach.
- Avoid forced retrograde contrast medium injections through a sheath in patients with severely diseased iliac arteries.
- Even apparently simple cases can unexpectedly result in more complex procedures.

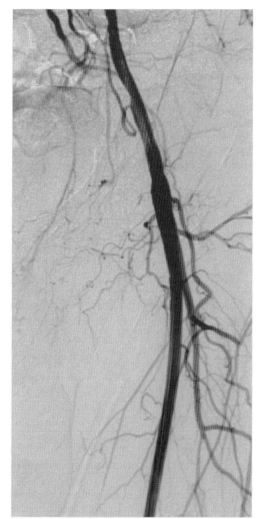

Fig. 4.187 After PTA the dissection is no longer present; there is no residual stenosis.

Further Reading

Fanelli F, Cannavale A, Gazzetti M, D'Adamo A. Commentary: how do we deal with dissection after angioplasty? J Endovasc Ther 2013;20(6):801–804

Funovics MA, Lackner B, Cejna M, et al. Predictors of long-term results after treatment of iliac artery obliteration by transluminal angioplasty and stent deployment. Cardiovasc Interv Radiol 2002;25(5):397–402

Onal B, Ilgit ET, Yücel C, Ozbek E, Vural M, Akpek S. Primary stenting for complex atherosclerotic plaques in aortic and iliac stenoses. Cardiovasc Interv Radiol 1998;21(5):386–392

Treiman GS, Schneider PA, Lawrence PF, Pevec WC, Bush RL, Ichikawa L. Does stent placement improve the results of ineffective or complicated iliac artery angioplasty? J Vasc Surg 1998;28(1):104–112

Tsetis D. Endovascular treatment of complications of femoral arterial access. Cardiovasc Interv Radiol 2010;33(3):457–468

Distal embolization after lesion crossing treated with thrombolysis

Patient History

A 68-year-old man suffered from claudication of his right leg with a pain-free walking distance of 50 m. Symptoms had been worsening over the previous 4 weeks. Noninvasive imaging proved peripheral vascular disease with a short-segment occlusion of the superficial femoral artery (SFA). The patient was scheduled for percutaneous transluminal angioplasty (PTA).

Initial Treatment Received

Antegrade puncture of the right common femoral artery (CFA) was performed and a 6F sheath was introduced. Heparin 5,000 IU was given intrarterially. The short SFA occlusion (**Fig. 4.188a**) was passed with a 0.018-inch wire (V18, Boston Scientific) and a 4F diagnostic catheter. Angioplasty was performed with a 5-mm balloon. Following angioplasty there was no relevant residual stenosis; however, distal embolization was present (**Fig. 4.188b, c**).

Problems Encountered during Treatment

Control angiography revealed diffuse distal embolization into the proximal aspect of all three below-the-knee (BTK) arteries (**Fig. 4.189**).

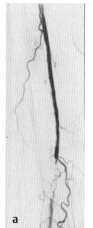 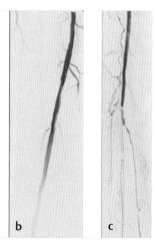

Fig. 4.188 (a) Angiography of the occluded SFA segment. **(b)** The short SFA occlusion was passed with a 0.018" wire (V18, Boston Scientific) and a 4F diagnostic. After angioplasty there was no relevant residual stenosis visible. **(c)** Distal embolization is shown at the level of the trifurcation involving the anterior tibial artery and the proneal trunk as well into the peroneal artery.

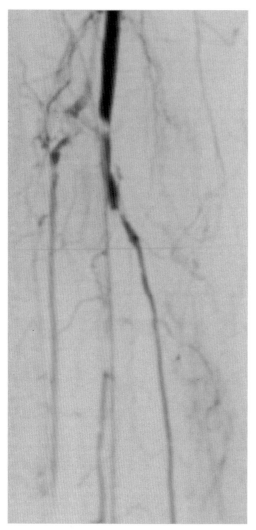

Fig. 4.189 Magnified angiography showing the difusse distal embolization in the proximal below the knee arteries.

Imaging Plan

Selective angiography.

Resulting Complication

Diffuse distal embolization into all three BTK arteries.

Possible Strategies for Complication Management

- Percutaneous aspiration thrombectomy.
- Locoregional catheter thrombolysis.
- Mechanical thrombolysis.
- Open surgical thrombectomy.

Final Complication Management

Locoregional low-dose thrombolysis was performed. The distal popliteal artery was cannulated with a 4F multipurpose catheter and a bolus of 5 mg of recombinant tissue plasminogen activator (rtPA) (Actilyse, Boehringer Ingelheim) was given. Then, 10 mg of rtPA was administered in small fractions over a period of 30 minutes. Control angiography showed the beginning of thrombolysis in all affected arteries. Locoregional lysis was continued until the next day with 1 mg rtPA per hour and patency was fully restored.

Complication Analysis

This case shows a typical complication of a recanalization procedure in a patient with peripheral vascular disease. Depending on plaque composition and age of occlusion, different types of debris from a lesion may dislodge during catheter manipulation. Caught in the bloodstream, plaque material or thrombus will be carried distally and block the outflow vessel(s). In order to secure the outcome of the initial procedure this material must be removed immediately. In this case there was diffuse embolization into all three BTK arteries with relatively high thrombus burden. Worsening of clinical symptoms during the previous 4 weeks led to the assumption that there was subacute thrombosis involved in the underlying lesion. Locoregional low-dose thrombolysis of emboli was initiated and showed marked improvement of flow after 30 minutes (**Fig. 4.190**).

Prevention Strategies and Take-home Message

- Distal embolization is a common complication of peripheral angioplasty.
- Use of low-profile catheter techniques may lead to lower rates of distal embolization.
- Patients should receive antiplatelet and anticoagulation medication before recanalization procedures.
- Patency of distal outflow vessels must be documented before and after recanalization procedures to detect and treat distal embolization.
- Interventionists should be familiar with endovascular clot removal techniques.

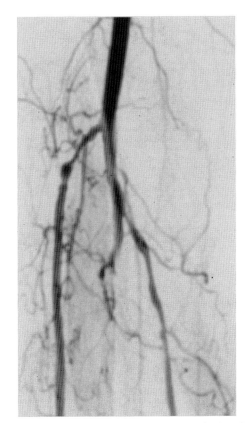

Fig. 4.190 Selective angiography showing the final result after short-term local fibrinolysis therapy. The anterior and posterior tibial arteries are patent again as the main feeding arteries for the foot, whereas the peroneal artery remains partially occluded.

Further Reading

Banerjee S, Sarode K, Brilakis ES. Protected PTA in the lower limbs: a step forward in preventing distal embolization. J Endovasc Ther 2013;20(3):420–421

De Luca G, Navarese EP, Suryapranata H. A meta-analytic overview of thrombectomy during primary angioplasty. Int J Cardiol 2013;166(3):606–612

Jahnke T, Schäfer JP, Bolte H, et al. Retrospective study of rapid-exchange monorail versus over-the-wire technique for femoropopliteal angioplasty. Cardiovasc Intervent Radiol 2008;31(5):854–859

Morrissey NJ. When is embolic protection needed in lower extremity interventions and how should it be done. J Cardiovasc Surg (Torino) 2012;53(2):173–175

Razavi MK. Detection and treatment of acute thromboembolic events in the lower extremities. Tech Vasc Interv Radiol 2011;14(2):80–85

Reeves R, Imsais JK, Prasad A. Successful management of lower extremity distal embolization following percutaneous atherectomy with the JetStream G3 device. J Invasive Cardiol 2012;24(6):E124–E128

Spiliopoulos S, Theodosiadou V, Koukounas V, et al. Distal macro- and microembolization during subintimal recanalization of femoropopliteal chronic total occlusions. J Endovasc Ther 2014;21(4):474–481

Zeller T, Schmidt A, Rastan A, Noory E, Sixt S, Scheinert D. Initial experience with the 5 × 300-mm Proteus embolic capture angioplasty balloon in the treatment of peripheral vascular disease. J Endovasc Ther 2012;19(6):826–833

Zhang F, Zhang H, Luo X, Liang G, Feng Y, Zhang WW. Catheter-directed thrombolysis-assisted angioplasty for chronic lower limb ischemia. Ann Vasc Surg 2014;28(3):590–595

Renal injury from a hydrophylic-coated guidewire

Patient History

A 72-year-old man with a long history of renovascular disease and status post bilateral renal stents was transferred to the vascular surgery department for evaluation of worsening arterial hypertension, not adequately controlled by antihypertensive triple medication. Duplex ultrasound revealed signs of in-stent restenosis (ISR), more on the right than on the left side. The patient was scheduled for angiographic evaluation of restenosis and possible treatment.

Initial Treatment Received

The patient was on dual antiaggregation medication with 75 mg clopidogrel and 100 mg ASA (aspirin). Following puncture of the right common femoral artery (CFA) and insertion of a 6F 45-cm-long sheath, which was positioned into the infrarenal aorta, ISR of both renal arteries was confirmed. There was high-grade stenosis of the right renal stent and moderate stenosis of the left renal stent (**Fig. 4.191a, b**). Cannulation of the right renal artery with 0.014-inch atraumatic wire (Spartacore, Abbott Vascular) and a 4F cobra-shaped catheter was attempted but failed. In order to gain access to the right kidney, a 0.018-inch wire with a straight hydrophylic-coated tip (V18 ControlWire, Boston Scientific) was used. The wire easily passed the stenosis and enabled advancement of the diagnostic catheter. The wire was then exchanged for the 0.014-inch guidewire and cutting-balloon angioplasty (CBA) was performed for treatment of ISR. Angiographic control showed a good result without significant residual stenosis.

Problems Encountered during Treatment

Following removal of catheters and wires, and closure of the puncture site in the right groin the patient started to complain of worsening right-sided flank pain, which had started a few minutes after initial lesion recanalization. The patient was immediately transferred for native computed tomography (CT) imaging to rule out retroperitoneal hematoma.

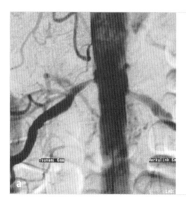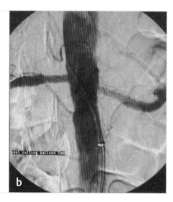

Fig. 4.191 (a) Angiography shows a high-grade stenosis of the right renal stent and moderate stenosis of the left renal stent. (b) Control angiography after balloon angioplasty showed a good result without significant residual stenosis.

Imaging Plan

CT.

Resulting Complication

CT imaging showed a large subcapsular hematoma of the right dorsal kidney (**Fig. 4.192**). No retroperitoneal hemorrhage was present.

Possible Strategies for Complication Management

- Wait and see. Symptomatic treatment of pain.
- Angiographic evaluation of a bleeding source in the right kidney and endovascular treatment.
- Surgery.

Final Complication Management

The patient was immediately transferred back to the Angio Suite. The right groin was repunctured

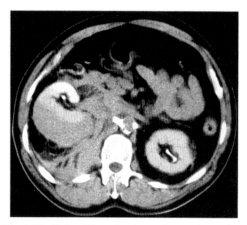

Fig. 4.192 Native CT imaging shows a large subcapsular hematoma of the right dorsal kidney.

and a 5F standard sheath was inserted. Using a cobra-shaped catheter and a 0.035-inch guidewire, the right renal artery was cannulated and selective contrast injections were made. Angiography (**Fig. 4.193a, b**) showed active arterial bleeding from a segmental capsular renal artery branch. A 2.7F microcatheter was advanced into the bleeding branch and the artery was successfully embolized with a 3-mm microcoil (**Fig. 4.194**).

CT angiography 1 day after the procedure showed a nonexpanding subcapsular renal hematoma and no signs of active bleeding. Note the artifacts from the placed micro-coil (**Fig. 4.195**). The patient was asymptomatic at this time and could be ambulated.

Complication Analysis

It can be assumed that the straight hydrophilic-coated 0.018-inch guidewire used for cannulation of the right renal artery injured the capsular branch of the kidney, leading to a potentially life-threatening bleeding complication. Endovascular treatment was possible and the kidney could be saved.

Prevention Strategies and Take-home Message

- Exclusively use atraumatic low-profile wires for selective catheterization of visceral arteries.
- If hydrophylic-coated wires are used to recanalize lesions of visceral arteries, the wire tip must be fluoroscopically controlled at any time.
- Flank pain after endovascular procedures in renal arteries must prompt diagnostic imaging to rule out active bleeding.

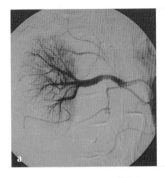
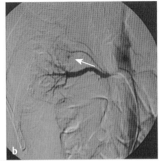

Fig. 4.193 (a, b) Selective angiography shows active arterial bleeding from a segmental capsular renal artery branch (*arrow*).

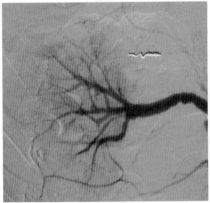

Fig. 4.194 Final angiography after successful placement a 3mm microcoil for complete embolization of the bleeding branch.

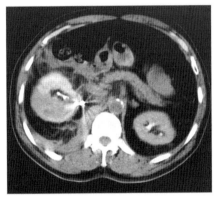

Fig. 4.195 Native control CT after successful embolization indicating artifacts from the micro-coil at the level of embolization. Note, the hematoma stayed stable.

Further Reading

Lee SY, Kim SM, Bae JW, et al. Renal artery perforation related with hydrophilic guidewire during coronary intervention: successful treatment with polyvinyl alcohol injection. Can J Cardiol 2012;28(5):612.e5–e7

Axelrod DJ, Freeman H, Pukin L, Guller J, Mitty HA. Guidewire perforation leading to fatal perirenal hemorrhage from transcortical collaterals after renal artery stent placement. J Vasc Interv Radiol 2004;15(9):985–987

Soriano-Pérez AM, Baca-Morilla Y, Galindo-de Blas B, Bejar-Palma MP, Martín-Ortiz M, Bueno-Millán MP. Renal artery rupture during complicated recovery from angioplasty to treat renal stenosis. Nefrologia 2012;32(2):258–260

Distal embolization after lesion crossing treated with aspiration

Patient History

A 77-year-old woman presented with critical limb ischemia of her left leg. There was a short-segment occlusion of the superficial femoral artery (SFA). The patient was scheduled for percutaneous transluminal angioplasty (PTA).

Initial Treatment Received

Antegrade puncture of the right common femoral artery (CFA) was performed and a 6F sheath was introduced. Heparin 5,000 IU was administered intrarterially. The short SFA occlusion was recanalized with a hydrophilic-wire and a diagnostic catheter. Angioplasty with a 5-mm balloon was uneventful and the result was technically good.

Problems Encountered during Treatment

Control angiography of the arterial outflow revealed an occlusion of the distal fibular artery, which represented the only patent below-the-knee (BTK) artery before the intervention (**Fig. 4.196**). The patient did not complain of rest pain at this point.

Imaging Plan

Selective angiography.

Resulting Complication

Iatrogenic embolization of a single BTK artery.

Possible Strategies for Complication Management

- Percutaneous aspiration thrombectomy (PAT).
- Locoregional catheter thrombolysis.
- Mechanical thrombolysis.
- Open surgical thrombectomy.

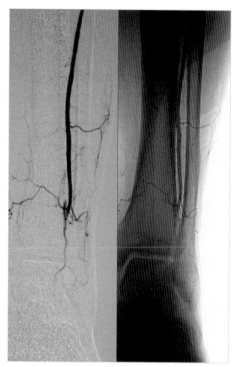

Fig. 4.196 Control digital subtraction angiography and fluoroscopy image after recanalization of a short-segment SFA occlusion showing distal occlusion.

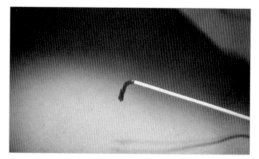

Fig. 4.197 5F guiding catheter with embolus.

Final Complication Management

PAT was performed. The distal occlusion was cannulated with a diagnostic catheter and a hydrophylic-coated 0.035-inch guidewire. A 5F 100-cm guiding catheter was introduced over the wire and placed with the catheter tip in the beginning of the occlusion. The wire was removed and suction was applied with a 50 mL syringe to the catheter. Under constant negative pressure the catheter was retracted and flushed. Two catheter passes were needed to recover an embolus (**Fig. 4.197**). Control angiography showed the reopened single BTK artery (**Fig. 4.198**).

Complication Analysis

This case shows a typical complication of a recanalization procedure in patients with peripheral vascular disease. Depending on plaque composition and age of occlusion, different types of debris from a lesion may dislodge during catheter manipulation. Caught in the bloodstream the material or thrombus will be carried distally and block the outflow vessel(s). In order to secure the outcome of the procedure this material should be removed immediately. In this case aspiration of a blood clot was easy and vessel patency was restored.

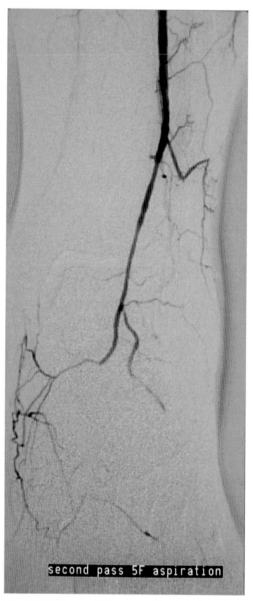

Fig. 4.198 Following PAT, reopened distal single outflow vessel.

Prevention Strategies and Take-home Message

- Distal embolization is a common complication of peripheral angioplasty.
- Use of low-profile catheter techniques may lead to lower rates of distal embolization.
- Patients should receive antiplatelet and anticoagulation medication before recanalization procedures.
- Patency of distal outflow vessels must be documented before and after recanalization procedures to detect and treat distal embolization.
- Interventionists should be familiar with endovascular clot removal techniques.

Further Reading

Banerjee S, Sarode K, Brilakis ES. Protected PTA in the lower limbs: a step forward in preventing distal embolization. J Endovasc Ther 2013;20(3):420–421

De Luca G, Navarese EP, Suryapranata H. A meta-analytic overview of thrombectomy during primary angioplasty. Int J Cardiol 2013;166(3):606–612

Morrissey NJ. When is embolic protection needed in lower extremity interventions and how should it be done. J Cardiovasc Surg (Torino) 2012;53(2):173–175

Razavi MK. Detection and treatment of acute thromboembolic events in the lower extremities. Tech Vasc Interv Radiol 2011;14(2):80–85

Reeves R, Imsais JK, Prasad A. Successful management of lower extremity distal embolization following percutaneous atherectomy with the JetStream G3 device. J Invasive Cardiol 2012;24(6):E124–E128

Spiliopoulos S, Theodosiadou V, Koukounas V, et al. Distal macro- and microembolization during subintimal recanalization of femoropopliteal chronic total occlusions. J Endovasc Ther 2014;21(4):474–481

Zeller T, Schmidt A, Rastan A, Noory E, Sixt S, Scheinert D. Initial experience with the 5 × 300-mm Proteus embolic capture angioplasty balloon in the treatment of peripheral vascular disease. J Endovasc Ther 2012;19(6):826–833

Zhang F, Zhang H, Luo X, Liang G, Feng Y, Zhang WW. Catheter-directed thrombolysis-assisted angioplasty for chronic lower limb ischemia. Ann Vasc Surg 2014;28(3):590–595

4.3.3 Balloon Inflation

Embolic event into the dorsal pedal artery during percutaneous transluminal angioplasty of multilevel diseased superficial femoral artery and popliteal artery

Patient History

A 75-year-old patient presented with left leg claudication; magnetic resonance imaging (MRI) depicted multilevel arterial disease of the left femoropopliteal artery. Antegrade angiography prior to endovascular therapy proved multiple superficial femoral artery (SFA) stenoses and a distal SFA and popliteal artery occlusion involving the first popliteal artery segment (**Figs. 4.199** and **4.200**). The proximal part of the anterior tibial artery presented a moderate short-segment stenosis; the anterior tibial artery was the main feeder artery for the foot, while the peroneal and posterior tibial artery displayed a small caliber (**Fig. 4.201**). The patient was scheduled for a ballooning procedure from an ipsilateral antegrade access route, coming from the common femoral artery (CFA).

Initial Treatment Received

Under local anesthesia, a 6F 10-cm-long sheath was placed in an antegrade manner into the left CFA. A hydrophilic-coated 0.018-inch guidewire combined with 4F angle-tip catheter crossed the SFA stenosis and the popliteal artery occlusion. Following recanalization, long-term PTA (5 × 200 mm at 6 atmospheres [atm]) was performed.

Problems Encountered during Treatment

The patient complained of sudden onset of dysesthesia and pain in the foot.

Imaging Plan

Angiographic check of the run-off.

Resulting Complication

Embolic occlusion of the distal anterior tibial artery (main feeder artery), resulting in insufficient blood supply to the foot (**Fig. 4.202**).

Possible Strategies for Complication Management

- Endovascular treatment from the established transfemoral approach via a 65-cm-long 6F sheath placed in the distal SFA or if possible in the popliteal artery. Percutaneous aspiration thrombectomy (PAT) using a dedicated aspiration or guiding catheter. In lengthy procedures, activated clotting time (ACT) should be checked and additional heparin applied accordingly.
- Endovascular management with a mechanical thrombectomy device (e.g., hydromechanical thrombolysis; stent retriever).
- Short-term fibrinolysis therapy.
- Surgery (if endovascular approach fails).

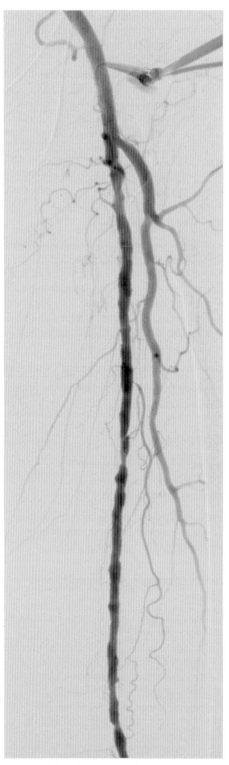

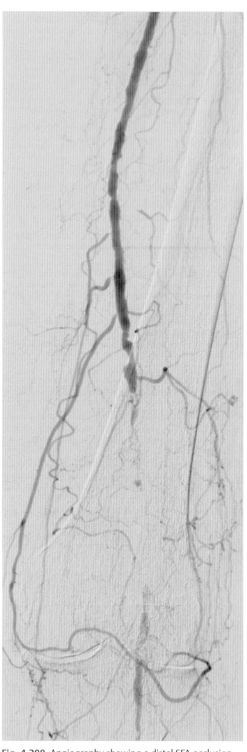

Fig. 4.199 Digital subtraction angiography presenting multiple wall irregularities and moderate stenosis of the SFA's mid- and distal part.

Fig. 4.200 Angiography showing a distal SFA occlusion reaching into the first popliteal artery segment. Note some supragenual collaterals.

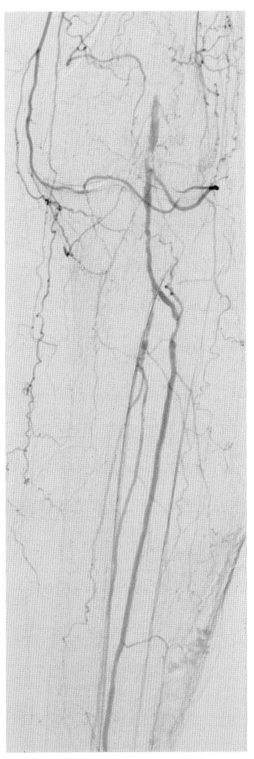

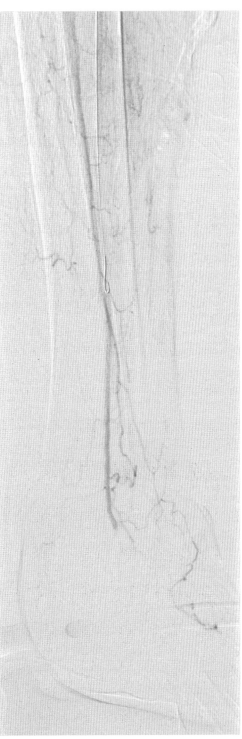

Fig. 4.201 At the knee joint level, the popliteal artery seems stenosed, and the proximal part of the anterior tibial artery is also narrowed. The anterior tibial artery is the main feeder vessel for the foot.

Fig. 4.202 Angiography after long-term PTA and plain old balloon angioplasty (POBA) of the SFA and the popliteal artery. The blood supply for the foot is severely compromised due to an embolic occlusion of the distal, supramalleolar anterior tibial artery. The collateral flow is rather poor.

Final Complication Management

Endovascular treatment was performed via the existing access. The short sheath was exchanged with a long 65-cm-long 6F sheath. A 125-cm-long 4F multipurpose (MP) catheter was placed over a 0.014-inch wire with hydrophilic tip across the occlusion and into the distal dorsal pedal artery. After removal of the MP catheter an aspiration catheter with so-called rapid-exchange/mono-rail technology (Fetch 2, 135-cm, distal shaft 4F, Medrad) was placed into the occlusion and a first aspiration maneuver was begun, keeping the wire in place during removal of the aspiration catheter under suction.

A first angiographic control showed a significant improvement of flow; previously blocked collaterals are now patent (**Fig. 4.203**). After two additional aspiration maneuvers, the flow into the foot was entirely restored (**Fig. 4.204**). Thromboembolic material was collected in a filter (**Fig. 4.205**).

Complication Analysis

Simple PTA resulted in downstream embolization into the calf arteries.

Prevention Strategies and Take-home Message

- Lesion passing and PTA should be performed with great care!

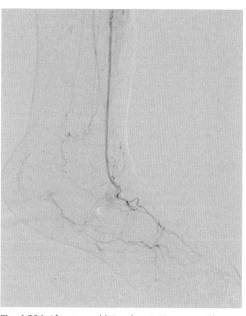

Fig. 4.204 After two additional aspiration runs with so-called rapid-exchange/monorail technology, the final angiography shows completely restored flow into the foot via the main feeder vessel, the dorsal pedal artery.

- Consider using smaller profiles for both lesion crossing and lesion treatment, like 0.018-inch wire and 0.018-inch-compatible balloons (as done in this case!).
- Embolization events are unpredictable—lesions that look prone to embolism often don't result

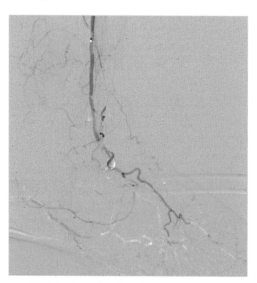

Fig. 4.203 Angiography after a first aspiration maneuver; collaterals are reopened. However, the main part of the dorsal pedal artery still shows prolonged flow.

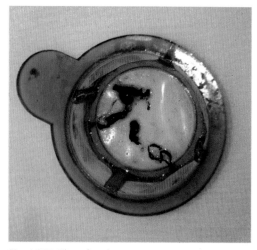

Fig. 4.205 Filter after three aspiration maneuvers; a huge amount of fresh emboli was collected. Aspiration was performed with 20 mL Luer lock syringe, keeping the guidewire in a stable position, which is possible due to the catheter's monorail technology.

in dislodgement of debris (although this lesion looked bad and resulted in this complication) and lesions that look safe might result in embolism!

- When embolic events occur, do not hesitate. Proceed with PAT or other pharmacomechanical clearing techniques!

Further Reading

Spiliopoulos S, Theodosiadou V, Koukounas V, et al. Distal macro- and microembolization during subintimal recanalization of femoropopliteal chronic total occlusions. J Endovasc Ther 2014;21(4):474–481

Zhang F, Zhang H, Luo X, Liang G, Feng Y, Zhang WW. Catheter-directed thrombolysis-assisted angioplasty for chronic lower limb ischemia. Ann Vasc Surg 2014;28(3):590–595

Below-the-knee embolic event during infrainguinal percutaneous transluminal angioplasty via transbrachial approach

Patient History

A 65-year-old patient suffered from lifestyle-limiting peripheral artery disease. The underlying lesion was a high-grade, short-distance stenosis at the origin of both the deep femoral artery and the superficial femoral artery (SFA) (**Fig. 4.206**). The patient was scheduled for a ballooning procedure from a left transbrachial approach due to a previous kissing stent procedure at the level of the aortic bifurcation, which made a crossover procedure from the contralateral groin impossible.

Initial Treatment Received

Under local anesthesia, a 5F, 90-cm-long sheath was placed in a retrograde manner into the left brachial artery. A first 0.018-inch guidewire crossed the SFA lesion followed by immediate long-term PTA of the SFA origin (5 × 60 mm at 10 atmospheres [atm]) (**Fig. 4.207**). A second wire was placed into the deep femoral artery, leaving the SFA wire in place. PTA of the deep femoral artery lesion was performed (4 × 60 mm)

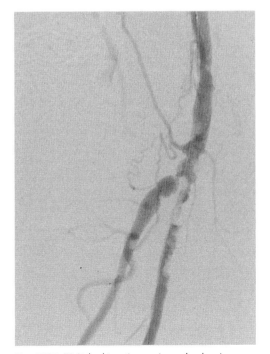

Fig. 4.206 Digital subtraction angiography showing a high-grade short-distance stenosis at the origin of both the deep femoral artery and the SFA.

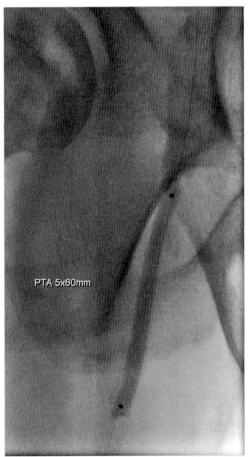

Fig. 4.207 An 0.018-inch guidewire crossed the SFA lesion followed by immediate long-term PTA (5 × 60 mm at 10 atm) of the SFA origin.

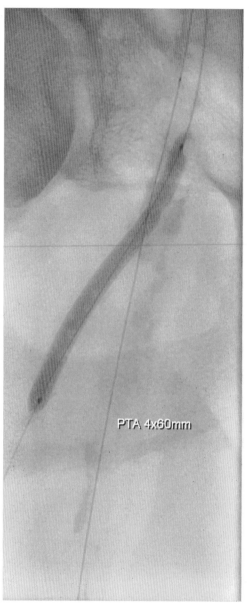

Fig. 4.208 A second wire into the deep femoral artery, with the SFA wire left in place. PTA of the deep femoral artery lesion (4 × 60 mm).

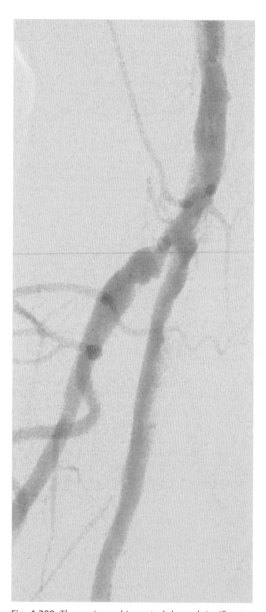

Fig. 4.209 The angiographic control showed significant residual stenosis of the deep femoral artery, whereas the result of the SFA's PTA was acceptable.

(**Fig. 4.208**). The angiographic control showed significant residual stenosis of the deep femoral artery, whereas the result of the SFA's PTA was acceptable (**Fig. 4.209**).

Problems Encountered during Treatment

The patient complained of sudden onset of dysesthesia of the calf.

Imaging Plan

Angiography to check the run-off.

Resulting Complication

Embolic occlusion of the peroneal trunk; only the anterior tibial artery remained patent (**Fig. 4.210**).

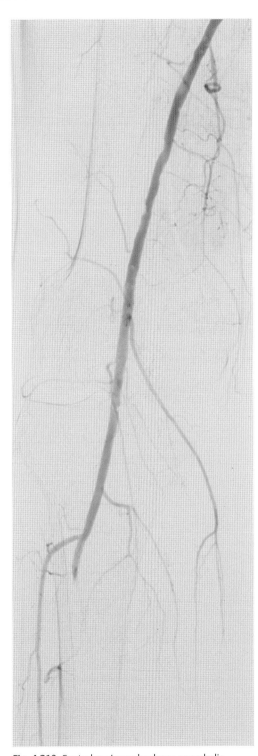

Fig. 4.210 Control angiography shows an embolic occlusion of the peroneal trunk; only the anterior tibial artery was patent.

Possible Strategies for Complication Management

- Endovascular treatment via established transbrachial approach and the 90-cm-long sheath placed in the infrarenal aorta. Further advancement of the sheath as far down as possible. Percutaneous aspiration thrombectomy (PAT). In lengthy procedures activated clotting time (ACT) should be checked and additional heparin can be given accordingly.
- If needed, an antegrade puncture of the ipsilateral common femoral artery (CFA) should be considered (not the primary option in this case).
- Initiation of short-term fibrinolysis therapy.
- Surgery (if an endovascular approach fails).

Final Complication Management

Endovascular treatment was performed via the established transbrachial approach and the 90-cm-long sheath placed in the infrarenal aorta. The 0.018-inch wire was exchanged for a 125-cm-long 4F multipurpose catheter over a 0.014-inch wire with hydrophilic tip. The wire was navigated towards the lesion; the occlusion was crossed without any resistance, the wire was placed in the peroneal artery first (**Fig. 4.211**). An aspiration catheter with so-called rapid-exchange/monorail technology (Fetch 2, 135-cm, distal shaft 4F, Medrad) was positioned in the occlusion and a first aspiration maneuver began, keeping the wire in place while removing the aspiration catheter under suction.

After successful aspiration the guidewire was placed in the posterior tibial artery for a final aspiration procedure for some residual debris (**Fig. 4.212**). The final angiography showed a patent trifurcation without any residual thromboembolic material (**Fig. 4.213**).

Complication Analysis

Simple PTA resulted in downstream embolization to the calf arteries.

Prevention Strategies and Take-home Message

- Lesion passing and PTA should be performed with great care!

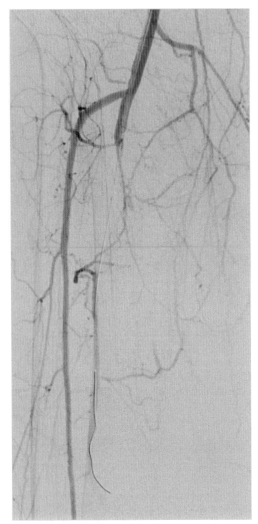

Fig. 4.211 Angiography showing an 0.014-inch wire already navigated into the peroneal artery; the occlusion was crossed without any resistance.

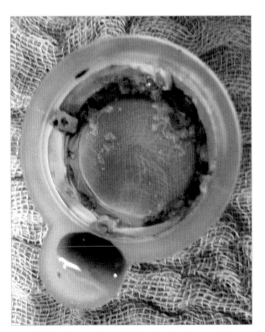

Fig. 4.212 The resulting debris after the first aspiration maneuver collected in a filter.

- Use smaller profiles for both lesion crossing and lesion treatment, like 0.018-inch wire and 0.018-inch-compatible balloons (as was done in this case)!
- Embolization events are unpredictable—lesions that look prone to embolism often don't result in dislodgement of debris, and lesions that look safe might result in embolism! When embolic events occur, do not hesitate. Proceed with PAT!

Further Reading

Spiliopoulos S, Theodosiadou V, Koukounas V, et al. Distal macro- and microembolization during subintimal recanalization of

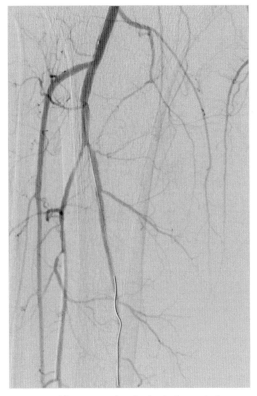

Fig. 4.213 After a second aspiration in the posterior tibial artery, final angiography shows a patent trifurcation without any residual thromboembolic material.

femoropopliteal chronic total occlusions. J Endovasc Ther 2014;21(4):474–481

Zhang F, Zhang H, Luo X, Liang G, Feng Y, Zhang WW. Catheter-directed thrombolysis-assisted angioplasty for chronic lower limb ischemia. Ann Vasc Surg 2014;28(3):590–595

Damage to a self-expanding stent during repeated percutaneous transluminal angioplasty

Patient History

An 87-year-old man with Parkinson's disease and peripheral vascular disease presented with limited walking distance of 100 m. At that time he was treated successfully by plain old balloon angioplasty (POBA) and stent placement (6 × 200 mm and 6 × 39 mm) in the distal superficial femoral artery (SFA). One year later repeat percutaneous transluminal angioplasty was considered because of reoccurrence of symptoms. Pre-interventional color duplex ultrasound detected a high-grade stenosis in the mid-part of the still unstented part of the SFA.

Initial Treatment Received

Access route was via the ipsilateral common femoral artery (CFA) using a regular 6F sheath. Groin puncture and treatment of index lesion was without event. POBA (5 × 200 mm) was performed after passing the high-grade stenosis with a 0.018-inch hydrophilic-tip wire (**Figs. 4.214** and **4.215**).

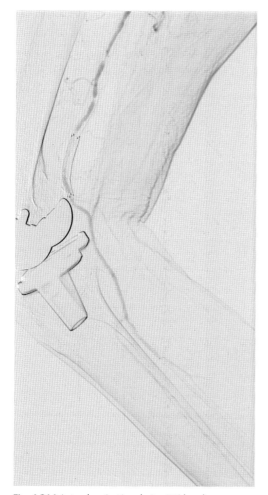

Fig. 4.214 Lateral projection during 90° bending; angiography of the distal SFA depicts high-grade in-stent restenosis at two levels in the adductor canal due to intimal hyperplasia.

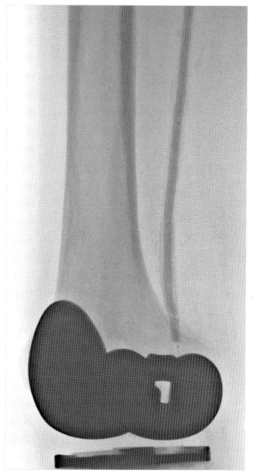

Fig. 4.215 Fluoroscopic view during percutaneous transluminal angioplasty (PTA) (5 × 200 mm at 12 atmospheres [atm] for 180 s).

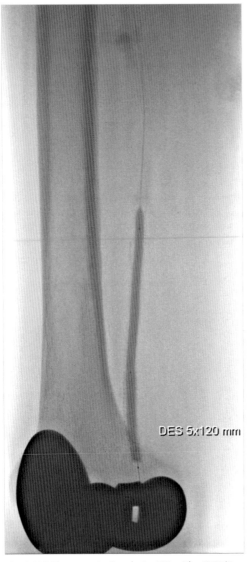

Fig. 4.216 Fluoroscopic view during PTA with a DCB (5 × 120 mm at 8 atm for 60 s).

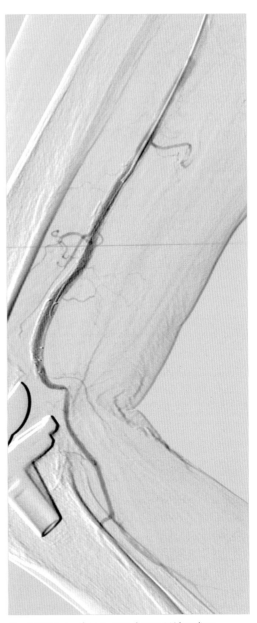

Fig. 4.217 Lateral projection during 90° bending; angiography of the distal SFA depicts no further ISR.

Due to the fact that an in-stent restenosis (ISR) was treated, 0.035-inch-compatible drug-coated balloons (DCBs) (paclitaxel) were used for final drug-eluting balloon angioplasty (**Fig. 4.216**).

Problems Encountered during Treatment

Final angiography in two planes presented no signs of residual stenosis; the distal run-off was fine without any signs of distal embolization. However, careful evaluation of the stents showed an irregularity of the distal marker positions of the stent placed distally in the first popliteal segment (**Fig. 4.217**). The flow of injected contrast media was not compromised, whereas the stent outflow area was narrowed by dislodged, elongated stent struts resulting in at least 50% stenosis.

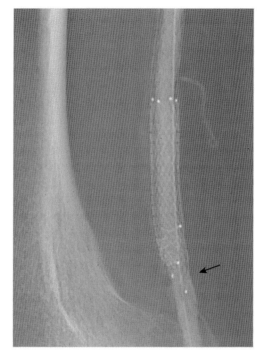

Fig. 4.218 Magnified fluoroscopic view showing the elongated distal stent strut rows indicated by position of the radiopaque marker at different levels (*arrow*) compared to the proximal markers, which are positioned at the same horizontal level.

Imaging Plan

Magnified angiography and fluoroscopy for further evaluation (**Fig. 4.218**).

Resulting Complication

Dislodged, elongated stent struts resulted in at least 50% stenosis. How did that happen? The following might be a possible explanation: initial PTA was performed over a 0.018-inch wire with a 0.018-inch-compatible balloon. The subsequently used DCB was 0.035-inch compatible; this resulted in a mismatch and gap between wire and distal balloon tip. The gap might have interacted with the stent struts in that struts were engaged, which resulted in stent elongation.

Possible Strategies for Complication Management

- Long-term PTA to try to refix the dislodged stent struts (unlikely to be successful).

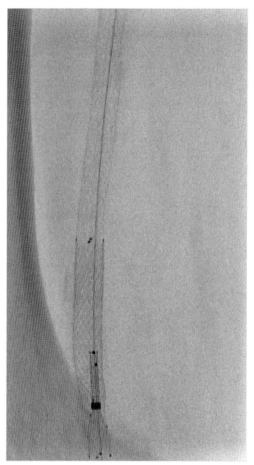

Fig. 4.219 Fluoroscopy of the partially deployed additional SES (6 × 20 mm).

- Additional placement of a self-expanding stent (SES) (**Fig. 4.219**) in order to fixate the dislodged stent elements (**Figs. 4.220** and **4.221**).

Final Complication Management

Additional placement of an SES.

Complication Analysis

Despite careful handling of instruments, there was interaction (supposed engagement) between stent struts and the balloon catheter during advancement and removal of the device. Possible explanations are (1) advancement of an insufficiently deflated balloon (after previous use for PTA), which became caught in the struts; (2) a gap between the 0.018-inch wire

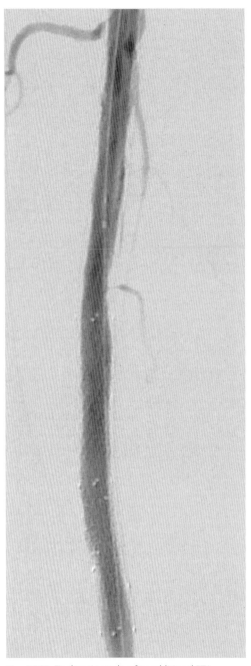

Fig. 4.220 Final angiography after additional PTA (5 mm) showing a contrast media filling without any residual stenosis or narrowing due to the dislodged stent elements.

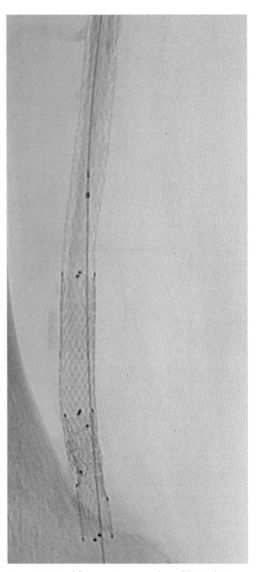

Fig. 4.221 Final fluoroscopic view after additional PTA (5 mm) showing no residual narrowing due to elongated stent struts.

and 0.035-inch-compatible balloon, which might have damaged the stent; or (3) the passage of a guidewire through the distal rows of the stent struts. The latter, however, was not recognized during PTA in this case.

Prevention Strategies and Take-home Message

- Handle instruments with care. Push or pull all instruments with controlled power and never against resistance.
- Deflate balloons carefully, especially when they have been used for treatment of other lesions.
- Handle devices with great care when the guidewire used is smaller than the available guidewire lumen of the device.

Further Reading

Nikanorov A, Schillinger M, Zhao H, Minar E, Schwartz LB. Assessment of self-expanding nitinol stent deformation after chronic implantation into the femoropopliteal arteries. EuroIntervention 2013;9(6):730–737

Nikanorov A, Smouse HB, Osman K, Bialas M, Shrivastava S, Schwartz LB. Fracture of self-expanding nitinol stents stressed in vitro under simulated intravascular conditions. J Vasc Surg 2008;48(2):435–440.

Vessel perforation during renal angioplasty

Patient History

A 55-year-old man had undergone right renal artery stenting in 2005 and, 6 years later, left renal artery stenting for severe atherosclerotic stenosis.

In the last month he had observed increased blood pressure (190/95 mm Hg). Color Doppler ultrasound showed an in-stent restenosis (ISR) in the left renal artery.

An endovascular reintervention was scheduled.

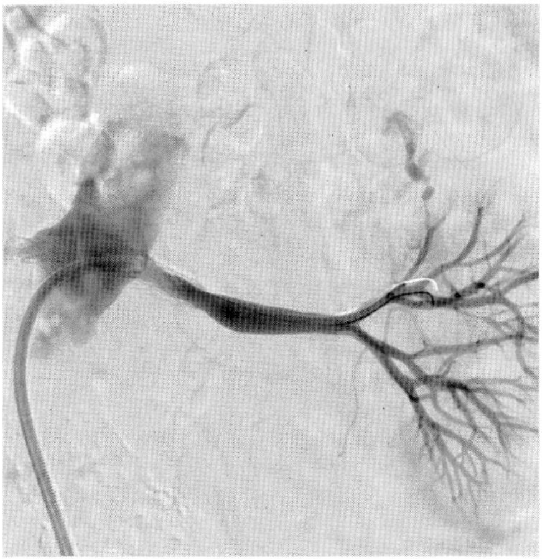

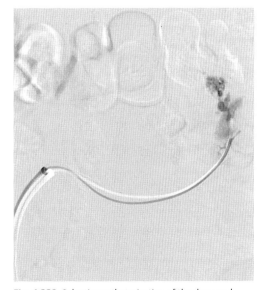

Fig. 4.222 Selective angiography performed after dilatation of the ISR. A good flow was evident within the stent. In the upper pole of the left kidney an extravasation of contrast media was evident.

Initial Treatment Received

Digital subtraction angiography (DSA) of the left renal artery confirmed a severe intrastent stenosis. The stenotic tract was managed with a 0.014-inch guidewire and dilatated initially with a 4-mm balloon and after that with a 4-mm cutting balloon.

Problems Encountered during Treatment

The final DSA confirmed a good flow within the stent and the renal artery with complete resolution of the stenosis. However, contrast media extravasation was clearly evident at the level of the upper pole of the kidney arising from a little branch (**Fig. 4.222**). After selective catheterization with a 2.7F microcatheter (Progreat, Terumo) of the upper branch of the left kidney, DSA confirmed the site of bleeding. (**Fig. 4.223**)

Fig. 4.223 Selective catheterization of the damaged branch performed with a 2.7F microcatheter. DSA confirmed the damage of the distal branch.

Imaging Plan

Selective angiography of the left renal artery.

Resulting Complication

Perforation of a polar branch with bleeding and hematoma formation. Moreover, vasospasm of other vessels was observed.

Possible Strategies for Complication Management

- Endovascular approach with selective embolization.
- Surgery (if endovascular approach fails).

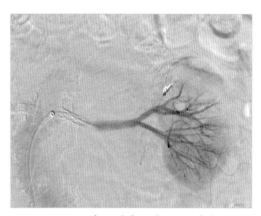

Fig. 4.224 DSA performed after selective embolization with detachable microcoils confirms the absence of further contrast media extravasation.

Final Complication Management

Embolization was carried out using detachable microcoils (Concerto, Ev3) (**Fig. 4.224**).

Complication Analysis

Arterial damage (perforation) during renal intervention represents a common complication; it can occur when the tip of the guidewire is distal in a branch. In some cases multifocal bleeding has occurred.[1,2]

Involuntary movements of the guidewire, for example during stent or balloon insertion, can lacerate a distal vessel, resulting in bleeding.

Prevention Strategies and Take-home Message

- Always use 0.014-inch nonhydrophilic guidewires in order to minimize the risk of perforation of distal branches.
- During the intervention always keep the tip of the guidewire visible.
- It is very important to keep the guidewire as firm as possible.
- At the end of the procedure always perform DSA, looking at all parts of the kidney.
- In a case of bleeding, selective catheterization of the diseased branch using a microcatheter is required.
- Coils and microcoils should be always available in the cath lab during renal artery procedures.[3]

References

1. Axelrod DJ, Freeman H, Pukin L, Guller J, Mitty HA. Guidewire perforation leading to fatal perirenal hemorrhage from transcortical collaterals after renal artery stent placement. J Vasc Interv Radiol 2004;15(9):985–987
2. Aytekin C, Yildirim UM, Ozyer U, Harman A, Boyvat F. Emergency renal ablation for life-threatening hemorrhage from multiple capsular branches during renalartery stenting. Cardiovasc Intervent Radiol 2010;33(3):663–666
3. Ierardi AM, Floridi C, Fontana F, et al. Transcatheter embolization of iatrogenic renal vascular injuries. Radiol Med 2014;119(4):261–268

Distal embolization after balloon angioplasty treated with aspiration

Patient History

A 68-year-old woman was diagnosed with an occlusion of the proximal aspect of the right superficial femoral artery (SFA). She was referred for endovascular treatment.

Initial Treatment Received

Antegrade puncture of the right common femoral artery (CFA) was performed and a 6F sheath was introduced. Heparin 5,000 IU was applied intrarterially. The SFA occlusion (**Fig. 4.225**) was recanalized with a hydrophilic-coated 0.018-inch guidewire and a diagnostic catheter. Angioplasty with a 5-mm balloon was uneventful and showed a good local technical result (**Fig. 4.226**).

Problems Encountered during Treatment

Control angiography of the arterial outflow after angioplasty revealed a new short-segment occlusion of the tibioperoneal trunk from an embolus with consecutive slow flow in the fibular artery and an occlusion of the posterior tibial artery (**Fig. 4.227**). The patient did not complain of rest pain at this point.

Imaging Plan

Selective angiography.

Resulting Complication

Percutaneous transluminal angioplasty (PTA)–associated iatrogenic embolization.

Possible Strategies for Complication Management

- Percutaneous aspiration thrombectomy (PAT).
- Locoregional catheter thrombolysis.
- Mechanical thrombolysis.
- Open surgical thrombectomy.

Final Complication Management

PAT was performed. The distal occlusion was cannulated with a diagnostic catheter and a hydrophylic-coated 0.035-inch guidewire. A 6F 100-cm guiding catheter (Vista Brite Tip, Cordis/Johnson & Johnson) was introduced over the wire and placed with the tip in the occlusion. The wire was removed and suction was applied with a 50-mL syringe. Under constant negative pressure the catheter was retracted and flushed. After one catheter pass an embolus was recovered. Control angiography showed a reopened tibioperoneal trunk (**Fig. 4.228**).

Complication Analysis

This case shows a common complication of angioplasty. Depending on plaque composition and age of occlusion, different types of debris from a lesion may dislodge during ballooning. Caught in the bloodstream the material or thrombus will be carried distally and block the outflow vessel(s). In order to secure the outcome of the procedure this material should be removed immediately. In this case aspiration of an embolus was successful and vessel patency was restored.

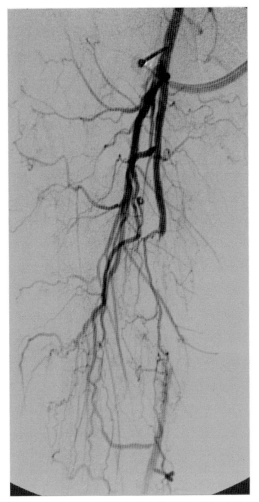

Fig. 4.225 Occlusion of the proximal aspect of the right SFA.

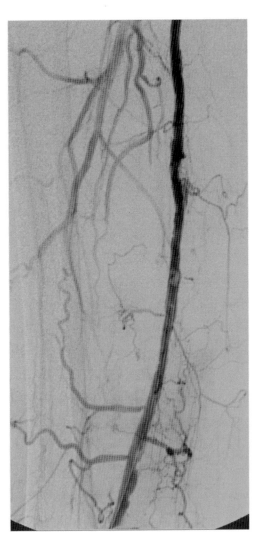

Fig. 4.226 Following percutaneous transluminal angioplasty with a 5-mm balloon no significant residual stenosis is present.

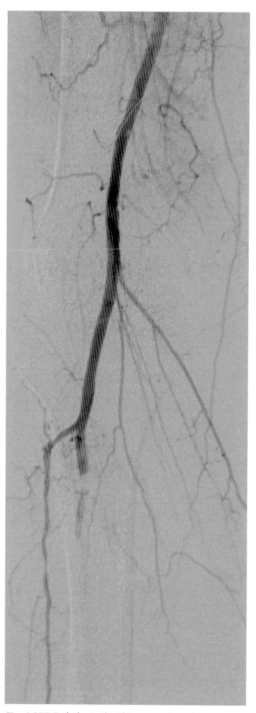

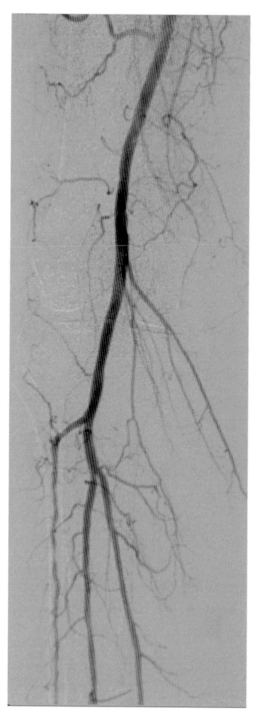

Fig. 4.227 Embolus in the tibioperoneal trunk.

Fig. 4.228 Final angiography after one catheter pass with successful embolus aspiration. The tibio-peroneal trunk is reopened completely.

Prevention Strategies and Take-home Message

- Distal embolization is a common complication of peripheral angioplasty.
- Patients should receive antiplatelet and anticoagulation medication before recanalization procedures.
- Patency of distal outflow vessels must be documented before and after recanalization procedures to detect and treat distal embolization.
- Interventionists should be familiar with endovascular clot removal techniques.

Further Reading

Banerjee S, Sarode K, Brilakis ES. Protected PTA in the lower limbs: a step forward in preventing distal embolization. J Endovasc Ther 2013;20(3):420–421

De Luca G, Navarese EP, Suryapranata H. A meta-analytic overview of thrombectomy during primary angioplasty. Int J Cardiol 2013;166(3):606–612

Morrissey NJ. When is embolic protection needed in lower extremity interventions and how should it be done. J Cardiovasc Surg (Torino) 2012;53(2):173–175

Razavi MK. Detection and treatment of acute thromboembolic events in the lower extremities. Tech Vasc Interv Radiol 2011;14(2):80–85

Reeves R, Imsais JK, Prasad A. Successful management of lower extremity distal embolization following percutaneous atherectomy with the JetStream G3 device. J Invasive Cardiol 2012;24(6):E124–E128

Spiliopoulos S, Theodosiadou V, Koukounas V, et al. Distal macro- and microembolization during subintimal recanalization of femoropopliteal chronic total occlusions. J Endovasc Ther 2014;21(4):474–481

Zeller T, Schmidt A, Rastan A, Noory E, Sixt S, Scheinert D. Initial experience with the 5 × 300-mm Proteus embolic capture angioplasty balloon in the treatment of peripheral vascular disease. J Endovasc Ther 2012;19(6):826–833

Zhang F, Zhang H, Luo X, Liang G, Feng Y, Zhang WW. Catheter-directed thrombolysis-assisted angioplasty for chronic lower limb ischemia. Ann Vasc Surg 2014;28(3):590–595

Renal artery rupture by cutting balloon

Patient History

A 46-year-old woman with a history of renovascular hypertension due to fibromuscular dysplasia (FMD) and worsening of symptoms, despite triple antihypertensive medication, is readmitted for suspected restenosis.

Initial Treatment Received

The patient had been treated by angioplasty 8 months earlier. Duplex ultrasound now detected high-grade restenosis. Following retro-grade puncture of the right common femoral artery (CFA) a 5F sheath was introduced. A pigtail catheter was used for angiography, which showed two separate segmental arteries of the right kidney with high-grade restenosis in the proximal aspect of the upper segment vessel (**Fig. 4.229**). Access in the right groin was exchanged for a 45-cm-long 6F sheath and the renal artery was recanalized using a 4F cobra catheter over a 0.014-inch guidewire (Spartacore, Abbott Vascular). A 4 × 20-mm cutting balloon was used for "off-label" paclitaxel-coated balloon (PCB) angioplasty of the renal artery. The rationale was to limit barotrauma of the vessel and likelihood of restenosis.

Problems Encountered during Treatment

The initial result of PCB angioplasty was good with lack of significant residual stenosis in the treated vessel. There was a dissection in a major segmental branch, for which angioplasty with a smaller balloon was considered as the next step (**Fig. 4.230**). Before the second angioplasty could be performed, the patient complained of onset of severe right-sided flank pain. Using the sheath, selective angiography was performed immediately, showing rupture of the treated renal artery with massive contrast extravasation (**Fig. 4.231**).

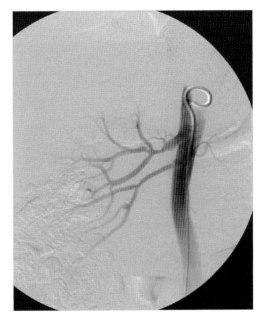

Fig. 4.229 FMD restenosis of the right upper segmental renal artery.

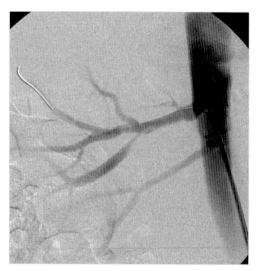

Fig. 4.230 Initial result after PCB angioplasty.

Imaging Plan

Selective angiography.

Resulting Complication

Cutting-balloon angioplasty resulted in perforation of the renal artery vessel.

Possible Strategies for Complication Management

- Balloon occlusion to control bleeding.
- Stent graft implantation.

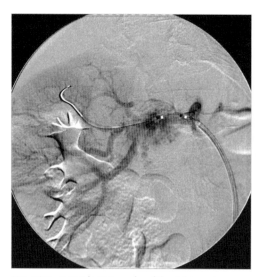

Fig. 4.231 Control angiography of the right renal artery after onset of right flank pain showing contrast extravasation.

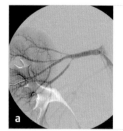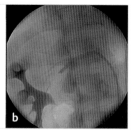

Fig. 4.232 (a) Control angiography after 6 minutes of vessel occlusion without any signs of continuous bleeding. (b) Angioplasty of the dissected middle segmental branch.

- Embolization of the entire kidney.
- Emergency surgery (if endovascular measures fail).

Final Complication Management

A standard 4-mm balloon catheter was inserted over the guidewire already in place. The balloon was inflated in the main trunk of the right renal artery and left in place for 6 minutes. Control angiography then showed hemostasis without signs of continuous bleeding (**Fig. 4.232a**). There was no stent graft of a suitable size available. The dissection of the middle segmental branch was treated with a smaller angioplasty balloon (**Fig. 4.232b**). The patient was observed in the Intensive Care Unit overnight, but remained clinically stable. Computed tomography angiography (CTA) was performed the next day, showing only a mild retroperitoneal hematoma (**Fig. 4.233**).

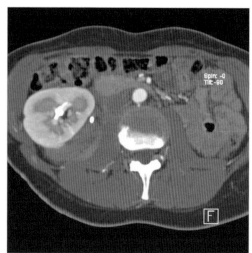

Fig. 4.233 CTA showed mild retroperitoneal hematoma; no signs of active bleeding.

Complication Analysis

The diameter of the cutting balloon was inadequate and/or the vessel was too fragile due to the underlying disease. The cutting blades of the balloon perforated the vessel, leading to a potentially fatal hemorrhage. Immediate occlusion of the rupture site using a standard balloon was able to control the bleeding.

Prevention Strategies and Take-home Message

- Avoid "off-label" use of cutting balloons in visceral arteries.
- Start PCB with markedly undersized balloon diameters.
- Have stent grafts available for a broad range of vessel sizes to treat rupture.

Further Reading

Brountzos EN, Ptohis N, Triantafyllidi H, et al. Renal artery rupture following cutting-balloon angioplasty for fibromuscular dysplasia: a case report. Cases J 2009;2:8881

Oguzkurt L, Tercan F, Gulcan O, Turkoz R. Rupture of the renal artery after cutting-balloon angioplasty in a young woman with fibromuscular dysplasia. Cardiovasc Interv Radiol 2005;28(3):360–363

Towbin RB, Pelchovitz DJ, Cahill AM, et al. Cutting balloon angioplasty in children with resistant renal artery stenosis. J Vasc Interv Radiol 2007;18(5):663–669

Dissection from balloon malsizing due to communication error

Patient History

A 62-year-old man with known peripheral vascular disease presented with claudication of his left leg. He complained about a limited pain-free walking distance of 20 m and occasional episodes of rest pain at night. The patient had a history of previous angioplasty with stent implantation in his left iliac artery. Noninvasive imaging showed restenosis in the external iliac artery (EIA) stent in combination with a chronic total occlusion of the superficial femoral artery (SFA).

Initial Treatment Received

Following puncture of the right common femoral artery (CFA) a 4F sheath was inserted. The stent in the left EIA was passed with a diagnostic catheter and a hydrophilic-coated guidewire. The wire was exchanged with a standard steel type over which a 45-cm-long 6F sheath was introduced. After heparinization with 5,000 IU the restenosis in the iliac stent was dilatated using a standard balloon with good result. As a next step the left SFA was recanalized with a 0.018-inch guidewire in combination with a tapered 3F support catheter.

Problems Encountered during Treatment

The wire passed the SFA occlusion intraluminally (**Fig. 4.234a, b**); the true lumen of the popliteal

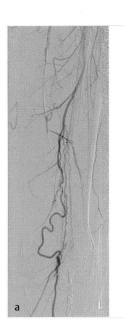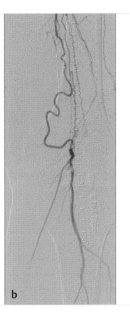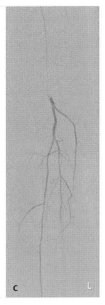

Fig. 4.234 Intraluminal recanalization of a chronic occlusion of the left SFA with a 0.018-inch guidewire and support catheter **(a, b)**. Intraluminal position of the support catheter verified by contrast injection **(c)**.

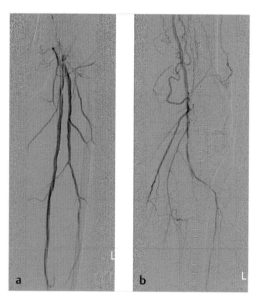

Fig. 4.235 (a) Control angiography following long-segment stent placement shows a widely patent SFA. (b) Distally there is outflow obstruction due to an embolus in the tibioperoneal trunk.

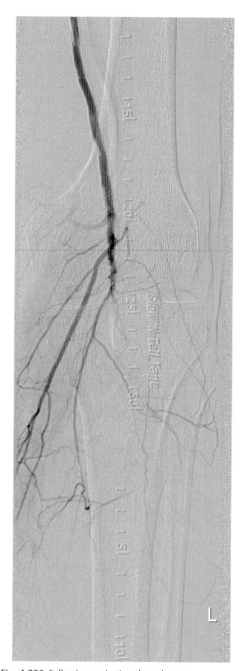

Fig. 4.236 Following aspiration thrombectomy thrombosis worsened.

artery was reached successfully (**Fig. 4.234c**). Following angioplasty there was extensive dissection, so that long-segment stenting was performed. After stent placement there was a widely patent SFA (**Fig. 4.235a**); however, distal embolization had occurred with occlusion of the tibioperoneal trunk (**Fig. 4.235b**). Aspiration thrombectomy was performed using a 5F guide catheter, but thrombosis of the peripheral outflow worsened with development of an occlusion extending into the popliteal artery (**Fig. 4.236**). A bolus of 5 mg recombinant tissue plasminogen activator (rtPa) was applied and the posterior tibial artery was intubated with the guidewire.

The operator then asked the technician for a 3.5 × 150-mm balloon catheter for additional angioplasty. A balloon was handed to the operator and percutaneous transluminal angioplasty (PTA) of the popliteal artery and tibioperoneal trunk was performed. During fluoroscopy the operator noticed that the inflated balloon showed a significant size mismatch in relation to the diameter of the treated vessel; the balloon appeared much larger. After questioning the technician, it was realized that the balloon given was in fact a balloon with diameter of 5 mm, not 3.5 mm. The technician had not heard the operator state the correct diameter. Control angiography after angioplasty did show a patent popliteal artery; however, there was extensive dissection, most likely due to overdilatation of the treated vessel (**Fig. 4.237a, b**). In addition, control angiography at this point revealed acute

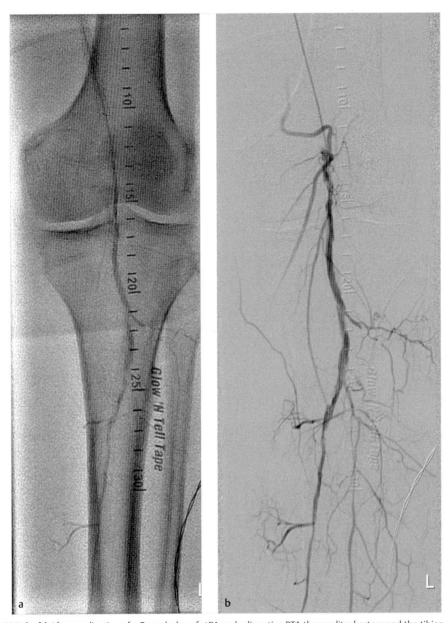

Fig. 4.237 (a, b) After application of a 5-mg bolus of rtPA and adjunctive PTA the popliteal artery and the tibioperoneal trunk was recanalized. Note the iatrogenic dissection of popliteal artery, trunk and posterior tibial artery after use of an oversized 5-mm balloon in a 3.5-mm vessel.

"on-table" thrombosis of the previously stented SFA (**Fig. 4.238**).

Imaging Plan

Selective control angiography.

Resulting Complication

Distal embolization, iatrogenic dissection, and "on-table" thrombosis.

Possible Strategies for Complication Management

- Endovascular management with locoregional long-term lysis, stent placement of the popliteal artery and tibioperoneal trunk.
- Abort procedure; surgical thrombectomy and femoropopliteal or infragenual bypass with or without reconstruction of the tibial trifurcation.

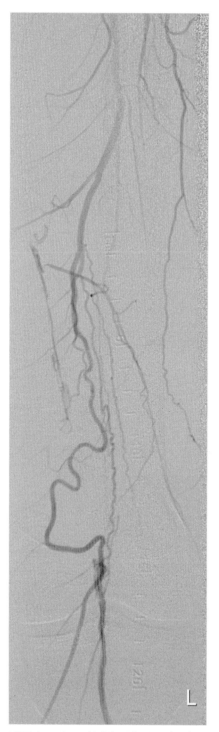

Fig. 4.238 Acute "on-table" thrombosis within the previously stented SFA.

Final Complication Management

A side-hole catheter was positioned into the proximal SFA and—following application of a bolus of 5 mg rtPA—locoregional lysis was initiated with 1 mg rtPa per hour for a total of 16 hours. The patient was also continued on IV heparin at 1,000 IU per hour. Control angiography the next morning showed a successfully recanalized previously stented SFA with residual stenosis in the second popliteal artery segment (**Fig. 4.239a–c**). There was still dissection present in the distal popliteal artery/tibioperoneal trunk; however, it did not seem flow relevant. The popliteal artery was stented to secure outflow, while the iatrogenic dissection was left untreated (**Fig. 4.240**).

The patient now had palpable foot pulses and was asymptomatic. He was medicated with aspirin 100 mg and apixaban (Eliquis, Bristol-Myers Squibb and Pfizer) 2 × 5 mg daily.

Complication Analysis

This case represents a very complex intervention, with multiple obstacles arising during the procedure. Distal embolization after stent implantation prompted the need for aspiration, thrombolysis, and angioplasty. Despite successful reopening of distal outflow, "on-table" thrombosis of the SFA occurred during the procedure, instigating the need for low-dose locoregional thrombolysis. What this complex case also

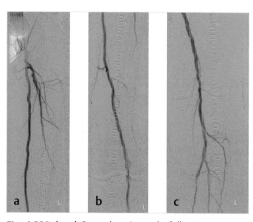

Fig. 4.239 (a–c) Control angiography following 16 hours of locoregional lysis. Restored patency in the long-segment stent. Residual stenosis and persistence of dissection in popliteal artery.

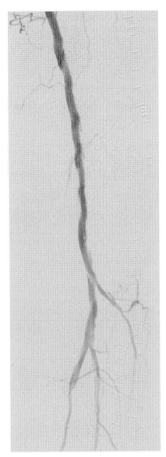

Fig. 4.240 Angiography after stent implantation in the popliteal artery. The iatrogenic dissection was left untreated.

highlights is the importance of communication between team members during interventional procedures. The dissection of the below-the-knee arteries was a result of miscommunication between operator and technician. Instead of a low-profile balloon, a device with the wrong diameter was used.

Prevention Strategies and Take-home Message

- Even long-segment occlusions of the SFA can be treated by endovascular means; however, these procedures can be complex and may be further complicated by embolization, thrombosis, and dissection.
- The operator is responsible for the use of interventional equipment. They must ensure that they are given the correct tools.

Implementation of standard operating procedures (SOPs) may be helpful in this respect.
- When requesting equipment, the technician/nurse should repeat loudly what he or she has understood, so that both sides of the team can be sure that the information has been perceived correctly.
- Operators should check packages of devices requested before they are opened.

Further Reading

Biffl WL, Gallagher AW, Pieracci FM, Berumen C. Suboptimal compliance with surgical safety checklists in Colorado: a prospective observational study reveals differences between surgical specialties. Patient Saf Surg 2015;9(1):5

Katsanos K, Tepe G, Tsetis D, Fanelli F. Standards of practice for superficial femoral and popliteal artery angioplasty and stenting. Cardiovasc Interv Radiol 2014;37(3):592–603

Pugel AE, Simianu VV, Flum DR, Patchen Dellinger E. Use of the surgical safety checklist to improve communication and reduce complications. J Infect Public Health 2015;8(3):219–225

Tiferes J, Bisantz AM, Guru KA. Team interaction during surgery: a systematic review of communication coding schemes. J Surg Res 2015;195(2):422–432

Wade P. Developing a culture of collaboration in the operating room: more than effective communication. ORNAC J 2014;32(4):16–20, 22–23, 32–38

Iliac embolization after repeat percutaneous transluminal angioplasty of subacute occlusion

Patient History

A 72-year-old man with a known history of peripheral vascular disease presented with recurrence of right-sided buttock claudication 6 weeks after recanalization with long-segment aortoiliac kissing stent implantation for TASC II D (TransAtlantic Inter-Society Consensus II class D) disease. The patient was scheduled for repeat PTA for suspected restenosis.

Initial Treatment Received

After puncture of the right common femoral artery (CFA) a 6F standard sheath was introduced. The stents in the right iliac artery could easily be passed with a 0.035-inch hydrophilic-coated guidewire and a pigtail catheter. Digital subtraction angiography showed total occlusion of the right iliac axis with reconstitution of flow near the inguinal ligament. The left side was widely patent (**Fig. 4.241**). Balloon angioplasty of the right iliac axis was performed with a standard balloon catheter.

Problems Encountered during Treatment

Following dilatation of the right iliac axis there was restored patency of the proximal aspect of the stented region. However, control angiography via the pigtail now revealed an occlusion of the external iliac artery (EIA) (**Fig. 4.242**). Contrast injection through the sheath showed that there was an approximately 3-cm-long thrombus that had apparently embolized into the EIA and was caught near the end of the 6F sheath (**Fig. 4.243**). No residual stenosis in the right iliac artery was detected.

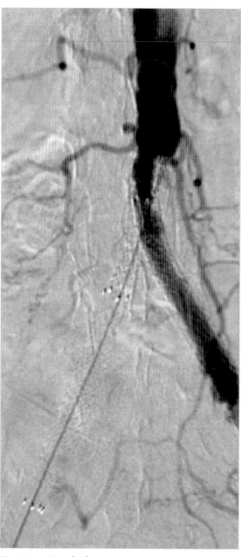

Fig. 4.241 Digital substraction angiography showing total occlusion of the right iliac axis. Reconstitution of flow was near the inguinal ligament (not shown).

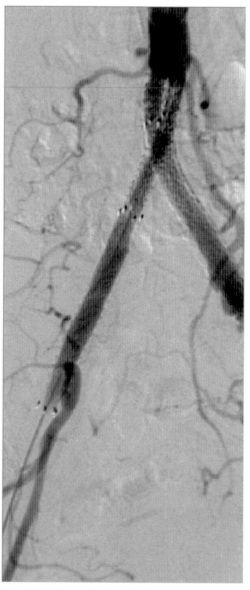

Fig. 4.242 After angioplasty, the lumen was patent again in the previously stented region. However, in the external iliac artery, thromboembolic occlusion was documented.

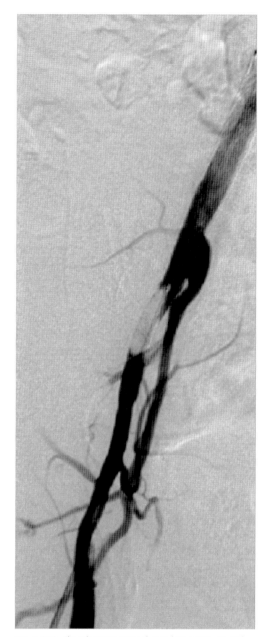

Fig. 4.243 Sheath angiogram showed an approximately 3-cm long thrombus caught near the end of the 6F sheath.

Imaging Plan

Angiography.

Resulting Complication

PTA triggered distal embolization with a "floating" embolus in the EIA.

Possible Strategies for Complication Management

- Aspiration thrombectomy.
- Locoregional thrombolysis.
- Mechanical thrombectomy (e.g., Trellis, Covidien; AngioJet, Boston Scientific; Rotarex, Straub Medical).
- Surgical thrombectomy.

Final Complication Management

The embolus was removed surgically with a Fogarty maneuver and direct atherectomy of the CFA.

Complication Analysis

The occlusion of the stented iliac artery had occurred 6 weeks after the initial procedure, indicating presence of subacute thrombosis. Due to the high plaque burden, parts of thrombotic debris embolized distally, but were caught by the sheath in the groin. There was no attempt to remove the clot endovascularly because of the risk of embolization further downstream with development of critical limb ischemia.

Prevention Strategies and Take-home Message

- A thorough history can lead to an estimation of age of occlusion.
- If there is acute/subacute recurrence of symptoms after stent placement, the presence of fresher clot should be considered.
- In the case of acute/subacute reocclusion of peripheral stents, mechanical thrombectomy and/or thrombolysis should be considered as primary treatment strategy.

Further Reading

Berczi V, Thomas SM, Turner DR, Bottomley JR, Cleveland TJ, Gaines PA. Stent implantation for acute iliac artery occlusions: initial experience. J Vasc Interv Radiol 2006;17(4):645–649

Erzurum VZ, Sampram ES, Sarac TP, et al. Initial management and outcome of aortic endograft limb occlusion. J Vasc Surg 2004;40(3):419–423

Lewis DR, Bullbulia RA, Murphy P, et al. Vascular surgical intervention for complications of cardiovascular radiology: 13 years' experience in a single centre. Ann R Coll Surg Engl 1999;81(1):23–26

Ozkan U, Oguzkurt L, Tercan F, Gumus B. Endovascular treatment strategies in aortoiliac occlusion. Cardiovasc Interv Radiol 2009;32(3):417–421

External iliac artery angioplasty with retroperitoneal hemorrhage

Patient History

A 75-year-old man with claudication in his right leg was scheduled for angioplasty of a right external iliac artery (EIA) stenosis.

Initial Treatment Received

None.

Problems Encountered during Treatment

After retrograde distal puncture of the right common femoral artery (CFA) and insertion of a 6F sheath, a stenosis in the EIA was passed with a guidewire and dilatated with a standard over-the-wire (OTW) balloon catheter. The diameter of the EIA was 7 mm as measured using digital calipers. The balloon was 7 × 40 mm. During angioplasty, which was performed with nominal balloon pressure, the patient complained of pain in his pelvis. Angiography showed contrast extravasation at the origin of the superficial circumflex iliac artery (**Fig. 4.244**).

Imaging Plan

Angiography via the sheath.

Resulting Complication

Iliac artery vessel rupture.

Possible Strategies for Complication Management

- Balloon tamponade.
- Stent graft implantation.
- Embolization of the feeder artery with coils or plugs (not possible because of rupture directly at vessel origin).
- Surgical repair (if endovascular treatment fails).

Final Complication Management

The balloon used for angioplasty was reinserted and inflated to limit the extent of the hematoma. Then a stent graft (8 × 60 mm Fluency, Bard PV) was implanted and the origin of the superficial circumflex iliac artery was covered (**Fig. 4.245**). The patient was hemodynamically stable during the procedure. The patient recovered uneventfully and no further clinical sequelae were noted.

Complication Analysis

Even in simple cases of iliac angioplasty vessel rupture can complicate the procedure. Here rupture of an iliac side branch occurred during

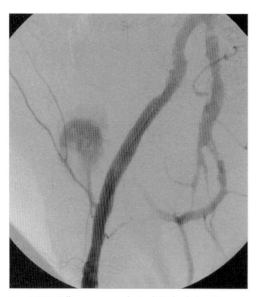

Fig. 4.244 Following angioplasty digital substraction angiography showed contrast extravasation at the origin of the superficial circumflex iliac artery.

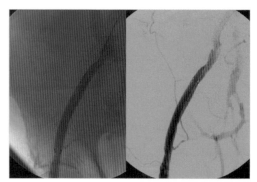

Fig. 4.245 Non-substracted and digitally substracted angiography image after stent graft implantation (Fluency 8/60mm) showed successful sealing of the rupture site with the stent graft.

balloon inflation for unknown reasons. Instant balloon tamponade prevented significant hemorrhage and arterial injury was successfully treated with a stent graft.

Prevention Strategies and Take-home Message

- Iliac artery rupture is a potentially fatal complication of angioplasty and stenting.
- Always be prepared for vessel rupture and have stent grafts available.
- Carefully choose the size of balloons and particularly stents.
- Start with an undersized balloon and ask the patient about their pain during inflation, which may be an indicator for balloon oversizing.

Further Reading

Allaire E, Melliere D, Poussier B, Kobeiter H, Desgranges P, Becquemin JP. Iliac artery rupture during balloon dilatation: what treatment? Ann Vasc Surg 2003;17(3):306–314

Chong WK, Cross FW, Raphael MJ. Iliac artery rupture during percutaneous angioplasty. Clin Radiol 1990;41(5):358–359

Cooper SG, Sofocleous CT. Percutaneous management of angioplasty-related iliac artery rupture with preservation of luminal patency by prolonged balloon tamponade. J Vasc Interv Radiol 1998;9(1 pt 1):81–83

Formichi M, Raybaud G, Benichou H, Ciosi G. Rupture of the external iliac artery during balloon angioplasty: endovascular treatment using a covered stent. J Endovasc Surg 1998;5(1):37–41

Hamdan MF, Maguire BG, Walker MA. Balloon-expandable stent deformation during deployment into the iliac artery: a procedural complication managed conservatively. Vascular 2012;20(4):233–235

Kufner S, Cassese S, Groha P, et al. Covered stents for endovascular repair of iatrogenic injuries of iliac and femoral arteries. Cardiovasc Revasc Med 2015;16(3):158–162

Molpus WM, McCowan TC, Eidt JF. External iliac artery rupture during angioplasty: control by balloon tamponade. South Med J 1991;84(9):1138–1139

Ozkan U, Oguzkurt L, Tercan F. Technique, complication, and long-term outcome for endovascular treatment of iliac artery occlusion. Cardiovasc Interv Radiol 2010;33(1):18–24

Park JK, Oh SJ, Shin JY. Delayed rupture of the iliac artery after percutaneous angioplasty. Ann Vasc Surg 2014;28(2):491.e1–e4

Redman A, Cope L, Uberoi R. Iliac artery injury following placement of the memotherm arterial stent. Cardiovasc Interv Radiol 2001;24(2):113–116

Reed H, Shandall A, Ruttley M. Iliac artery rupture during percutaneous angioplasty. Clin Radiol 1991;43(2):142–143

Sato K, Orihashi K, Hamanaka Y, Hirai S, Mitsui N, Chatani N. Treatment of iliac artery rupture during percutaneous transluminal angioplasty: a report of three cases. Hiroshima J Med Sci 2011;60(4):83–86

Scheinert D, Ludwig J, Steinkamp HJ, Schröder M, Balzer JO, Biamino G. Treatment of catheter-induced iliac artery injuries with self-expanding endografts. J Endovasc Ther 2000;7(3):213–220

Trehan V, Nigam A, Ramakrishnan S. Iatrogenic iliac artery rupture: emergency management by longer stent graft on a shorter balloon. Cardiovasc Interv Radiol 2007;30(1):108–110

Vorwerk D, Günther RW. Percutaneous interventions for treatment of iliac artery stenoses and occlusions. World J Surg 2001;25(3):319–326

Yeo KK, Rogers JH, Laird JR. Use of stent grafts and coils in vessel rupture and perforation. J Interv Cardiol 2008;21(1):86–99

Zollikofer CL, Salomonowitz E, Castaneda-Zuniga WR, Brühlmann WF, Amplatz K. The relation between arterial and balloon rupture in experimental angioplasty. AJR Am J Roentgenol 1985;144(4):777–779

4.3.4 Stent Placement

Stent malpositioning during superficial femoral artery stent placement

Patient History

A 58-year-old woman with a slow-healing ulcer of the foot due to an occlusion of the femoropopliteal artery was scheduled for recanalization. The decision for endovascular treatment was reached by interdisciplinary consensus. A senior fellow was the primary operator.

Initial Treatment Received

After antegrade puncture of the left common femoral artery (CFA) and insertion of a 6F sheath, recanalization of the 2.5-cm-long occlusion was performed with a 0.018-inch hydrophilic-coated wire in combination with a 4F angle-tip end-hole catheter (**Fig. 4.246**). A 5 × 30-mm monorail balloon was used for initial angioplasty with inflation times of up to 3 minutes. After angioplasty, there was a flow-limiting dissection at the treatment site (**Fig. 4.247**). Therefore, stent placement was performed using a 6 × 60-mm self-expanding stent (SES). Control angiography in the working plane initially showed adequate flow after stent deployment (**Fig. 4.248**). However, the distal part of the stent did not reach its full diameter and seemed malaligned to the wall of the popliteal artery. An oblique projection revealed that the distal part of the stent had been deployed into a side branch (**Fig. 4.249**).

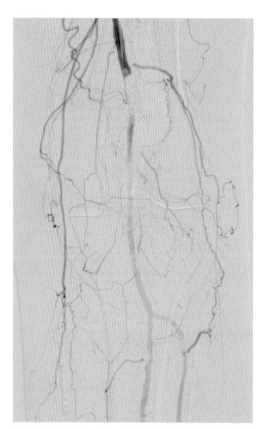

Fig. 4.246 Angiography of the still-occluded artery after successful guidewire passage.

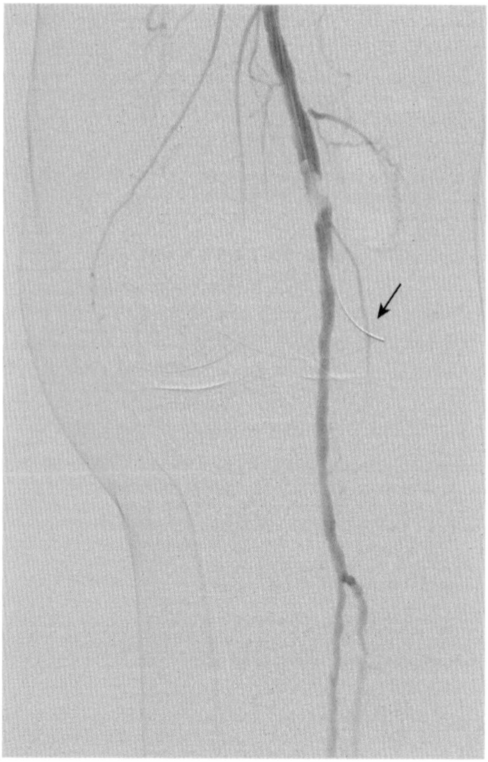

Fig. 4.247 Angiography following two long-term dilatations of 180 seconds each; the flow-limiting dissection was regarded as an indication for stent placement. Note the distal hydrophilic part of the guidewire placed in a side branch (*arrow*).

Problems Encountered during Treatment

The malpositioned stent with "narrowing" of the distal segment resulted in flow impairment of the popliteal artery.

Imaging Plan

Magnified angiography and fluoroscopy for further evaluation (i.e., determination of the exact stent position).

Complication Analysis

Failure to check the correct position of the guidewire in two planes resulted in deployment of the distal end of the stent into a side branch running parallel to the popliteal artery in the anteroposterior (AP) projection.

Possible Strategies for Complication Management

- Leave it as it is. Initiation of double antiplatelet therapy for at least 8 weeks or even longer.
- Additional placement of an SES after correction of the guidewire position, by passing the stent struts and placing the guidewire into the popliteal artery; crush stenting with additional stent.

Final Complication Management

Placement of a second SES (6 × 30 mm), after successfully passing the popliteal artery with the guidewire through the stent struts and percutaneous transluminal angioplasty (PTA) of the entire stented area (**Fig. 4.250**).

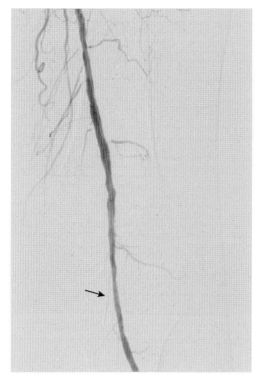

Fig. 4.248 Initial angiogram after deployment of an SES (6 × 60 mm). The distal 1.5 cm of the stent appears malaligned to the wall of the popliteal artery; 2 cm further distally the guidewire is still positioned in a side branch (*arrow*).

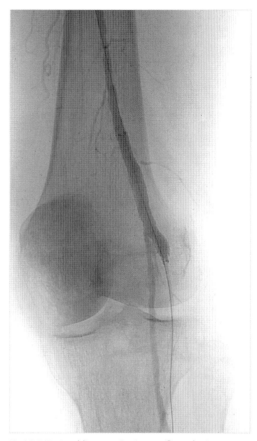

Fig. 4.249 An oblique projection confirms the incorrect position of the guidewire running into the side branch. Unfortunately, this resulted in stent malplacement as depicted in this unsubtracted angiography.

Complication Analysis

Hydrophylic-coated guidewires have the tendency to run into side branches. Sometimes the wrong position is easily visible and is therefore easy to correct, but sometimes, as in this case, the position appears correct in the working plane, especially when the side branch "runs parallel" to the target vessel in a certain image projection. In order to rule out this pitfall, the working plane needs to be changed during the procedure. Only by doing this, and by looking at things from a different view/projection, can this complication be avoided.

One of the editors had reported a quite similar complication some weeks earlier. Everybody during that time was aware of this case from a personal communication. Nevertheless, a similar complication happened again!

Prevention Strategies and Take-home Message

- Handle instruments with care. Always be familiar with the distal position of the guidewire.
- Change your angiographic plane during the procedure to make sure the guidewire position is correct for its entire course.
- Be aware that complications do occur even with experienced operators.

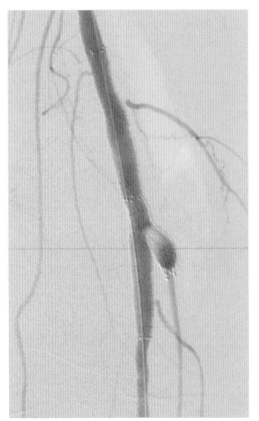

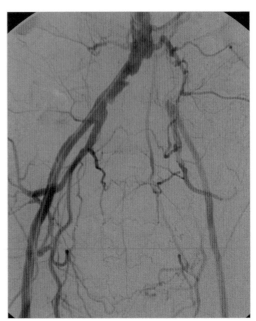

Fig. 4.251 Angiography prior to treatment showed a complete occlusion of the left CIA with lumbar collaterals. Note the eccentric plaque material located at the mid- and distal part of the right CIA. There is also attenuation of contrast filling in the proximal aspect of the right CIA, indicative of heavy wall calcification.

Fig. 4.250 Final angiography after crush stenting of the malpositioned stent and final PTA of the femoropopliteal segment. The "stented" side branch still shows flow of contrast media.

Further Reading

Cho YJ, Han SS, Lee SC. Guidewire malposition during central venous catheterization despite the use of ultrasound guidance. Korean J Anesthesiol 2013;64(5):469–471

Dawson DL, Terramani TT, Loberman Z, Lumsden AB, Lin PH. Simple technique to ensure coaxial guidewire positioning for placement of iliac limb of modular aortic endograft. J Interv Cardiol 2003;16(3):223–226

Unexpected plaque shift after direct stenting of the contralateral common iliac artery

Patient History

A 60-year-old man suffered from claudication due to a complete occlusion of the left common iliac artery (CIA) (**Fig. 4.251**). Based on interdisciplinary consensus, the patient was scheduled for an endovascular procedure. Direct stenting was intended as the primary treatment option.

Initial Treatment Received

Under local anesthesia, retrograde access to the ipsilateral common femoral artery (CFA) was established and a 6F sheath was inserted. In combination with a 4F multipurpose catheter, a 0.035-inch guidewire was used to cross the occluded lesion. The operator planned to place a 9 × 60-mm balloon-expandable stent. Lesion crossing with the balloon–stent device was without severe resistance. Once in the correct position, the stent was deployed (**Fig. 4.252**).

Problems Encountered during Treatment

Stent advancement and stent delivery seemed uneventful; however, severe plaque shifting and protrusion to the contralateral CIA was observed during control angiography (**Fig. 4.253**).

Imaging Plan

Angiography in different planes to identify extent and location of the protruding plaque material.

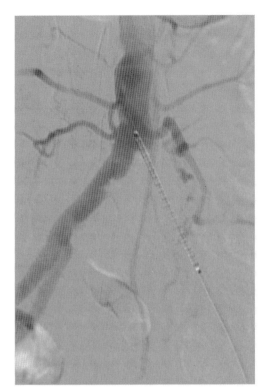

Fig. 4.252 Control angiography via the balloon–stent guidewire lumen (guidewire is removed). The stent position is appropriate, the device ready for deployment. For the deployment procedure, the 0.035-inch guidewire was reinserted again.

Complication Analysis

In aortic bifurcation lesions, percutaneous transluminal angioplasty (PTA) and/or stent placement can result in plaque shift with protrusion of calcified material from the treatment side into the contralateral CIA, which may lead to secondary stenosis of the previously unaffected side.

Possible Strategies for Complication Management

- Crossover maneuver via the left access route with placement of a second balloon-expandable stent into the right CIA stenosis.
- Endovascular treatment with a retrograde approach via the contralateral right CFA with placement of a balloon-expandable stent into the CIA stenosis.
- Kissing stent–balloon procedure with stent placement into the right CIA from right groin and simultaneous inflation of a balloon in the left CIA in order to avoid plaque shift and/or material embolization.

Final Complication Management

After successful puncture and access creation to the contralateral right groin, a 9 × 37-mm balloon-expandable stent was deployed into the proximal CIA; a balloon catheter was placed into the already stented left CIA with simultaneous balloon inflation in kissing stent–balloon technique (**Fig. 4.254**).

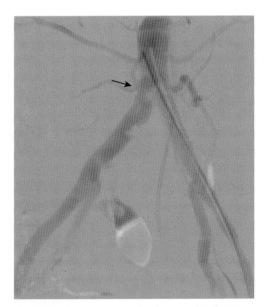

Fig. 4.253 Control angiography after completed stent deployment. Plaque material protrudes (*arrow*) toward the origin of the contralateral CIA and leads to moderate- to high-grade stenosis.

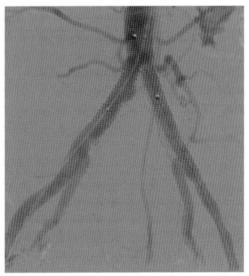

Fig. 4.254 Final angiography after completion of the kissing stent procedure; no peripheral embolization is observed in the infrainguinal or infragenual arteries.

Complication Analysis

In this case the operator underestimated the plaque burden of the aortic bifurcation and both common iliac arteries. Particularly in patients in whom both iliac arteries are diseased, and the origin of at least one side is involved, planning and performing a direct kissing stent procedure for aortic bifurcation disease treatment seems more appropriate. Plaque shifting as seen in this case may not only result in secondary stenosis of the contralateral side, which is easily treated by stents, but may also lead to distal embolization of material into the contralateral peripheral arterial circulation.

Prevention Strategies and Take-home Message

- Direct stenting of the iliac arteries seems warranted in order to fixate plaque material. However, when operating close to the aortic bifurcation, a direct kissing stent procedure should be considered.
- For kissing stent procedures with balloon-expandable stents the inflation of the balloons should be performed simultaneously with equal dilatation pressures. When self-expanding stents are used (not the first choice in this case), deployment and postdilatation should both be performed simultaneously!

Further Reading

Xu J, Hahn JY, Song YB, et al. Carina shift versus plaque shift for aggravation of side branch ostial stenosis in bifurcation lesions: volumetric intravascular ultrasound analysis of both branches. Circ Cardiovasc Interv 2012;5(5):657–662

Unexpected stent elongation during superficial femoral artery stent placement

Patient History

A 60-year-old man with lifestyle-limiting claudication (200 m) was scheduled for superficial femoral artery (SFA) recanalization. The decision for endovascular treatment was based on interdisciplinary consensus. A resident was the primary operator and was supervised by a well-experienced fellow.

Initial Treatment Received

After successful antegrade puncture of the right common femoral artery (CFA) and sheath insertion,

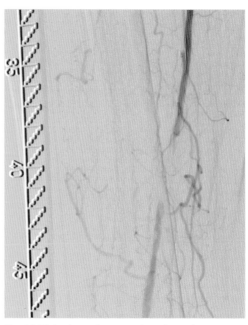

Fig. 4.255 Angiography presenting a 3-cm short-distance occlusion of the mid-part SFA.

recanalization of a 3-cm-long occlusion was performed with a 0.018-inch hydrophilic-coated wire in combination with a 4F angle-tip end-hole catheter (**Fig. 4.255**). Primary balloon angioplasty was performed using a 5 × 40-mm monorail balloon catheter with an inflation time of 3 minutes. The index lesion changed from an occlusion to a flow-limiting dissection with signs of elastic recoil (**Fig. 4.256**). Therefore, immediate stent placement was performed using a 5 × 80-mm self-expanding stent (SES). The stent diameter of 5 mm was chosen after a calibrated measurement of the unaffected vessel segment. A stent length of 80 mm was considered appropriate to also cover some proximal eccentric plaque material. Stent deployment was performed according to instructions for use.

Problems Encountered during Treatment

During stent deployment, which was done cautiously in order to avoid malpositioning, both operators noted elongation beside constriction of parts of the stent; the delivery system was kept stable—neither uncontrolled push nor pull was exerted. The remaining segment of the stent deployed correctly. The deployed stent length was exactly 70 mm, instead of 80 mm as indicated by the ruler (**Fig. 4.257**). The delivery catheter was removed, keeping the guidewire in a stable position.

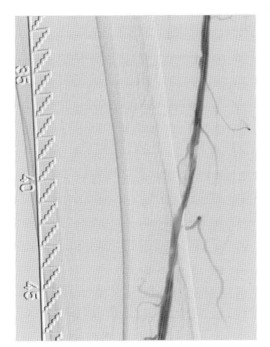

Fig. 4.256 Control angiography after long-term percutaneous transluminal angioplasty (5 × 40 mm) showing dissection and elastic recoil.

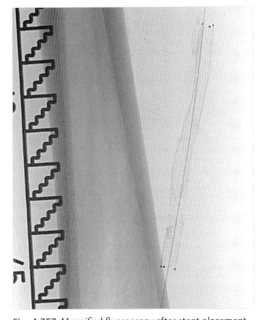

Fig. 4.257 Magnified fluoroscopy after stent placement showing an area of elongation of the distal aspect of the implanted stent. The stent struts in this area are disintegrated from the original design and protrude into the vessel lumen. Instead of 80 mm in length, the total final stent length was 70 mm due to stent infolding and elongation.

Imaging Plan

Magnified angiography and fluoroscopy for further evaluation (i.e., determination of the exact location of stent elongation and looking for further areas of deployment failure).

Complication Analysis

Stent elongation during deployment without any detectable error by the operators when activating the stent delivery system.

Possible Strategies for Complication Management

- Leave it as it is. Ongoing double platelet therapy for at least 8 weeks or even longer.
- Percutaneous transluminal angioplasty (PTA) of the stent and hope for wall apposition.
- Additional placement of an SES, meaning deploying one stent inside another (sandwich stenting) in order to achieve a wall apposition of the protruding stent elements.
- Call the vascular surgeon and ask for explant procedure and bypass surgery.

Final Complication Management

First, PTA was performed in order to correct the stent strut protrusion. This maneuver failed, the position of the stent struts remained unchanged; however, the flow was uncompromised during angiographic control (**Fig. 4.258**). Therefore, an

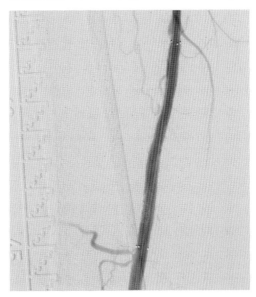

Fig. 4.258 Angiography after stent deployment without any signs of a compromised flow.

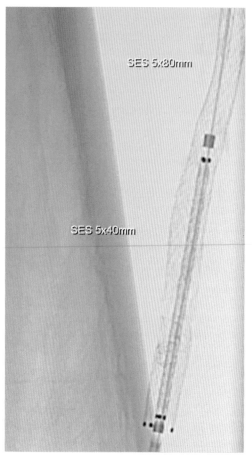

Fig. 4.259 Magnified fluoroscopy shows the infolded and elongated distal stent part covered by a second 5 × 40-mm SES in place ready for delivery.

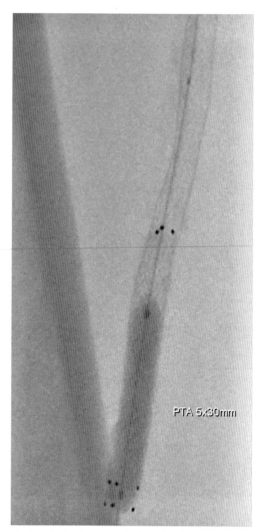

Fig. 4.260 PTA (5 × 30 mm) of the double-layer stented area.

additional placement of a 5 × 30-mm SES via the wire still in place was performed (**Fig. 4.259**), followed by PTA (5 × 30 mm) of the entire stented area (**Fig. 4.260**). The final fluoroscopy showed the double-layer stented area (**Fig. 4.261**), and final angiography once more showed an uncompromised flow (**Fig. 4.262**). After the procedure, the patient was put on double antiplatelet therapy for 3 months.

Complication Analysis

Incorrect stent deployment resulting in stent infolding and elongation of stent struts protruding into the vessel lumen, most likely due to operator failure. During deployment there was probably some pushing or pulling force for correction, even if both operators deny such a mistake. A failure of the delivery mechanism might also be a potential explanation. In order to rule out this technical problem, the stent delivery device was sent to the manufacturer for further evaluation.

Prevention Strategies and Take-home Message

• Handle instruments with care. Be familiar with the instructions for use.

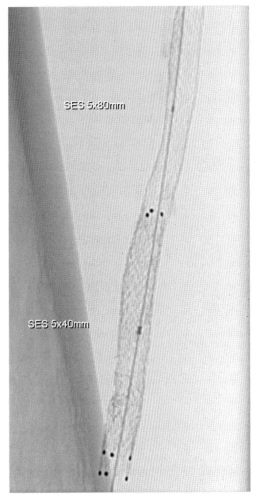

Fig. 4.261 Fluoroscopy after PTA. The distal half of the stented area looks denser due to double layer of two SESs.

• Take your time in stent deployment, especially when working with open-cell design stents—open-cell stent design is a predictor for stent elongation or infolding during the delivery procedure.
• Be aware that even experienced operators are prone to errors.

Further Reading

Hamdan MF, Maguire BG, Walker MA. Balloon-expandable stent deformation during deployment into the iliac artery: a procedural complication managed conservatively. Vascular 2012;20(4):233–235

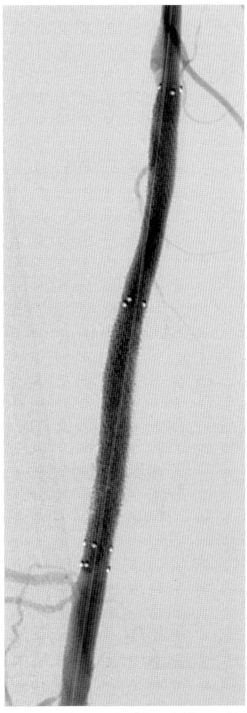

Fig. 4.262 Final angiography of the sandwich stent with a good flow without any signs of restenosis. Note some residual plaque at the inflow area of the stent without any significant narrowing.

Inaba S, Weisz G, Kobayashi N, et al. Prevalence and anatomical features of acute longitudinal stent deformation: an intravascular ultrasound study. Catheter Cardiovasc Interv 2014;84(3):388–396

Ormiston JA, Webber B, Webster MW. Stent longitudinal integrity bench insights into a clinical problem. JACC Cardiovasc Interv 2011;4(12):1310–1317

Taniguchi N, Mizuguchi Y, Takahashi A. Longitudinal stent elongation during retraction of entrapped jailed guidewire in a side branch with balloon catheter support: a case report. Cardiovasc Revasc Med 2015;16(1):52–54

Stent detachment from carrier balloon during catheter advancement

Patient History

A 75-year-old man with multilevel atherosclerotic disease and stenoses of the left external iliac artery (EIA) and the left superficial femoral artery (SFA) suffered from claudication (**Figs. 4.263** and **4.264**). It was decided to improve arterial inflow into the left extremity by treating the EIA lesion first before addressing the more distal lesions. Direct stenting was planned as the initial treatment strategy.

Initial Treatment Received

Under local anesthesia, retrograde access to the ipsilateral common femoral artery (CFA) was established and a 6F sheath was inserted. A hydrophilic-coated 0.035-inch guidewire was used

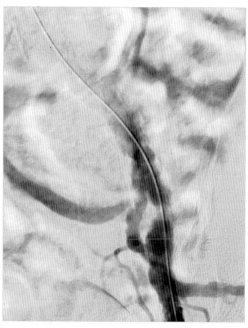

Fig. 4.264 A magnified digital subtraction angiogram in a right oblique projection; a guidewire had already crossed the short-distance stenosis.

in combination with a 4F multipurpose catheter to cross the stenosis. After successfully crossing the lesion the operator intended to place an 8 × 27-mm balloon-expandable stent into the lesion.

Problems Encountered during Treatment

During advancement of the delivery catheter mild resistance was encountered. While trying to further advance the device into the target lesion the stent detached from its carrier balloon. The operator was able to remove the balloon while the stent kept its position on the wire distally to the lesion (**Fig. 4.265**). Secondary attempts to advance the stent into the lesion with the carrier balloon failed. The stent could also not be removed with the balloon and stayed in a stable position.

Imaging Plan

Fluoroscopic guidance.

Resulting Complication

Stent detachment from the carrier balloon; primary attempts at stent repositioning or removal failed.

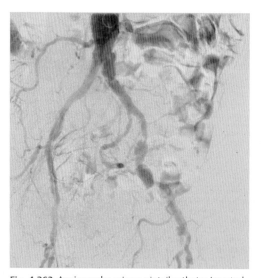

Fig. 4.263 Angiography using a pigtail catheter inserted from the right groin showing multilevel disease of the left limb with a focal, eccentric high-grade stenosis at the proximal level of the left EIA.

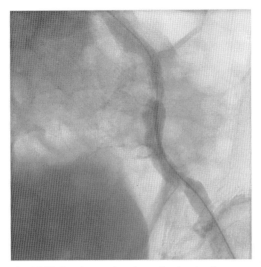

Fig. 4.265 Unsubtracted angiography showing the detached stent close to the target lesion; the carrier balloon catheter is still inside the stent. However, the balloon is not adhering to the stent and can be removed easily.

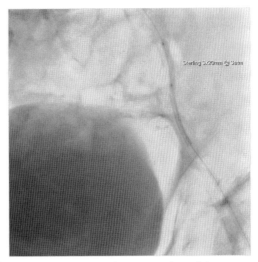

Fig. 4.266 Fluoroscopy during angioplasty of the target lesion after passage of the detached stent using a low-profile 0.018-inch-compatible 3 × 20-mm balloon catheter. This balloon was used for predilatation of both the stent and, in a second step, the stenosis at low pressure.

Possible Strategies for Complication Management

- Deployment of the stent in its current location and outside the intended treatment site. This is generally possible when the position of the stent is not in a biomechanically challenging area, that is, in a moving vessel segment. This would be a viable option in this case.
- Snaring the stent with removal through the sheath. This would be possible in this case. However, before attempting a snaring maneuver and to ensure easy and complete stent removal, the sheath should be exchanged for a sheath at least 2F larger (8F in the current case).
- Repositioning of the stent into the target lesions by trying to reattach it to a balloon.
- Surgical removal of the stent if the above procedures fail.

Final Complication Management

With the stent still intact and secure on the guidewire, a 0.035-inch-compatible 4F diagnostic catheter could be threaded over the wire through the stent. This was used to exchange for a 0.018-inch guidewire that allowed insertion of a low-profile 0.018-inch-compatible 3 × 20-mm balloon catheter for predilatation of both the stent and the stenosis at low pressure (**Fig. 4.266**). This balloon was then carefully removed and exchanged for a larger low-profile balloon (6 × 20 mm). This

was used to dilatate the target lesion with high pressure (**Fig. 4.267**).

Now the 0.035-inch guidewire was reinserted again in the same manner. A 0.035-inch-compatible over-the-wire (OTW) balloon (5 × 20 mm) was then positioned in the malpositioned stent and inflated mildly without expanding the stent, but with enough force to advance both the bal-

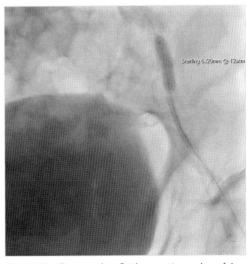

Fig. 4.267 After complete fluid evacuation and careful removal of the balloon, a larger-diameter low-profile balloon (6 × 20 mm) was inserted and used to dilatate the target lesion with high pressure.

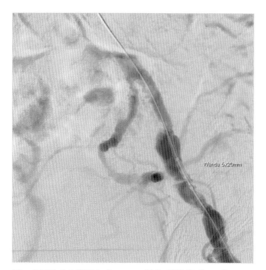

Fig. 4.268 A 0.035-inch-compatible OTW balloon is positioned within the stent and mildly inflated without expanding the stent, but giving enough force to advance both the balloon and the stent into the lesion.

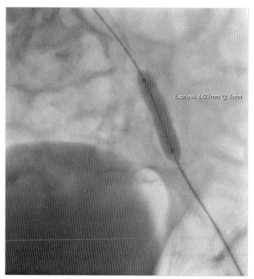

Fig. 4.270 The 8 × 27-mm stent carrier balloon was used again and inflated at 8 atmospheres (atm) for complete stent expansion.

loon and the stent into the predilatated lesion (**Figs. 4.268** and **4.269**). Once in a proper position, the 5-mm balloon was inflated to its maximum diameter, then exchanged for the original 8 × 27-mm stent carrier balloon, which was also inflated (**Fig. 4.270**).

The final angiography showed a sufficiently treated lesion with a remaining distal lesion, which was dilatated using the same balloon (**Fig. 4.271**).

Complication Analysis

A balloon-expandable stent is mounted on a carrier balloon catheter. When pushed through a stenosis or a tortuous vessel segment the forces acting on the stent may be high enough to scale it from its balloon. In this case resistance was felt during advancement of the stent delivery catheter, but the device was further advanced, leading to detachment of the stent from the carrier balloon.

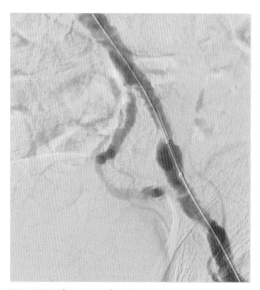

Fig. 4.269 The proximal stent segment was covering the index lesion at this point.

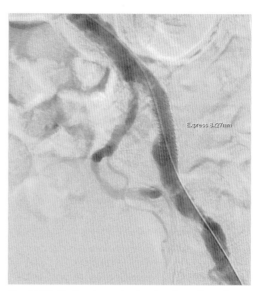

Fig. 4.271 Final angiography showing the sufficiently treated lesion with a remaining distal stenosis, which was dilatated using the same balloon.

Prevention Strategies and Take-home Message

- All endovascular instruments should be handled with great care. Devices and implants should always be guided by fluoroscopy!
- Especially when steering devices outside of guiding catheters and/or sheaths, or when vessels are narrow and/or elongated, visual feedback is key to controlling pulling or pushing forces and to avoiding complications.
- If any resistance is encountered during placement of a device the reason for this should be evaluated. Never push or pull anything against resistance.
- When balloon-expandable stents do not cross a stenosis or occlusion without resistance, the lesion should be predilatated or a longer sheath should be used for protected positioning of the stent.
- Never "give up" your guidewire until you find a way to manage a complication!

Further Reading

Blackman D, Dzavik V. Inadvertent detachment of an entrapped cutting balloon from the balloon catheter during treatment of in-stent restenosis. J Invasive Cardiol 2005;17(11): E27–E29

Hussain F, Rusnak B, Tam J. Retrieval of a detached partially expanded stent using the SpideRX and EnSnare devices—a first report. J Invasive Cardiol 2008;20(2):E44–E47

Pappy R, Gautam A, Abu-Fadel MS. AngioSculpt PTCA Balloon Catheter entrapment and detachment managed with stent jailing. J Invasive Cardiol 2010;22(10):E208–E210

Shiojima I, Ikari Y, Abe J, et al. Thrombotic occlusion of the coronary artery associated with accidental detachment of undeployed Palmaz-Schatz stent. Cathet Cardiovasc Diagn 1996;38(4):360–362

Unexpected stent migration during stenting of the superior vena cava for upper venous obstruction due to tumor compression

Patient History

A 69-year-old woman suffered from non–small cell lung cancer with tumor compression of the superior superior vena cava (SVC) and consecutive upper vein obstruction syndrome. The patient was scheduled for stent placement into the SVC (**Fig. 4.272**).

Initial Treatment Received

Under local anesthesia, retrograde puncture of the right common femoral vein (CFV) was per-

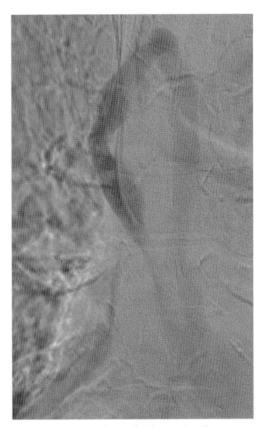

Fig. 4.272 Angiography via the diagnostic catheter placed beyond the lesion. A severe obstruction localized in the SVC is visible. Note the enlarged hemiazygos vein serving as a collateral.

formed and a 12F sheath was inserted. Using a combination of a 4F multipurpose catheter with a 0.035-inch guidewire, the high-grade stenosis of the SVC was successfully crossed. Placement of a 10 × 60-mm self-expanding nitinol stent was attempted. Size of the stent was chosen on the basis of a computed tomography (CT) scan performed recently indicating a residual open diameter of 7 mm.

Problems Encountered during Treatment

Stent advancement and stent delivery were uneventful at first; however, during placement of the stent, the device dislodged towards the right atrium.

Imaging Plan

Fluoroscopy/angiography for identification of the exact position of the stent and potential damage to the stent, that is, the stent struts.

Resulting Complication

Stent migration into the right atrium.

Possible Strategies for Complication Management

- Endovascular treatment via the ipsilateral retrograde approach using the existing access to the CFV. Securing the stent with a balloon inserted over the guidewire still in place. Pulling the stent down into external iliac vein when possible; trying to remove the entire stent via the 12F sheath. In the case of a smaller sheath initially placed, sheath upsizing to 12F. Snaring maneuver in order to remove the entire stent carefully.
- Surgery (if an endovascular approach fails).

Final Complication Management

Endovascular management used an ipsilateral retrograde approach via the existing access to the CFV. The original guidewire was left in place in order to "catch" the stent with a balloon (10 × 60 mm). The stent was pulled into the external iliac vein. When catching the stent with a snare, it elongated and due to the self-expanding outback force and the open-cell design, the stent did not enter the sheath properly (**Fig. 4.273**). The proximal parts of the stent were removed through the sheath, but major parts of the device did not enter the sheath. The sheath was severely damaged due to repeated snaring and pulling attempts. The sheath was finally removed, leaving an 0.035-inch wire in place. Fluoroscopy showed a partially removed stent in the subcutis, whereas parts of the stent still remained intraluminally (**Fig. 4.274**).

A new sheath was inserted through the stent and a 14 × 60-mm self-expanding stent (SES) was placed at the target lesion (**Fig. 4.275**). The remaining stent parts were removed entirely by the vascular surgeons.

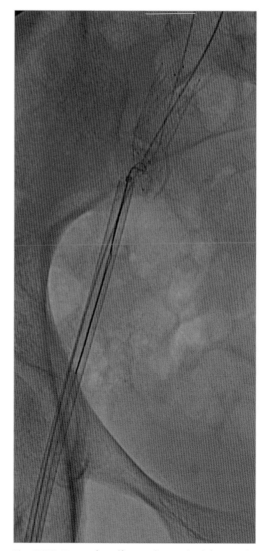

Fig. 4.273 Due to the self-expanding outback force and the open-cell design, the stent did not enter the sheath properly. Therefore, a maneuver to snare the stent through the sheath failed.

Complication Analysis

For venous stenting procedures, marked oversizing should be considered in order to avoid immediate stent migration.

Prevention Strategies and Take-home Message

- Cross-sectional imaging should be obtained before every venous stenting procedure.

- Stent sizing has to be done with great care before and/or intraoperatively!
- Any mismatch between vessel diameter and measured size should be evaluated before stent deployment starts!
- In unsafe situations, withhold stent deployment and consult a colleague!
- Stent advancement should be controlled under permanent fluoroscopy!

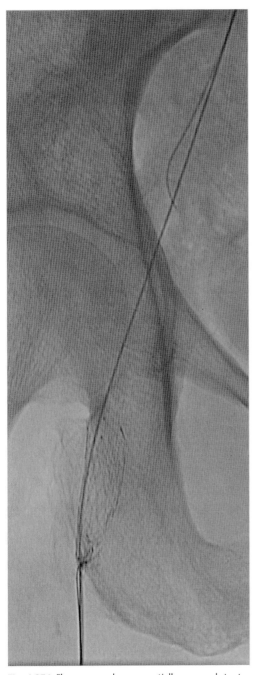

Fig. 4.274 Fluoroscopy shows a partially removed stent in the subcutis, whereas parts of the stent still remain intraluminally.

Further Reading

Anand G, Lewanski CR, Cowman SA, Jackson JE. Superior vena cava stent migration into the pulmonary artery causing fatal pulmonary infarction. Cardiovasc Interv Radiol 2011;34(2 suppl):S198–S201

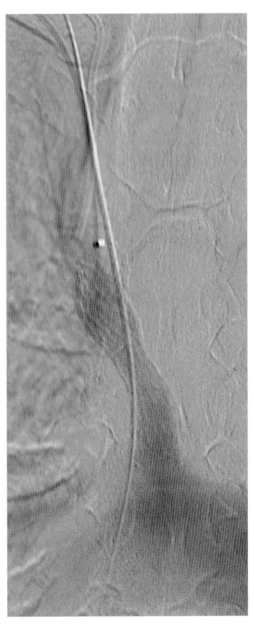

Fig. 4.275 Final angiography after placement of a 14 × 60-mm SES showing a sufficient opacification of the SVC.

Bobylev D, Meschenmoser L, Boethig D, Horke A. Migration of an endovascular stent into the right ventricle following deployment in the inferior vena cava after liver transplantation. Eur J Cardiothorac Surg 2015;48(2):308

Lin X, Fang L, Wang Y. Multiple heart injuries caused by fracture and migration of the inferior vena stent. Eur Heart J 2013;34(8):625

Rana MA, Oderich GS, Bjarnason H. Endovenous removal of dislodged left renal vein stent in a patient with nutcracker syndrome. Semin Vasc Surg 2013;26(1):43–47

Sakhri L, Pirvu A, Toffart A-C, Thony F, Moro-Sibilot D. Unusual migration of a vena cava stent into the pulmonary artery because of tumor reduction after chemotherapy. J Thorac Oncol 2013;8(12):1585–1586

Toyoda N, Torregrossa G, Itagaki S, Pawale A, Reddy R. Intracardiac migration of vena caval stent: decision-making and treatment considerations. J Card Surg 2014;29(3):320–322

Trehan VK, Jain G, Pandit BN. Hepatic vein anchor-wire technique to prevent stent migration during inferior vena cava stenting for Budd-Chiari syndrome. J Invasive Cardiol 2014;26(5):225–227

Stent migration during balloon inflation at the aortoiliac level

Patient History

A 56-year-old man suffered from claudication due to an occlusion of the right common iliac artery (CIA). These findings were based on ultrasound examination and verified by contrast-enhanced magnetic resonance angiography (MRA) (**Fig. 4.276**). Based on interdisciplinary consensus, it was decided to treat the CIA lesions by endovascular means. Direct stenting was planned as the primary treatment strategy.

Initial Treatment Received

Under local anesthesia, retrograde access to the ipsilateral right common femoral artery (CFA)

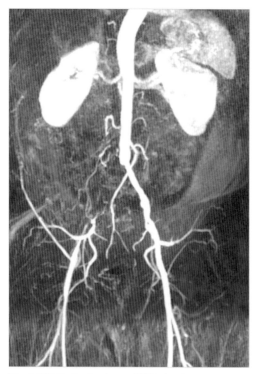

Fig. 4.276 Contrast-enhanced MRA showing an occlusion of the right CIA.

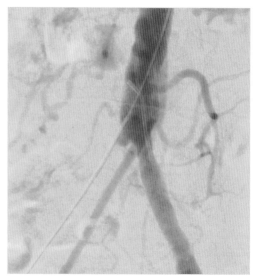

Fig. 4.277 A short, proximal stump of the CIA was confirmed by DSA.

was performed and a 6F sheath was inserted. In combination with a 4F multipurpose catheter, a 0.035-inch hydrophilic-coated guidewire was used to cross the occlusion. As seen on MRA, a short, proximal stump of the CIA was confirmed by digital subtraction angiography (DSA) (**Fig. 4.277**). Based on this finding, the intended strategy of direct stenting within the right CIA was pursued. Lesion crossing with the balloon–stent catheter was uneventful. The operator implanted an 8 × 59-mm balloon-expandable stent. The angiographic control showed significant residual stenosis of the right CIA due to ostial calcification and plaque (**Fig. 4.278**). A secondary kissing stent procedure was therefore planned. Two 8 × 29-mm balloon-expandable stents were positioned (**Fig. 4.279**) and slowly inflated.

Problems Encountered during Treatment

During balloon inflation, the stent on the left side detached from the carrier balloon and migrated to a more distal location. Fluoroscopy revealed that only the proximal part of the stent was partially expanded, whereas the mid- and distal parts remained unfolded (**Fig. 4.280**). Any attempts to remove and reposition the stent towards target lesion failed.

Imaging Plan

Fluoroscopy/angiography.

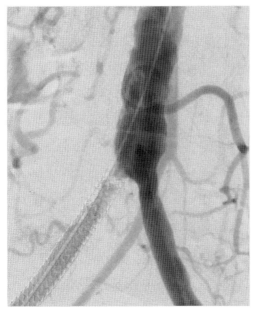

Fig. 4.278 An 8 × 59-mm balloon-expandable stent in position. A first angiographic control shows reduced opacification and flow to the right CIA in comparison to the contralateral side.

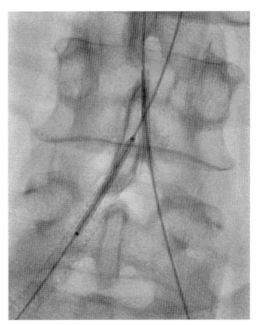

Fig. 4.280 Fluoroscopy indicating that only the proximal part of the stent was partially expanded, whereas the mid- and distal parts remained unfolded.

Resulting Complication

Detachment of balloon-expandable stent from carrier balloon.

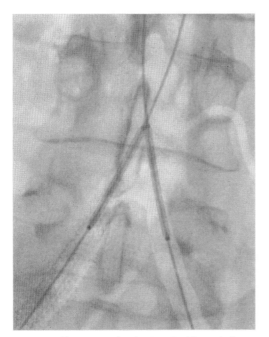

Fig. 4.279 Fluoroscopy showing two 8 × 29-mm balloon-expandable stents prior to deployment.

Possible Strategies for Complication Management

- Deployment of the stent in its current location outside the intended treatment site. This is possible when the stent is not impairing blood flow and the location is biomechanically unchallenging. In this particular case the unsecured stent in the distal aorta could lead to changed flow dynamics with the potential of thromboembolic complications. Thus, additional stents would have to be implanted.
- Snaring the stent and removal of the device through the sheath. This would be possible in this case. However, before attempting a snaring maneuver, the sheath would need to be exchanged for a larger inner diameter (at least 2F).
- Repositioning of the stent into the target lesions by trying to reattach it to a balloon.
- Surgical removal of the stent (if endovascular techniques fail).

Final Complication Management

Knowing that the stent (which is still undamaged but partially unfolded) is still secure on the wire, a 0.035-inch-compatible 2.7F 4 × 40-mm balloon catheter was threaded over the wire through the

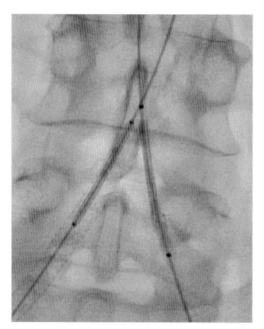

Fig. 4.281 Fluoroscopy after successful stent retrieval towards target lesion. A 4 × 40-mm balloon catheter was threaded over the wire through the stent. This allowed a mild balloon dilatation, sufficient to fix the predilatated stent onto the balloon and pull it back into the target location.

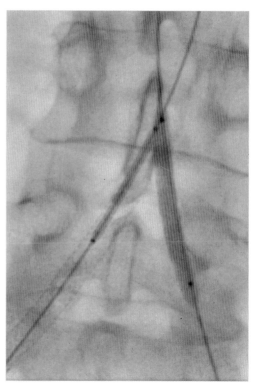

Fig. 4.282 The 4-mm balloon was inflated up to its rated burst pressure of 14 atm.

stent. This allowed a mild balloon dilatation, sufficient to fix the predilatated stent on the balloon. The balloon was pulled slowly towards the target location. When it was noted that the stent did not follow, the inflation pressure was increased without further dilatating the stent. With this maneuver, the stent could be repositioned into the target lesion (**Fig. 4.281**). The 4-mm balloon was then inflated up to its rated burst pressure of 14 atmospheres (atm) (**Fig. 4.282**).

Finally the 4-mm balloon was exchanged for the original carrier balloon and both stents were deployed as primarily intended (**Fig. 4.283**).

The final angiography showed a sufficiently treated lesion with a remaining distal lesion, which was dilatated with the same balloon. Final angiography also showed the completed kissing stent procedure (**Fig. 4.284**).

Complication Analysis

In this case a balloon-expandable stent dislocated from its carrier balloon. The most likely cause was a mismatch of the stent–balloon diameter in comparison to the lumen of the distal aorta. Also there was only mild stenosis in the left CIA and the stent

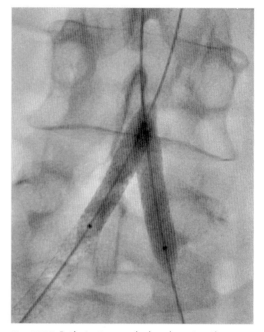

Fig. 4.283 Both stents were deployed as primarily intended in kissing stent technique.

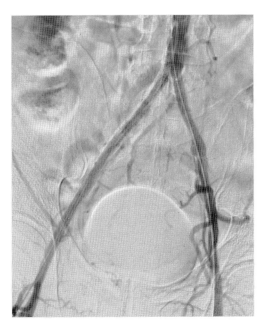

Fig. 4.284 Final angiography of the completed kissing stent procedure.

could not immediately attach to the lesion or the wall of the CIA. In such a case it is important that the implantation of the stent is performed rapidly and simultaneously with its "kissing" counterpart to prevent dislodgement from the balloon. Constant visual control during the implantation procedure using high-quality fluoroscopy is mandatory to ensure that a stent is delivered correctly and not moving during implantation

Prevention Strategies and Take-home Message

- Constantly control your devices and implants during positioning and deployment of stents using high-quality fluoroscopy! Switch to higher pulse rates if necessary.
- Do not rely merely on DSA reference images or drawings on the monitor for positioning, as patients or the table may have moved. Instead use anatomical landmarks for exact positioning of stents.
- Never "give up" your guidewire until you find a way to manage the complication!

Further Reading

Ahmed S, Ratanapo S, Srivali N, Cheungpasitporn W. Stent dislodgement: a rare complication of subclavian artery angioplasty and stenting. N Am J Med Sci 2013;5(3):251

Aydin M, Sayin MR. Successful coronary stent retrieval from the saphenous vein graft to right coronary artery. Case Rep Med 2009;2009:718685

Broadbent LP, Moran CJ, Cross DT III, Derdeyn CP. Management of neuroform stent dislodgement and misplacement. AJNR Am J Neuroradiol 2003;24(9):1819–1822

Chiu KM, Chu SH, Chan CY. Dislodged caval stent in right pulmonary artery. Catheter Cardiovasc Interv 2007;70(6):799–800

Cishek MB, Laslett L, Gershony G. Balloon catheter retrieval of dislodged coronary artery stents: a novel technique. Cathet Cardiovasc Diagn 1995;34(4):350–352

Deftereos S, Raisakis K, Giannopoulos G, Kossyvakis C, Pappas L, Kaoukis A. Successful retrieval of a coronary stent dislodged in the brachial artery by means of improvised snare and guiding catheter. Int J Angiol 2011;20(1):55–58

Gan HW, Bhasin A, Wu CJ. Complete stent dislodgement after successful implantation—a rare case. Catheter Cardiovasc Interv 2010;75(6):967–970

Grosso M, Spalluto F, Muratore P, Cristoferi M, Veltri A. Palmaz stent dislodgement into the left pulmonary artery complicating TIPS: percutaneous retrieval and extraction after venotomy. Cardiovasc Interv Radiol 1995;18(2):106–108

Hussain F, Kashour T, Philipp R. Old technique, new use: novel use of a buddy wire to deploy a detached stent. J Invasive Cardiol 2007;19(6):E160–E162

Jang JH, Woo SI, Yang DH, Park SD, Kim DH, Shin SH. Successful coronary stent retrieval from the ascending aorta using a gooseneck snare kit. Korean J Intern Med 2013;28(4):481–485

Kakisis JD, Vassilas K, Antonopoulos C, Sfyroeras G, Moulakakis K, Liapis CD. Wandering stent within the pulmonary circulation. Ann Vasc Surg 2014;28(8):1932.e9–e12

Kwan TW, Chaudhry M, Huang Y, et al. Approaches for dislodged stent retrieval during transradial percutaneous coronary interventions. Catheter Cardiovasc Interv 2013;81(6):E245–E249

Nishi M, Zen K, Kambayashi D, Asada S, Yamaguchi S, Tatsukawa H. Stent dislodgement induced by a vasodilator used for severe coronary artery spasm caused by Kounis syndrome. Cardiovasc Interv Ther 2015. [Epub ahead of print]

Oh Y, Hwang DH, Ko YH, Kang IW, Kim IS, Hur CW. Foreign body removal by snare loop: during intracranial stent procedure. Neurointervention 2012;7(1):50–53

Rozenman Y, Burstein M, Hasin Y, Gotsman MS. Retrieval of occluding unexpanded Palmaz-Schatz stent from a saphenous aorto-coronary vein graft. Cathet Cardiovasc Diagn 1995;34(2):159–161

Salinger-Martinović S, Stojković S, Pavlović M, et al. Successful retrieval of an unexpanded coronary stent from the left main coronary artery during primary percutaneous coronary intervention. Srp Arh Celok Lek 2011;139(9–10):669–672

Sentürk T, Ozdemir B, Yeşilbursa D, Serdar OA. Dislodgement of a sirolimus-eluting stent in the circumflex artery and its successful deployment with a small-balloon technique. Turk Kardiyol Dern Ars 2011;39(5):418–421

Yang DH, Woo SI, Kim DH, et al. Two dislodged and crushed coronary stents: treatment of two simultaneously dislodged stents using crushing techniques. Korean J Intern Med 2013;28(6):718–723

Dislodgement of a coronary stent during stenting of the ramus interventricularis anterior

Patient History

A 55-year-old man suffering from coronary heart disease received an initial coronary artery stent at the proximal ramus interventricularis anterior (RIVA) 6 years earlier. Due to reoccurrence of symptoms the patient was scheduled for coronary angiography.

Initial Treatment Received

Proven proximal 90% RIVA in-stent restenosis, which was treated by percutaneous transluminal angioplasty (PTA) followed by an attempt to stent a stenosis beyond the proximal stent. An initial right-side transradial approach failed, therefore the procedure was performed from a right groin approach.

Problems Encountered during Treatment

The stent–balloon catheter failed to pass the proximal stent, when the operator noted that the stent was dislodged from the balloon catheter. The stent position, before any snaring maneuver was started, was at the distal opening of the guide catheter (**Fig. 4.285**). Any attempt to snare the stent failed, before the stent finally dislodged from the left main coronary artery. Immediate fluoroscopy of the supra-aortic, visceral, and peripheral vessels identified the lost stent.

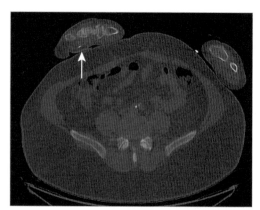

Fig. 4.286 Axial CT image showing a single migrated stent (*arrow*) into the left radial artery.

Imaging Plan

Whole-body low-dose computed tomography (CT) in order to identify and locate the stent. The stent was located at the distal level of the left radial artery (**Fig. 4.286**). Additional X-ray to visualize the stent (**Fig. 4.287**).

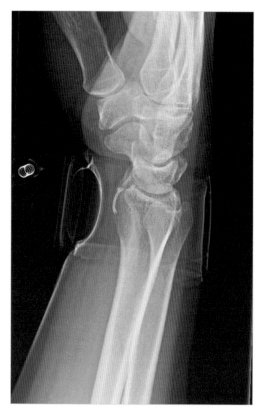

Fig. 4.287 An X-ray image proved the exact position of the stent for any further planning. Note the radial compression band, which is still in position.

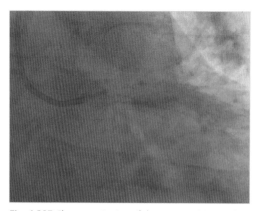

Fig. 4.285 Fluoroscopic view of the stent position at the distal opening of the guide catheter.

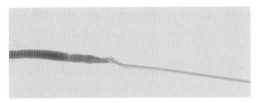

Fig. 4.288 Selective angiography of the distal radial artery in order to verify the exact position of the stent within the radial artery.

Resulting Complication

Coronary stent displacement in the left-side peripheral radial artery.

Possible Strategies for Complication Management

- Antegrade puncture of the brachial artery and try to snare the stent.
- Surgical cut-down at the level of the radial artery to remove the stent.

Final Complication Management

Antegrade puncture of the left brachial artery under local anesthesia and placement of a 4F sheath. Advancement of a 4F angle-tip catheter in front of the stent (**Fig. 4.288**), careful placement of a 5-mm snare beyond the proximal stent struts (**Fig. 4.289**). When the stent was successfully fixed by the snare, the retrieval maneuver was performed under continuous fluoroscopic control (**Fig. 4.290**). Finally, the stent was retrieved successfully (**Fig. 4.291**).

Complication Analysis

Stent migration and stent dislodgement are rare complications. In order to avoid them stent/balloon devices should be advanced with great care.

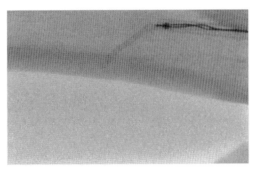

Fig. 4.290 Fluoroscopy of the snared stent at the level of the entrance of the 4F sheath.

If there is any resistance during advance and crossing maneuvers, the operator should stop immediately, reflect and evaluate potential reasons. In some cases a predilatation maneuver might overcome the problem.

Prevention Strategies and Take-home Message

- Never advance a stent against any resistance.
- Evaluate stent/balloon device removal. Especially be aware when moving it back into the guide catheter or sheath in order to avoid any stent dislodgement from the balloon.
- Perform predilatation of the critical area.
- If dislodgement and migration have already occurred, never, ever "give up" your guidewire. It guarantees any further displacement of the stent; try to advance the loop of the snare over the wire and try to remove everything when the stent is fixed—the wire and the snare with the engaged stent.

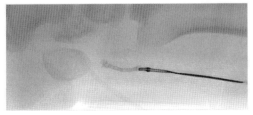

Fig. 4.289 Fluoroscopy of the snare at the level of the proximal stent. The compression device was still in position in order to avoid any further peripheral migration.

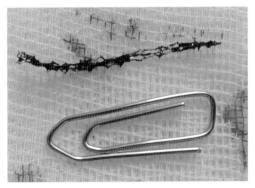

Fig. 4.291 Photograph of the successfully removed stent next to a paper clip.

Further Reading

Ahmed S, Ratanapo S, Srivali N, Cheungpasitporn W. Stent dislodgement: a rare complication of subclavian artery angioplasty and stenting. N Am J Med Sci 2013;5(3):251

Aydin M, Sayin MR. Successful coronary stent retrieval from the saphenous vein graft to right coronary artery. Case Rep Med 2009;2009:718685

Broadbent LP, Moran CJ, Cross DT III, Derdeyn CP. Management of neuroform stent dislodgement and misplacement. AJNR Am J Neuroradiol 2003;24(9):1819–1822

Chiu KM, Chu SH, Chan CY. Dislodged caval stent in right pulmonary artery. Catheter Cardiovasc Interv 2007;70(6): 799–800

Cishek MB, Laslett L, Gershony G. Balloon catheter retrieval of dislodged coronary artery stents: a novel technique. Cathet Cardiovasc Diagn 1995;34(4):350–352

Deftereos S, Raisakis K, Giannopoulos G, Kossyvakis C, Pappas L, Kaoukis A. Successful retrieval of a coronary stent dislodged in the brachial artery by means of improvised snare and guiding catheter. Int J Angiol 2011;20(1):55–58

Eeckhout E, Stauffer JC, Goy JJ. Retrieval of a migrated coronary stent by means of an alligator forceps catheter. Cathet Cardiovasc Diagn 1993;30(2):166–168

Gan HW, Bhasin A, Wu CJ. Complete stent dislodgement after successful implantation—a rare case. Catheter Cardiovasc Interv 2010;75(6):967–970

Hussain F, Kashour T, Philipp R. Old technique, new use: novel use of a buddy wire to deploy a detached stent. J Invasive Cardiol 2007;19(6):E160–E162

Jang JH, Woo SI, Yang DH, Park SD, Kim DH, Shin SH. Successful coronary stent retrieval from the ascending aorta using a gooseneck snare kit. Korean J Intern Med 2013;28(4): 481–485

Kakisis JD, Vassilas K, Antonopoulos C, Sfyroeras G, Moulakakis K, Liapis CD. Wandering stent within the pulmonary circulation. Ann Vasc Surg 2014;28(8):1932.e9–e12

Kwan TW, Chaudhry M, Huang Y, et al. Approaches for dislodged stent retrieval during transradial percutaneous coronary interventions. Catheter Cardiovasc Interv 2013;81(6):E245–E249

Meisel SR, DiLeo J, Rajakaruna M, Pace B, Frankel R, Shani J. A technique to retrieve stents dislodged in the coronary artery followed by fixation in the iliac artery by means of balloon angioplasty and peripheral stent deployment. Catheter Cardiovasc Interv 2000;49(1):77–81

Nishi M, Zen K, Kambayashi D, Asada S, Yamaguchi S, Tatsukawa H. Stent dislodgement induced by a vasodilator used for severe coronary artery spasm caused by Kounis syndrome. Cardiovasc Interv Ther 2015. [Epub ahead of print]

Oh Y, Hwang DH, Ko YH, Kang IW, Kim IS, Hur CW. Foreign body removal by snare loop: during intracranial stent procedure. Neurointervention 2012;7(1):50–53

Salinger-Martinović S, Stojković S, Pavlović M, et al. Successful retrieval of an unexpanded coronary stent from the left main coronary artery during primary percutaneous coronary intervention. Srp Arh Celok Lek 2011;139(9–10): 669–672

Sentürk T, Ozdemir B, Yeşilbursa D, Serdar OA. Dislodgement of a sirolimus-eluting stent in the circumflex artery and its successful deployment with a small-balloon technique. Turk Kardiyol Dern Ars 2011;39(5):418–421

Yang DH, Woo SI, Kim DH et al. Two dislodged and crushed coronary stents: treatment of two simultaneously dislodged stents using crushing techniques. Korean J Intern Med 2013;28(6):718–723

Dislocation and stent disintegration during iliac artery stenting

Patient History

A 72-year-old man with 4-cm-long high-grade stenosis of the left external iliac artery (EIA) was scheduled for iliac artery stent placement. Because of the proximity of the lesion to the inguinal ligament a contralateral right retrograde crossover approach was chosen as the initial treatment strategy.

Initial Treatment Received

Under local anesthesia, retrograde access to the right common femoral artery (CFA) was established and a 6F sheath was inserted. A hydrophylic-coated 0.035-inch guidewire was used in combination with a 4F Rösch inferior mesenteric (RIM; Cordis/Johnson & Johnson) catheter to navigate into the left iliac artery. After successfully crossing the lesion, the guide was exchanged for a standard steel core wire, over which it was attempted to place a 45-cm-long 6F sheath.

Problems Encountered during Treatment

Despite a favorable anatomy of the aortic bifurcation it was not possible to advance the sheath into the left iliac artery. This was attributed to the fact that there was scarring surrounding the right CFA after previous patch plasty. The operator left the sheath on the right side and tried to bring the delivery catheter of the balloon-expandable stent to the target lesion without the protective crossover sheath. Only mild resistance was encountered; however, the stent immediately detached from its balloon and got stuck on the aortic bifurcation. The guidewire was still in place; the balloon could be removed, but the stent did not follow (**Fig. 4.292**).

The operator now tried to catch the stent using a snare loop inserted over the wire. Unfortunately the stent could not be pulled out of the sheath. Fluoroscopy images revealed that the proximal part of the stent had disintegrated (**Fig. 4.293**). Furthermore, the snare maneuver had caused the proximal stent struts to become entangled with the guidewire. The wire–stent complex moved freely in the aorta and could be advanced and retracted but it was not possible to pull it into the right iliac artery without risking losing the stent (**Fig. 4.294**).

Imaging Plan

Fluoroscopic guidance.

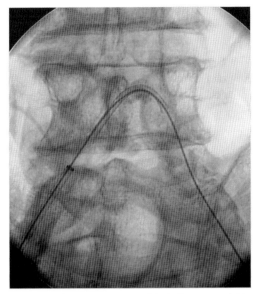

Fig. 4.292 Fluoroscopic image of the balloon expandable stent which had dislodged from the carrier balloon and is now "sitting" on the aortic bifurcation.

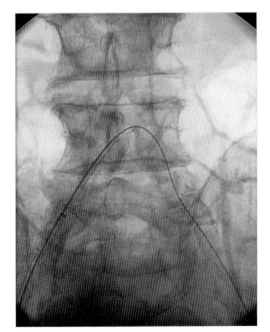

Fig. 4.293 Fluoroscopic image following attempts to snare the stent out of the sheath. The proximal stent-struts got entangled to the guidewire and its removal failed.

Resulting Complication

Stent detachment from the carrier balloon, disintegration of the proximal stent due to unsuccessful snaring maneuvers, fusion of the stent to the hydrophilic-coated wire.

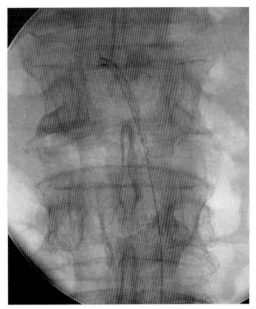

Fig. 4.294 The entangled wire/stent complex could be advanced into the aorta, but it was not possible to pull it into the right iliac artery without risking to loose the stent.

Possible Strategies for Complication Management

- Deployment of the stent outside the intended treatment site. This was not possible because the proximal part of the stent was disintegrated and attached to the wire. The carrier balloon could not be inserted any more.
- Snaring of the stent with removal of the device through the ipsilateral sheath. This had been tried; however, without upsizing the sheath the maneuver failed.
- Contralateral puncture, insertion of a large-bore sheath, and further attempts to remove the foreign body with a snare.
- Surgical removal of the stent (if endovascular approaches fail).

Final Complication Management

The left common iliac artery (CIA) was punctured in a retrograde fashion. A 12-cm-long 10F sheath was inserted over a guidewire. Using a snare the stent was grabbed at its distal end and could easily be removed through the large-bore sheath (**Fig. 4.295**). The puncture site was successfully closed using an 8F collagen-based vascular closure device.

Complication Analysis

Commercially available balloon-expandable stents are industrially premounted on their carrier

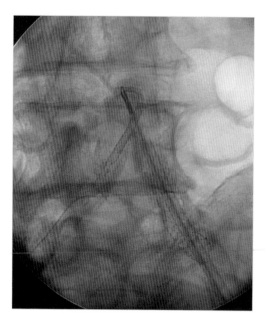

Fig. 4.295 Fluoroscopic image showing the snare maneuver of the stent via a large sheath from the contralateral groin.

balloon. While the connection between stent and balloon is commonly stable enough to engage simple ipsilateral lesions, detachment of a stent from its balloon is not uncommon when stents are advanced through high-grade calcified stenoses or anatomically challenging vessel segments. Advancement of a delivery catheter over the aortic bifurcation without sheath protection has a high probability of scaling the stent from its balloon and should be avoided. The second problem in this case was that the sheath was not upsized before snaring attempts for stent retrieval via the ipsilateral route were undertaken.

Prevention Strategies and Take-home Message

- When steering devices outside guiding catheters and/or sheaths, or when vessels are narrow and/or elongated, visual feedback is key to controlling pulling or pushing forces and to avoiding complications.
- Balloon-expandable stents should not be used across the aortic bifurcation if it is not possible to position a sheath for protected delivery.
- Never push or pull anything against resistance.
- When balloon-expandable stents are lost from their carrier balloon the sheath should be upsized at least 2F sizes before attempts at snaring and retrieval.

- When ipsilateral removal of a detached stent is not possible, consider a contralateral crossover approach with a large-bore sheath.

Further Reading

Blackman D, Dzavik V. Inadvertent detachment of an entrapped cutting balloon from the balloon catheter during treatment of in-stent restenosis. J Invasive Cardiol 2005;17(11): E27–E29

Hussain F, Rusnak B, Tam J. Retrieval of a detached partially expanded stent using the SpideRX and EnSnare devices—a first report. J Invasive Cardiol 2008;20(2):E44–E47

Pappy R, Gautam A, Abu-Fadel MS. AngioSculpt PTCA Balloon Catheter entrapment and detachment managed with stent jailing. J Invasive Cardiol 2010;22(10):E208–E210

Shiojima I, Ikari Y, Abe J, et al. Thrombotic occlusion of the coronary artery associated with accidental detachment of undeployed Palmaz-Schatz stent. Cathet Cardiovasc Diagn 1996;38(4):360–362

Migration of a self-expanding stent during treatment of malignant superior vena cava obstruction

Patient History

A 54-year-old man was planned for stenting of the superior vena cava (SVC) for central venous obstruction treatment.

Initial Treatment Received

SVC stenting from right groin approach via common femoral vein (CFV).

Problems Encountered during Treatment

Stent migration immediately after deployment of a 14 × 20-mm self-expanding stent (SES) down to infrarenal inferior vena cava (IVC) (**Fig. 4.296**).

Imaging Plan

Fluoroscopy to evaluate the exact stent position for further planning.

Resulting Complication

Incidental stent migration; the stent is still "on the wire."

Possible Strategies for Complication Management

- Exchange of the 8F sheath for a 12F sheath via the 0.035-inch guidewire. Advancement of snare to catch the stent for retrieval.

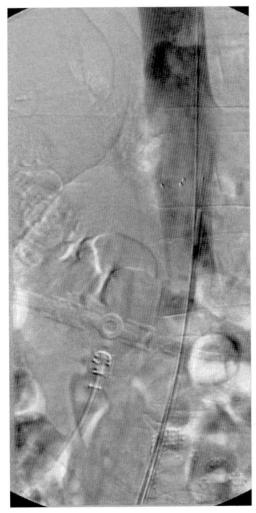

Fig. 4.296 Cavography showing the mismatch of stent diameter and IVC diameter; a straight diagnostic catheter and 0.035-inch guidewire are placed coaxially in the stents.

- To fix the stent at the current position by coaxially placing a larger SES in terms of diameter and length, that is, 18 × 60 mm.
- Surgery (if an endovascular approach fails).

Final Complication Management

Exchange of the 8F sheath for a 12F sheath via the 0.035-inch guidewire. Advancement of a 20-mm snare to catch the stent for retrieval (**Fig. 4.297**); while snaring the stent, the 12F sheath was gently advanced towards the stent (**Figs. 4.299** and **4.298**). After stent retrieval, a minor stent fragment remained in the IVC (**Fig. 4.300**). Final angiography revealed neither narrowing nor damage of the IVC (**Fig. 4.301**).

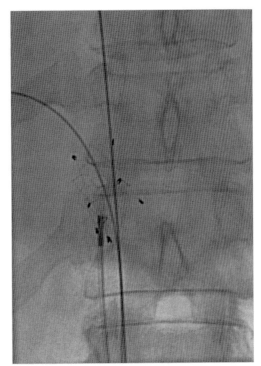

Fig. 4.297 Fluoroscopy of the snared stent. The stent was "fixed" by the snare and two coaxially running guidewires; one wire was placed in the right renal vein.

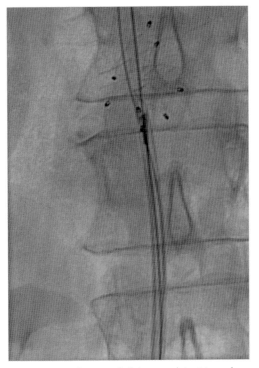

Fig. 4.298 Gentle removal of the snared stent towards the 12F sheath.

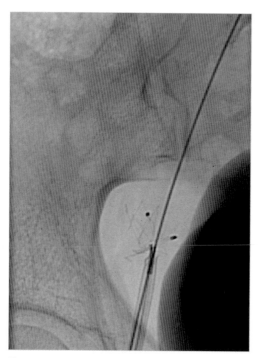

Fig. 4.299 Parts of the stent are already snared in the sheath, whereas some parts of the disrupted stent are still outside the sheath.

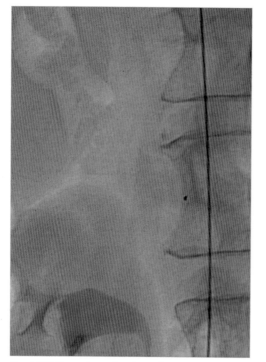

Fig. 4.300 Fluoroscopy of a migrated suprarenal stent fragment resistant to retrieval indicated by one radiopaque marker. An 0.035-inch guidewire was still in place.

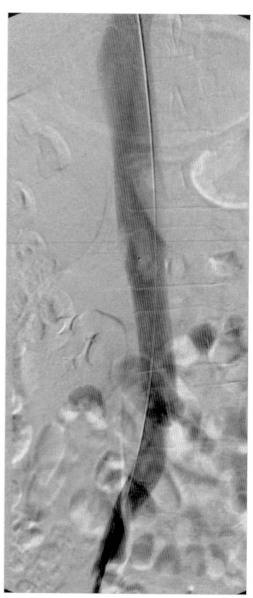

Fig. 4.301 Final cavography without any signs of narrowing or vessel damage (rupture).

Complication Analysis

Stent migration during SVC stenting due to mismatch of maximum stent diameter and length as well as SVC diameter.

Prevention Strategies and Take-home Message

- Determine the required stent length as well the diameter based on contrast-enhanced computed tomography (CT) images.

- Determine that the stent diameter is big enough in order to guarantee an adequate fixation by stent hoop strength and chronic outback force.

Further Reading

Bagul NB, Moth P, Menon NJ, Myint F, Hamilton G. Migration of superior vena cava stent. J Cardiothorac Surg 2008;3:12

Basu NN, Motallebzadeh R, Wendler O. A stranger in the heart: vena caval stent migration. Eur J Cardiothorac Surg 2005;28(5):770

Bobylev D, Meschenmoser L, Boethig D, Horke A. Migration of an endovascular stent into the right ventricle following deployment in the inferior vena cava after liver transplantation. Eur J Cardiothorac Surg 2015;48(2):308

Carroll MI, Ahanchi SS, Kim JH, Panneton JM. Endovascular foreign body retrieval. J Vasc Surg 2013;57(2):459–463

Chen S, Zhang H, Tian L, Li M, Zhou M, Wang Z. A stranger in the heart: LRV stent migration. Int Urol Nephrol 2009;41(2):427–430

Chiu KM, Chu SH, Chan CY. Dislodged caval stent in right pulmonary artery. Catheter Cardiovasc Interv 2007;70(6):799–800

Gabelmann A, Krämer SC, Tomczak R, Görich J. Percutaneous techniques for managing maldeployed or migrated stents. J Endovasc Ther 2001;8(3):291–302

Gan HW, Bhasin A, Wu CJ. Complete stent dislodgement after successful implantation—a rare case. Catheter Cardiovasc Interv 2010;75(6):967–970

Ghanem A, Tiemann K, Nickenig G. Gone with the flow: percutaneous retrieval of a migrated wallstent trapped in the right ventricle. Eur Heart J 2009;30(6):717

Goelitz BW, Darcy M. Longitudinal stent fracture and migration of a stent fragment complicating treatment of hepatic vein stenosis after orthotopic liver transplantation. Semin Interv Radiol 2007;24(3):333–336

Guimarães M, Uflacker R, Schönholz C, Hannegan C, Selby JB. Stent migration complicating treatment of inferior vena cava stenosis after orthotopic liver transplantation. J Vasc Interv Radiol 2005;16(9):1247–1252

Kakisis JD, Vassilas K, Antonopoulos C, Sfyroeras G, Moulakakis K, Liapis CD. Wandering stent within the pulmonary circulation. Ann Vasc Surg 2014;28(8):1932.e9–e12

O'Brien P, Munk PL, Ho SG, Legiehn GM, Marchinkow LO. Management of central venous stent migration in a patient with a permanent inferior vena cava filter. J Vasc Interv Radiol 2005;16(8):1125–1128

Oh Y, Hwang DH, Ko YH, Kang IW, Kim IS, Hur CW. Foreign body removal by snare loop: during intracranial stent procedure. Neurointervention 2012;7(1):50–53

Poludasu SS, Vladutiu P, Lazar J. Migration of an endovascular stent from superior vena cava to the right ventricular outflow tract in a patient with superior vena cava syndrome. Angiology 2008;59(1):114–116

Rana MA, Oderich GS, Bjarnason H. Endovenous removal of dislodged left renal vein stent in a patient with nutcracker syndrome. Semin Vasc Surg 2013;26(1):43–47

Sakhri L, Pirvu A, Toffart A-C, Thony F, Moro-Sibilot D. Unusual migration of a vena cava stent into the pulmonary artery because of tumor reduction after chemotherapy. J Thorac Oncol 2013;8(12):1585–1586

Schechter MA, O'Brien PJ, Cox MW. Retrieval of iatrogenic intravascular foreign bodies. J Vasc Surg 2013;57(1):276–281

Schefold JC, Krackhardt F. Dislocation of a metal stent to the right ventricle: an unusual finding in the heart. J Cardiovasc Med (Hagerstown) 2008;9(7):742–743

Slonim SM, Dake MD, Razavi MK, et al. Management of misplaced or migrated endovascular stents. J Vasc Interv Radiol 1999;10(7):851–859

Taylor JD, Lehmann ED, Belli AM, et al. Strategies for the management of SVC stent migration into the right atrium. Cardiovasc Interv Radiol 2007;30(5):1003–1009

Toyoda N, Torregrossa G, Itagaki S, Pawale A, Reddy R. Intracardiac migration of vena caval stent: decision-making and treatment considerations. J Card Surg 2014;29(3):320–322

Warren MJ, Sen S, Marcus N. Management of migration of a SVC Wallstent into the right atrium. Cardiovasc Interv Radiol 2008;31(6):1262–1264

Stent loss during inferior vena cava stenting

Patient History

A 45-year-old woman presented to the Emergency Department with acute left leg swelling over a period of 5 days involving the entire left leg. A venous duplex ultrasound demonstrated extensive deep vein thrombosis (DVT) in the left leg from the distal femoral vein to the external iliac vein. Given the proximal extension of the DVT a computed tomography (CT) scan of the abdomen and pelvis was requested. CT demonstrated DVT extending from the left common iliac vein (CIV) to the distal left femoral vein (**Fig. 4.302**) with marked soft tissue swelling of the entire left extremity. There was also a markedly enlarged multifibroid uterus that was felt to be compressing the left CIV.

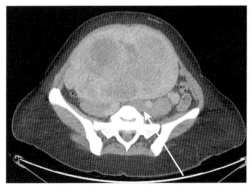

Fig. 4.302 CT Scan demonstrated extensive DVT (*arrow*) extending from the left CIV to the distal left femoral vein.

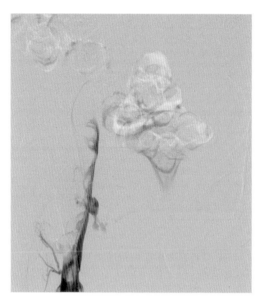

Fig. 4.303 Diagnostic venogram confirmed extensive DVT from the distal femoral vein to the external iliac vein.

Initial Treatment Received

Given the proximal extent of the DVT, pharmacomechanical thrombolysis was planned to decrease the probability of post-thrombotic syndrome. The patient was placed in a prone position on the angiographic table and ultrasound-guided micropuncture access was obtained into the left popliteal vein. A diagnostic venogram was obtained that confirmed extensive DVT from the distal femoral vein to the external iliac vein. There appeared to be an occlusion of the left CIV (**Fig. 4.303**). A Trellis (Covidien) pharmacomechanical device was placed from the left CIV to the common femoral vein (CFV) and pharmacomechanical thrombolysis was performed with 10 mg of recombinant tissue plasminogen activator (rtPA) (**Fig. 4.304**). After the pharmacomechanical thrombolysis significant residual thrombus remained in the left external iliac and CIV.

The patient was transferred to the Intensive Care Unit for a further 8 hours of infusion thrombolysis through a multiside-hole catheter. The following morning the patient was again brought down to the Angio Suite for a recheck. There was significant decrease in the thrombus burden; however a severe stenosis remained in the left CIV extending into the distal inferior vena cava

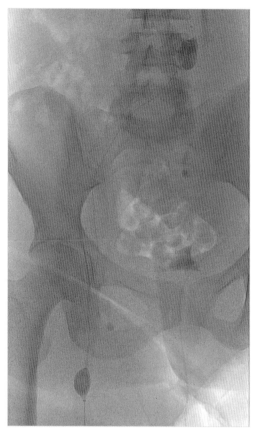

Fig. 4.304 A Trellis pharmacomechanical device was placed from the left CIV to the CFV for pharmacomechanical thrombolysis.

(IVC). Percutaneous ultrasound-guided micropuncture accessed the right popliteal vein. Bilateral 12 × 80-mm self-expanding Viabahn covered stents were deployed in the distal IVC extending into both CIVs.

Problems Encountered during Treatment

At the time of deployment, the left-sided covered stent dislodged and floated up into the heart while still on the wire (**Fig. 4.305**). A second covered stent was deployed on the left side, creating a "kissing stent configuration" (**Fig. 4.306**).

Resulting Complication

In this case a stent graft was lost during kissing stent placement from IVC extending into both CIVs and dislocated into the heart.

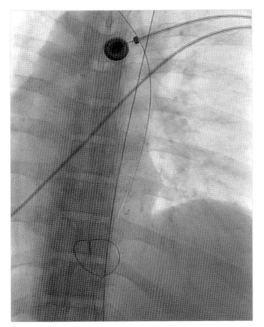

Fig. 4.305 Fluoroscopic image showing the dislodged and migrated covered stent at the level of the right heart.

Possible Strategies for Complication Management

- Endovascular treatment via right internal jugular vein to snare stent.
- Endovascular treatment via right CFV to snare catheter fragment.
- Sternotomy and open access to heart (if endovascular approaches fail).

Final Complication Management

Endovascular access was obtained via the left internal jugular vein under ultrasound guidance with the patient still in a prone position using a micropuncture kit. An 8F vascular sheath was inserted. Using a 0.035-inch diameter, 145-cm-long Rosen wire and an 80-cm-long MPA (multipurpose A) catheter cannulation into the right ventricle was obtained. A 25-mm loop snare was inserted and the venous stent was snared in the mid-portion of the stent within the right ventricle (**Fig. 4.307**). The stent was snared into the left brachiocephalic vein but could not be pulled out through the venous access site (**Fig. 4.308**). A vascular surgeon was consulted. The vascu-

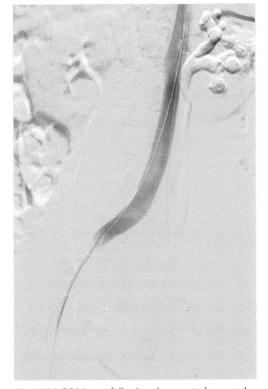

Fig. 4.306 DSA image following placement of a second covered stent on the left side, creating a "kissing stent configuration."

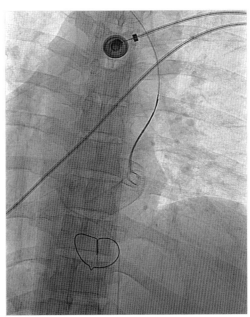

Fig. 4.307 Fluoroscopic image showing a snare maneuver with a 25-mm loop inserted from the right brachiocephalic vein. The venous stent was snared in mid portion of the stent within the right ventricle.

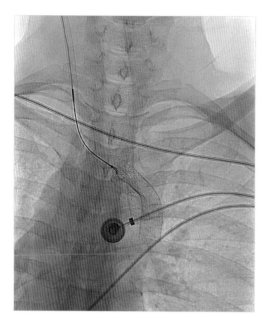

Fig. 4.308 The stent was snared into the left brachiocephalic vein but could not be pulled out through the venous access site.

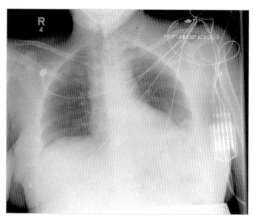

Fig. 4.310 Post stent removal, chest radiograph demonstrated no evidence of any retained stent fragments.

lar surgeon attempted a minisurgical cut-down in the neck; however the stent could still not be retrieved. The patient was brought to the operating room and placed in a supine position. A suprasternal venotomy was performed into the left brachiocephalic vein (**Fig. 4.309**). The stent

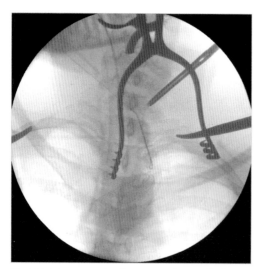

Fig. 4.309 Intraoperative fluoroscopy showing final removal of the stent via a suprasternal venotomy of the left brachiocephalic vein.

was removed by cutting the stent fabric and unwinding the stent metallic elements, which are one continuous piece in a Viabahn covered stent. Poststent removal a chest radiograph demonstrated no evidence of any retained stent fragments (**Fig. 4.310**).

Complication Analysis

In retrospect, placing kissing stents in the IVC was not the ideal strategy. Placing a larger-diameter appropriately sized IVC stent would have been prudent. When snaring the stent, the stent should have been snared at one end, which would have prevented the stent from folding onto itself and allowed much easier percutaneous removal. Also, it is very important to never lose wire access when you have a free-floating stent.

Prevention Strategies and Take-home Message

- Intravascular foreign bodies are a common occurrence. It is critical to have multiple techniques and access points for retrieval.
- It is also critical to carefully delineate the anatomy with endovascular contrast prior to any intervention.
- Always have alternative equipment and a plan in place if your initial access site or equipment is unsuccessful in retrieving the intravascular foreign body.

- Placing kissing stents in the IVC might not be an ideal strategy due to the flow direction toward the heart.
- When snaring a "lost" or "free" stent, try to snare at one end, which allows easier percutaneous removal.
- Always have a strong multidisciplinary team when performing endovascular procedures.

Further Reading

Bagul NB, Moth P, Menon NJ, Myint F, Hamilton G. Migration of superior vena cava stent. J Cardiothorac Surg 2008;3:12

Basu NN, Motallebzadeh R, Wendler O. A stranger in the heart: vena caval stent migration. Eur J Cardiothorac Surg 2005;28(5):770

Bobylev D, Meschenmoser L, Boethig D, Horke A. Migration of an endovascular stent into the right ventricle following deployment in the inferior vena cava after liver transplantation. Eur J Cardiothorac Surg 2015;48(2):308

Carroll MI, Ahanchi SS, Kim JH, Panneton JM. Endovascular foreign body retrieval. J Vasc Surg 2013;57(2):459–463

Chen S, Zhang H, Tian L, Li M, Zhou M, Wang Z. A stranger in the heart: LRV stent migration. Int Urol Nephrol 2009;41(2):427–430

Chiu KM, Chu SH, Chan CY. Dislodged caval stent in right pulmonary artery. Catheter Cardiovasc Interv 2007;70(6):799–800

Gabelmann A, Krämer SC, Tomczak R, Görich J. Percutaneous techniques for managing maldeployed or migrated stents. J Endovasc Ther 2001;8(3):291–302

Gan HW, Bhasin A, Wu CJ. Complete stent dislodgement after successful implantation—a rare case. Catheter Cardiovasc Interv 2010;75(6):967–970

Ghanem A, Tiemann K, Nickenig G. Gone with the flow: percutaneous retrieval of a migrated wallstent trapped in the right ventricle. Eur Heart J 2009;30(6):717

Goelitz BW, Darcy M. Longitudinal stent fracture and migration of a stent fragment complicating treatment of hepatic vein stenosis after orthotopic liver transplantation. Semin Interv Radiol 2007;24(3):333–336

Guimarães M, Uflacker R, Schönholz C, Hannegan C, Selby JB. Stent migration complicating treatment of inferior vena cava stenosis after orthotopic liver transplantation. J Vasc Interv Radiol 2005;16(9):1247–1252

Kakisis JD, Vassilas K, Antonopoulos C, Sfyroeras G, Moulakakis K, Liapis CD. Wandering stent within the pulmonary circulation. Ann Vasc Surg 2014;28(8):1932.e9–e12

O'Brien P, Munk PL, Ho SG, Legiehn GM, Marchinkow LO. Management of central venous stent migration in a patient with a permanent inferior vena cava filter. J Vasc Interv Radiol 2005;16(8):1125–1128

Oh Y, Hwang DH, Ko YH, Kang IW, Kim IS, Hur CW. Foreign body removal by snare loop: during intracranial stent procedure. Neurointervention 2012;7(1):50–53

Poludasu SS, Vladutiu P, Lazar J. Migration of an endovascular stent from superior vena cava to the right ventricular outflow tract in a patient with superior vena cava syndrome. Angiology 2008;59(1):114–116

Rana MA, Oderich GS, Bjarnason H. Endovenous removal of dislodged left renal vein stent in a patient with nutcracker syndrome. Semin Vasc Surg 2013;26(1):43–47

Sakhri L, Pirvu A, Toffart A-C, Thony F, Moro-Sibilot D. Unusual migration of a vena cava stent into the pulmonary artery because of tumor reduction after chemotherapy. J Thorac Oncol 2013;8(12):1585–1586

Schechter MA, O'Brien PJ, Cox MW. Retrieval of iatrogenic intravascular foreign bodies. J Vasc Surg 2013;57(1):276–281

Schefold JC, Krackhardt F. Dislocation of a metal stent to the right ventricle: an unusual finding in the heart. J Cardiovasc Med (Hagerstown) 2008;9(7):742–743

Slonim SM, Dake MD, Razavi MK, et al. Management of misplaced or migrated endovascular stents. J Vasc Interv Radiol 1999;10(7):851–859

Taylor JD, Lehmann ED, Belli AM, et al. Strategies for the management of SVC stent migration into the right atrium. Cardiovasc Interv Radiol 2007;30(5):1003–1009

Toyoda N, Torregrossa G, Itagaki S, Pawale A, Reddy R. Intracardiac migration of vena caval stent: decision-making and treatment considerations. J Card Surg 2014;29(3):320–322

Warren MJ, Sen S, Marcus N. Management of migration of a SVC Wallstent into the right atrium. Cardiovasc Interv Radiol 2008;31(6):1262–1264

Loss of self-expanding stent from delivery catheter during device placement

Patient History

A 79-year-old man with lifestyle-limiting claudication was scheduled for diagnostic angiography and angioplasty after ultrasound detected multilevel atherosclerotic disease with high-grade short-segment stenosis of the right superficial femoral artery (SFA).

Initial Treatment Received

Under local anesthesia, retrograde access to the left common femoral artery (CFA) was established and a 6F sheath was inserted. Diagnostic angiography revealed mild stenosis in the right CFA and confirmed a high-grade stenosis in the right SFA. A hydrophylic-coated 0.035-inch guidewire was used in combination with a 4F Rösch inferior mesenteric (RIM; Cordis/Johnson & Johnson) catheter to access the right iliac artery. A 6F crossover sheath was placed into the proximal external iliac artery (EIA). The lesion in the right SFA was recanalized using a 125-cm-long 5F multipurpose catheter and an 0.018-inch hydrophilic-coated wire. Following balloon angioplasty a hemodynamically relevant intimal dissection was present and stent placement was indicated (**Fig. 4.311**).

Problems Encountered during Treatment

A 0.035-inch wire-compatible 6 × 40-mm self-expanding stent (SES) was introduced through the

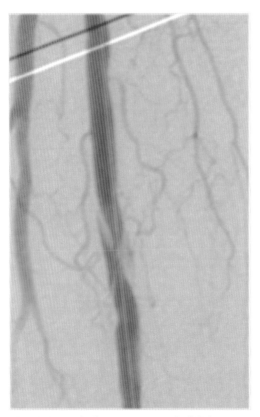

Fig. 4.311 Digital subtraction angiography (DSA) following percutaneous transluminal angioplasty (PTA) of a short-segment stenosis of the right SFA. Hemodynamically relevant dissection indicated stent placement.

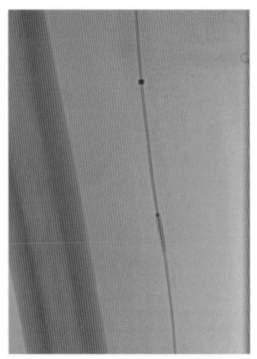

Fig. 4.312 Fluoroscopic image of the stent delivery catheter at the lesion site. However, no stent is visible.

sheath and advanced over the 0.018-inch wire. During advancement of the delivery catheter mild resistance was encountered; however, fluoroscopy was maintained at the position of the treated lesion and the catheter was advanced further. When the delivery catheter had reached the lesion the stent appeared to be missing from the catheter (**Fig. 4.312**).

Imaging Plan

Fluoroscopy/digital subtraction angiography to search for the missing stent.

Resulting Complication

Detachment of an SES from its delivery catheter resulted in stent malplacement into the right EIA (**Figs. 4.313** and **4.314**), which did not cause stenosis.

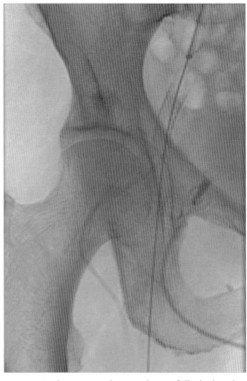

Fig. 4.313 Fluoroscopy showing the SES fully deployed in the EIA.

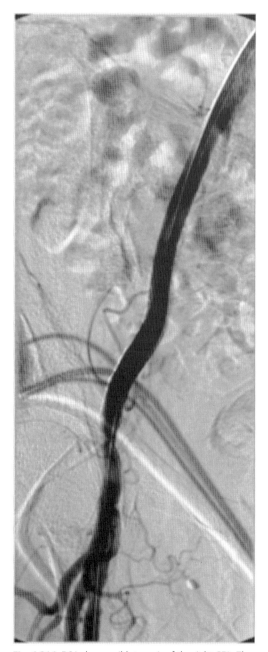

Fig. 4.314 DSA shows mild stenosis of the right CFA. The malplaced stent proximally to the lesion did not cause stenosis.

Possible Strategies for Complication Management

- Do nothing, as stent does not cause stenosis.
- Snare the stent to attempt removal through the sheath. This would not be possible in this case because of the large diameter of the stent

in relation to the small sheath size. The stent would most likely disintegrate.
- Surgical removal of the stent (if endovascular approaches fail).

Final Complication Management

With the stent in the EIA being intact and fully deployed without causing stenosis it was decided to leave the device in place and do nothing. The lesion of the right SFA was successfully treated with a second stent (images not shown).

Complication Analysis

SESs are mounted inside a delivery catheter and released by pulling back the outer sheath of the catheter. In this case there was resistance felt during advancement of the device, but it was still further advanced, leading to detachment of the stent from the delivery catheter. Since the incident was not observed during fluoroscopy the exact mechanism leading to this complication remains unclear. The delivery catheter was introduced over a 0.018-inch guidewire while it was 0.035-inch compatible. In this scenario there is a mismatch between the wire lumen of the catheter and the smaller guidewire, producing a step at the catheter tip that can interfere with vascular plaque.

Prevention Strategies and Take-home Message

- All endovascular instruments should be handled with great care. Devices and implants should always be guided by fluoroscopy!
- Especially when steering devices outside of guiding catheters and/or sheaths, or when vessels are narrow and/or elongated, visual feedback is key to control pulling or pushing forces and to avoid complications.
- If any resistance is encountered during placement of a device the reason for this should be evaluated. Never push or pull anything against resistance.
- Stent dislodgement not only happens with balloon-expandable stents, but also is also possible with SESs.
- "Off-label" use of smaller guidewires (0.018 inch and 0.014 inch) with 0.035-inch-compatible catheters is possible but can lead to complications.

Further Reading

Ahmed S, Ratanapo S, Srivali N, Cheungpasitporn W. Stent dislodgement: a rare complication of subclavian artery angioplasty and stenting. N Am J Med Sci 2013;5(3): 251

Aydin M, Sayin MR. Successful coronary stent retrieval from the saphenous vein graft to right coronary artery. Case Rep Med 2009;2009:718685

Broadbent LP, Moran CJ, Cross DT III, Derdeyn CP. Management of neuroform stent dislodgement and misplacement. AJNR Am J Neuroradiol 2003;24(9):1819–1822

Chiu KM, Chu SH, Chan CY. Dislodged caval stent in right pulmonary artery. Catheter Cardiovasc Interv 2007;70(6): 799–800

Cishek MB, Laslett L, Gershony G. Balloon catheter retrieval of dislodged coronary artery stents: a novel technique. Cathet Cardiovasc Diagn 1995;34(4):350–352

Deftereos S, Raisakis K, Giannopoulos G, Kossyvakis C, Pappas L, Kaoukis A. Successful retrieval of a coronary stent dislodged in the brachial artery by means of improvised snare and guiding catheter. Int J Angiol 2011;20(1):55–58

Eeckhout E, Stauffer JC, Goy JJ. Retrieval of a migrated coronary stent by means of an alligator forceps catheter. Cathet Cardiovasc Diagn 1993;30(2):166–168

Gan HW, Bhasin A, Wu CJ. Complete stent dislodgement after successful implantation—a rare case. Catheter Cardiovasc Interv 2010;75(6):967–970

Hussain F, Kashour T, Philipp R. Old technique, new use: novel use of a buddy wire to deploy a detached stent. J Invasive Cardiol 2007;19(6):E160–E162

Jang JH, Woo SI, Yang DH, Park SD, Kim DH, Shin SH. Successful coronary stent retrieval from the ascending aorta using a gooseneck snare kit. Korean J Intern Med 2013;28(4): 481–485

Kakisis JD, Vassilas K, Antonopoulos C, Sfyroeras G, Moulakakis K, Liapis CD. Wandering stent within the pulmonary circulation. Ann Vasc Surg 2014;28(8):1932.e9–e12

Kwan TW, Chaudhry M, Huang Y, et al. Approaches for dislodged stent retrieval during transradial percutaneous coronary interventions. Catheter Cardiovasc Interv 2013;81(6):E245–E249

Meisel SR, DiLeo J, Rajakaruna M, Pace B, Frankel R, Shani J. A technique to retrieve stents dislodged in the coronary artery followed by fixation by means of balloon angioplasty and peripheral stent deployment. Catheter Cardiovasc Interv 2000;49(1):77–81

Nishi M, Zen K, Kambayashi D, Asada S, Yamaguchi T, Tatsukawa H. Stent dislodgement induced by a vasodilator used for severe coronary artery spasm caused by Kounis syndrome. Cardiovasc Interv Ther 2015. [Epub ahead of print]

Oh Y, Hwang DH, Ko YH, Kang IW, Kim IS, Hur CW. Foreign body removal by snare loop: during intracranial stent procedure. Neurointervention 2012;7(1):50–53

Salinger-Martinović S, Stojković S, Pavlović M, et al. Successful retrieval of an unexpanded coronary stent from the left main coronary artery during primary percutaneous coronary intervention. Srp Arh Celok Lek 2011;139(9–10): 669–672

Sentürk T, Ozdemir B, Yeşilbursa D, Serdar OA. Dislodgement of a sirolimus-eluting stent in the circumflex artery and its successful deployment with a small-balloon technique. Turk Kardiyol Dern Ars 2011;39(5):418–421

Yang DH, Woo SI, Kim DH et al. Two dislodged and crushed coronary stents: treatment of two simultaneously dislodged stents using crushing techniques. Korean J Intern Med 2013;28(6):718–723

Venous complication—inferior vena cava stent

Patient History

A 42-year-old male presented with back pain and a long-standing inferior vena cava (IVC) occlusion with extensive paraspinal and azygos collateral veins. The pain was considered to be due to paraspinal venous engorgement over many years.

Initial Treatment Received

Angiography was performed from each femoral vein to outline the two large lumbar veins and confirm the hypoplasia of the IVC (**Fig. 4.315**).

It was decided to place a stent in the right ascending lumbar vein to improve venous drainage and relieve the spinal venous engorgement. A 5F catheter was inserted into the right lumbar vein but the vessel was extremely tortuous (**Fig. 4.316**).

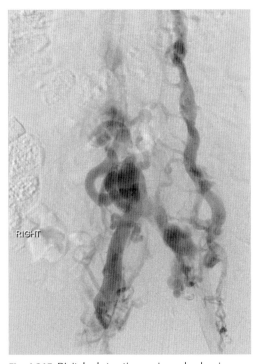

Fig. 4.315 Digital substraction angiography showing two large lumbar veins due to hypoplasia of the inferior vena cava.

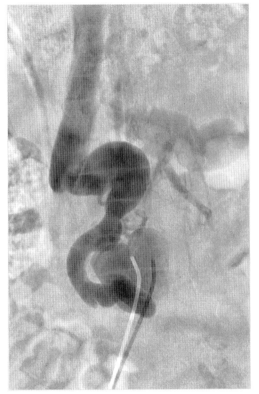

Fig. 4.316 Selective angiography during attempts to cannulate the right lumbar vein showing a highly tortuous vessel.

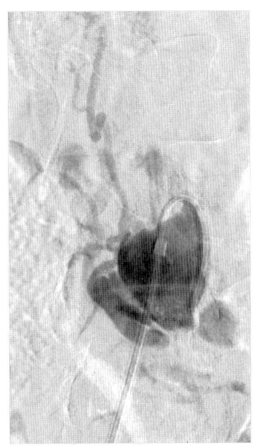

Fig. 4.317 Angiography following numerous cannulation attempts showed reduced flow in the target vein. The procedure was abandoned because of the risk of venous thrombosis.

Problems Encountered during Treatment

Much time was wasted using a succession of catheter shapes and wire guides before it became difficult to pass a wire guide into the vein and eventually the flow in the vein became very sluggish. The procedure was abandoned because of the risk of venous thrombosis (**Fig. 4.317**).

Imaging Plan

Angiography.

Resulting Complication

- Very high patient skin dose in excess of 5 millisieverts (mSv).
- Very poor flow in a major collateral with possible thrombosis and risk of pulmonary embolus.

Possible Strategies for Complication Management

- Refuse to attempt further angioplasty because of the radiation dose already received.
- Consider surgery with vein bypass.
- Wait an interval of several months and repeat the procedure with catheterization of the veins via the femoral and jugular approach.

Final Complication Management

From the right internal jugular vein and the right femoral vein catheters were placed into the right lumbar vein (**Fig. 4.318**). An endovascular snare

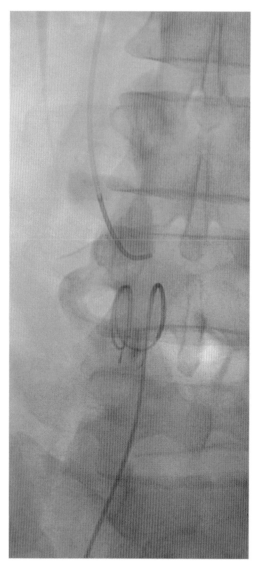

Fig. 4.318 Fluoroscopic image showing a rendezvouz maneuver with access from right internal jugular vein and right femoral vein.

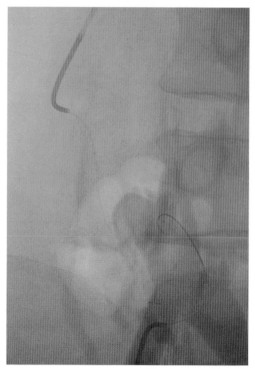

Fig. 4.319 An endovascular snare inserted from the jugular vein was used to catch the guide wire from the groin.

The final image (**Fig. 4.321**) shows a widely patent vessel. A self-expanding biliary Wallstent (Boston Scientific) was reinforced with a balloon-expandable stent.

Complication Analysis

There was a failure to realize that the strategy being used was not going to work. In this case persistence was not the answer. A fresh approach was what was needed and this became obvious when the case was discussed after the first procedure.

introduced from the jugular vein was deployed to rendezvous with a wire guide introduced from the femoral vein (**Fig. 4.319**). Once captured, the snare catheter was drawn through the tortuous region of vein and brought out through the femoral vein sheath. A Lunderquist (Cook Medical) 0.035 guidewire was inserted back through the snare catheter and a long 6-mm angioplasty catheter was inflated to create a channel to permit insertion of a series of stents (**Fig. 4.320**).

Prevention Strategies and Take-home Message

- Consider a top-down and a bottom-up approach where the possibility presents itself.
- A rendezvous procedure allows great control when crossing difficult regions.
- Locking the catheter to a guidewire will aid passage.
- Take time to consider alternative plans when the first plan fails.

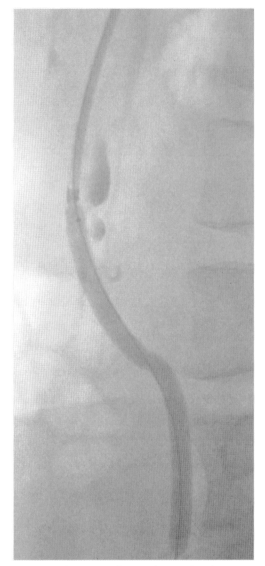

Fig. 4.320 Fluoroscopy showing the completed snaring maneuver and straightening of the lumbar vein with a stiff guide-wire. A long 6mm angioplasty catheter was used to create a channel to permit insertion of a series of stents.

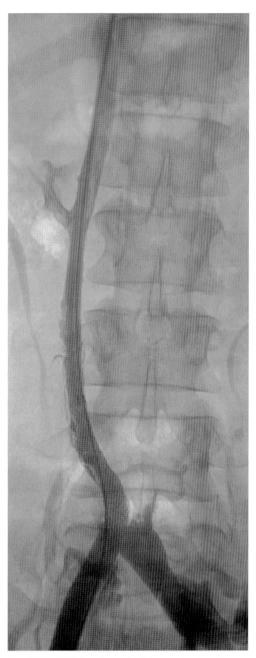

Fig. 4.321 Digital angiography following implantation of a self-expanding biliary Wallstent reinforced with a balloon expandable stent showed a widely patent vessel.

Further Reading

Massmann A, Rostam A, Fries P, Buecker A. A wire transposition technique for recanalization of chronic complex central venous occlusions. Phlebology 2014;pii:0268355514550260. [Epub ahead of print]

Migration of a Palmaz stent into the vena cava

Patient History

A 22-year-old woman presented with a stenosis in her left common iliac vein (CIV), which was found during an ultrasound examination for varicose veins. She was referred for angioplasty and stenting of the stenosis to prevent a May-Thurner iliofemoral thrombosis.

Initial Treatment Received

Angiography was performed from the left common femoral vein (CFV) (**Fig. 4.322**) and this revealed a typical stenosis at the origin of the left CIV caused by the crossing of the right common iliac artery (CIA).

Angioplasty was performed with a 10-mm-diameter angioplasty balloon and a Palmaz 4014 Maxi stent (Cordis/Johnson & Johnson) was inserted mounted on a 12-mm balloon angioplasty catheter. The intention was to inflate the Palmaz stent to a much larger diameter once the stent had been positioned across the stenosis. The large Palmaz stents are expandable to 25 mm while maintaining hoop strength but are not available premounted.

Problems Encountered during Treatment

The initial angioplasty was uneventful and the Palmaz stent was crimped by hand upon a 12-mm angioplasty catheter. However, during inflation at the site of the stenosis the stent expanded and migrated off the balloon into the inferior vena cava (IVC). The stent was then observed fluoroscopically as it continued up the IVC to the right atrium, crossed the tricuspid valve and lodged in the right ventricular outflow tract below the pulmonary valve.

Imaging Plan

Imaging in Angio/Interventional Suite.

Resulting Complication

Migrated expanded Palmaz stent lodged in the right ventricular outflow with risk of cardiac perforation and cardiac arrhythmia.

Possible Strategies for Complication Management

- Manipulate the stent so it enters the pulmonary artery.
- Retrieval and replacement of the stent to the cava.
- Call the cardiac surgery team for open retrieval under cardiac bypass.

Final Complication Management

Endovascular management with catheter-aided passage of a guidewire through the lumen of the stent followed by passage of an angioplasty balloon catheter over the guidewire (**Figs. 4.323** and **4.324**).

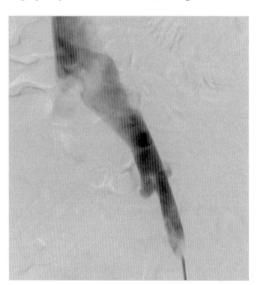

Fig. 4.322 Digital substraction venography showing a stenosis at the origin of the left common iliac vein.

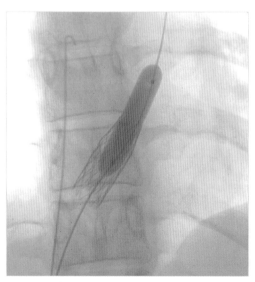

Fig. 4.323 Fluroscopy image depicting an inflated balloon in the dislodged stent after successfully passing the stent with a guidewire.

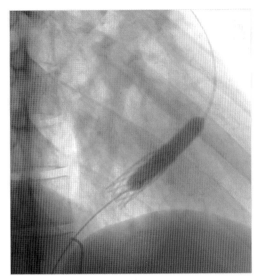

Fig. 4.324 Balloon mediated retrieval of the stent from the heart into the IVC was performed carefully under fluoroscopic control.

With the balloon inflated the stent was unable to progress further and it was gently withdrawn to the right atrium taking great care not to catch on the tricuspid valve attachments.

The stent was brought down to the iliac confluence but the partly expanded stent could not be positioned within the left iliac vein stenosis. A snare was passed around the stent in an attempt to reduce the diameter of the Palmaz stent but this failed (**Fig. 4.325**).

After discussion with the cardiac surgeons the stent was advanced to the upper superior vena cava (SVC) (**Fig. 4.326**) and expanded in place with an aortic valvuloplasty balloon to 25 mm diameter (**Figs. 4.327** and **4.328**). The same valvuloplasty balloon was used to perform definitive angioplasty of the left iliac vein stenosis (**Fig. 4.329**). No stent was placed in the iliac vein (**Fig. 4.330**).

A follow-up chest X-ray 3 years later showed that the stent was still in position. The patient was asymptomatic and has had no iliofemoral thrombosis (**Fig. 4.331**).

Complication Analysis

Positioning of large-diameter balloon-expandable stent is actually more difficult than using a

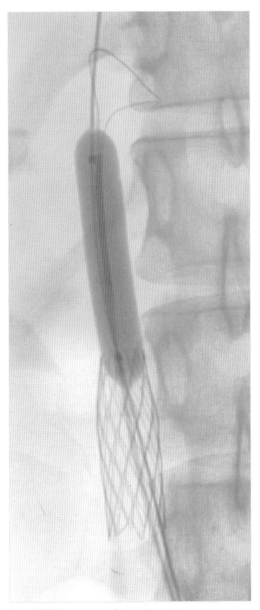

Fig. 4.325 Fluoroscopy during attempts to pass a snare around the dislodged stent.

self-expanding design as self-expanding stents can be recaptured and repositioned more easily.

In this case the stent did not fixate well enough to the vein wall during deployment and was free to migrate once the balloon was partly inflated.

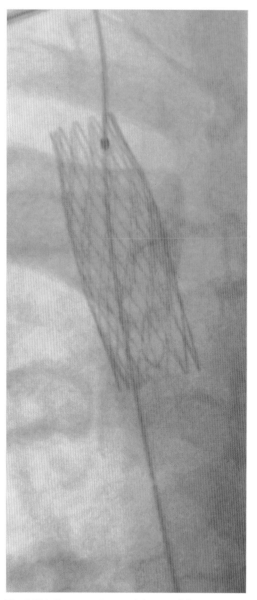

Fig. 4.326 Fluroscopy image of the stent following advancement into the upper superior vena cava.

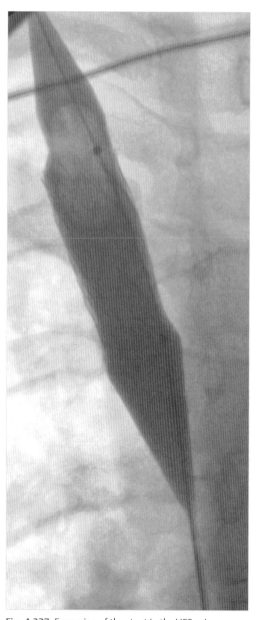

Fig. 4.327 Expansion of the stent in the VCS using a 25mm valvuloplasty balloon.

Prevention Strategies and Take-home Message

- When stenting the iliac veins or the vena cava use a long guidewire so that if the stent does migrate it will be contained by the wire to the cava and will not be free to enter the right ventricle.

- In very large veins, self-expanding nitinol stents are easier to position and control than balloon-mounted stents.
- Removal of stents across the tricuspid valve must be done with great caution to avoid damage to the valve leaflet attachments, which may result in severe tricuspid incompetence.

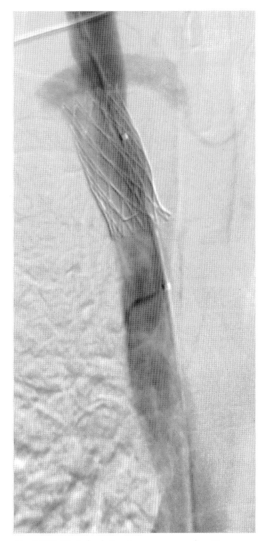

Fig. 4.328 Digital substraction venogram showing undisturbed flow in the SVC following stent expansion.

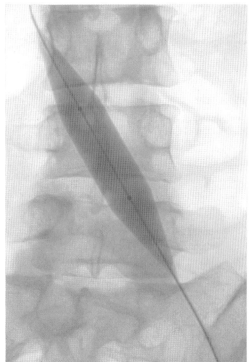

Fig. 4.329 Fluroscopy image showing the inflated valvuloplasty balloon in the left common iliac vein.

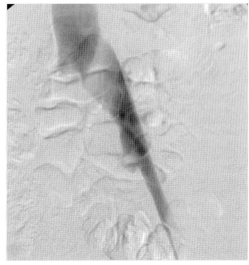

Fig. 4.330 Post procedure digital substraction venogram showing mildly enhanced flow in the left CIV.

Further Reading

Bagul NB, Moth P, Menon NJ, Myint F, Hamilton G. Migration of superior vena cava stent. J Cardiothorac Surg. 2008;3:12

Basu NN, Motallebzadeh R, Wendler O. A stranger in the heart: vena caval stent migration. Eur J Cardiothorac Surg 2005;28(5):770

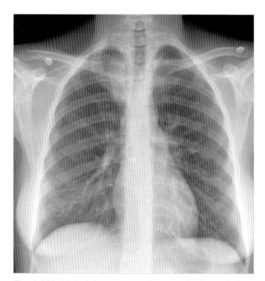

Fig. 4.331 Digital chest X-ray at 3 years F/U showed the stent in the SVC still in position.

Bobylev D, Meschenmoser L, Boethig D, Horke A. Migration of an endovascular stent into the right ventricle following deployment in the inferior vena cava after liver transplantation. Eur J Cardiothorac Surg 2015;48(2):308

Carroll MI, Ahanchi SS, Kim JH, Panneton JM. Endovascular foreign body retrieval. J Vasc Surg 2013;57(2):459–463

Chen S, Zhang H, Tian L, Li M, Zhou M, Wang Z. A stranger in the heart: LRV stent migration. Int Urol Nephrol 2009;41(2):427–430

Chiu KM, Chu SH, Chan CY. Dislodged caval stent in right pulmonary artery. Catheter Cardiovasc Interv 2007;70(6):799–800

Gabelmann A, Krämer SC, Tomczak R, Görich J. Percutaneous techniques for managing maldeployed or migrated stents. J Endovasc Ther 2001;8(3):291–302

Gan HW, Bhasin A, Wu CJ. Complete stent dislodgement after successful implantation—a rare case. Catheter Cardiovasc Interv 2010;75(6):967–970

Ghanem A, Tiemann K, Nickenig G. Gone with the flow: percutaneous retrieval of a migrated wallstent trapped in the right ventricle. Eur Heart J 2009;30(6):717

Goelitz BW, Darcy M. Longitudinal stent fracture and migration of a stent fragment complicating treatment of hepatic vein stenosis after orthotopic liver transplantation. Semin Interv Radiol 2007;24(3):333–336

Guimarães M, Uflacker R, Schönholz C, Hannegan C, Selby JB. Stent migration complicating treatment of inferior vena cava stenosis after orthotopic liver transplantation. J Vasc Interv Radiol 2005;16(9):1247–1252

Kakisis JD, Vassilas K, Antonopoulos C, Sfyroeras G, Moulakakis K, Liapis CD. Wandering stent within the pulmonary circulation. Ann Vasc Surg 2014;28(8):1932.e9–e12

O'Brien P, Munk PL, Ho SG, Legiehn GM, Marchinkow LO. Management of central venous stent migration in a patient with a permanent inferior vena cava filter. J Vasc Interv Radiol 2005;16(8):1125–1128

Oh Y, Hwang DH, Ko YH, Kang IW, Kim IS, Hur CW. Foreign body removal by snare loop: during intracranial stent procedure. Neurointervention 2012;7(1):50–53

Poludasu SS, Vladutiu P, Lazar J. Migration of an endovascular stent from superior vena cava to the right ventricular outflow tract in a patient with superior vena cava syndrome. Angiology 2008;59(1):114–116

Rana MA, Oderich GS, Bjarnason H. Endovenous removal of dislodged left renal vein stent in a patient with nutcracker syndrome. Semin Vasc Surg 2013;26(1):43–47

Sakhri L, Pirvu A, Toffart A-C, Thony F, Moro-Sibilot D. Unusual migration of a vena cava stent into the pulmonary artery because of tumor reduction after chemotherapy. J Thorac Oncol 2013;8(12):1585–1586

Schechter MA, O'Brien PJ, Cox MW. Retrieval of iatrogenic intravascular foreign bodies. J Vasc Surg 2013;57(1):276–281

Schefold JC, Krackhardt F. Dislocation of a metal stent to the right ventricle: an unusual finding in the heart. J Cardiovasc Med (Hagerstown) 2008;9(7):742–743

Slonim SM, Dake MD, Razavi MK, et al. Management of misplaced or migrated endovascular stents. J Vasc Interv Radiol 1999;10(7):851–859

Taylor JD, Lehmann ED, Belli AM, et al. Strategies for the management of SVC stent migration into the right atrium. Cardiovasc Interv Radiol 2007;30(5):1003–1009

Toyoda N, Torregrossa G, Itagaki S, Pawale A, Reddy R. Intracardiac migration of vena caval stent: decision-making and treatment considerations. J Card Surg 2014;29(3):320–322

Warren MJ, Sen S, Marcus N. Management of migration of a SVC Wallstent into the right atrium. Cardiovasc Interv Radiol 2008;31(6):1262–1264

External iliac artery rupture during primary stenting

Patient History

An 85-year-old woman, mobile and in good general health, presented to the vascular surgery department for treatment of claudication in her left leg. A standardized treadmill test documented a pain-free walking distance of 100 m; however, the patient also complained of pain occurring during her regular dance tea afternoons. Noninvasive imaging showed a long occlusion of the left external iliac artery (EIA). The patient was referred to the Interventional Radiology Department and scheduled for angioplasty.

Initial Treatment Received

None.

Problems Encountered during Treatment

Following retrograde puncture of the left common femoral artery (CFA) and insertion of a 6F, 10-cm-

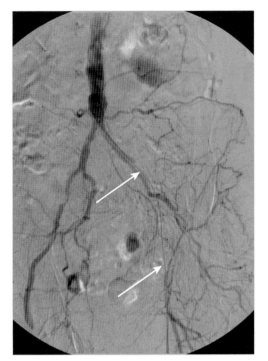

Fig. 4.332 DSA showing an occlusion of the left EIA (*arrows*) and a stenosis of the right EIA.

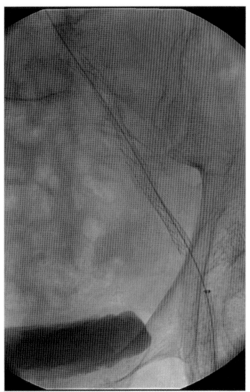

Fig. 4.333 Fluoroscopy image after balloon rupture showed a fully deployed stent with focal residual narrowing.

long standard sheath, the left EIA was passed with a 4F multipurpose catheter over a hydrophilic-coated 0.035-inch guidewire. Digital subtraction angiography (DSA) with a pigtail catheter in the infrarenal aorta confirmed the diagnosis of a 5-cm-long occlusion of the left EIA and a short-segment stenosis of the right EIA (**Fig. 4.332**). Because of the high plaque burden with heavy calcification it was decided to use primary stenting as the main treatment strategy. The diameter in the patent segment of the right EIA was 7 mm. Thus, a 7 × 60-mm balloon-expandable stent was positioned in the occluded vessel on the left side. The carrier balloon was inflated to its nominal pressure when suddenly the balloon burst and the patient complained of sharp and heavy pelvic pain. Fluoroscopy showed the stent deployed with mild residual narrowing (**Fig. 4.333**). DSA via the sheath revealed contrast extravasation into the retroperitoneal space (**Fig. 4.334**).

Imaging Plan

Angiography via the sheath.

Resulting Complication

Rupture of the left EIA.

Possible Strategies for Complication Management

- Balloon tamponade.
- Stent graft implantation.
- Embolization of the EIA with coils or plugs; and femorofemoral crossover bypass.
- Surgical repair (if endovascular approaches fail).

Final Complication Management

To seal the rupture site a 7-mm balloon was inflated instantly. A stent graft (covered nitinol 9 × 60 mm) was implanted and the rupture vessel was sealed (**Fig. 4.335**). The patient was hemodynamically compromised during the procedure, but responded well to fluid resuscitation. Postinterventional native computed tomography (CT) showed a moderate retroperitoneal hematoma reaching up to the left pararenal space (**Fig. 4.336**). The patient recovered and could resume her dance classes.

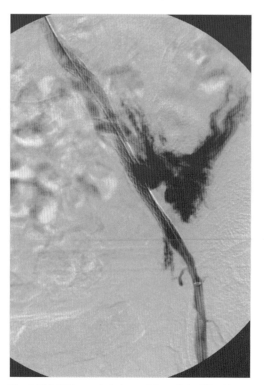

Fig. 4.334 DSA revealed a large defect of the EIA with extravasation.

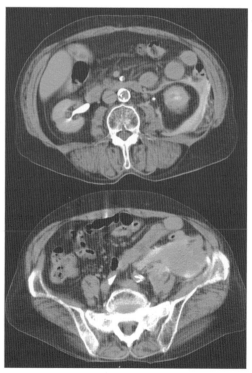

Fig. 4.336 Postinterventional native CT showed a moderate retroperitoneal hematoma reaching up to the left pararenal space.

Complication Analysis

Eccentric and heavily calcified lesions may lead to rupture of balloon catheters. When a balloon releases its nominal pressure of 8 atmospheres (atm; depending on the type of balloon) instantly into the vessel wall this can cause rupture. Modern high-pressure balloons feature very high-rated burst pressures of up to 18 atm and more. In clinical practice these pressures are sometimes reached for treatment of resistant lesions. In this case, rupture of a stent carrier balloon even at nominal pressure caused a large arterial defect and a potentially fatal hemorrhage. Instant balloon tamponade prevented serious cardiovascular compromise and the arterial injury was successfully sealed with a stent graft.

Prevention Strategies and Take-home Message

- Iliac artery rupture is a potentially fatal complication of angioplasty and stenting.
- Always be prepared for vessel rupture and have stent grafts available.
- Carefully choose the size of balloons and stents especially in heavily diseased arteries.

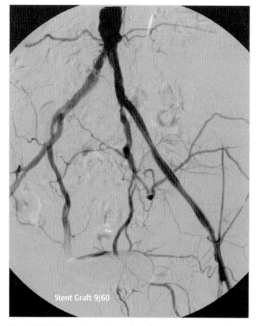

Stent Graft 9/60

Fig. 4.335 Control angiography after implantation of a stent graft; no active bleeding was detected.

Further Reading

Allaire E, Melliere D, Poussier B, Kobeiter H, Desgranges P, Becquemin JP. Iliac artery rupture during balloon dilatation: what treatment? Ann Vasc Surg 2003;17(3):306–314

Chong WK, Cross FW, Raphael MJ. Iliac artery rupture during percutaneous angioplasty. Clin Radiol 1990;41(5):358–359

Cooper SG, Sofocleous CT. Percutaneous management of angioplasty-related iliac artery rupture with preservation of luminal patency by prolonged balloon tamponade. J Vasc Interv Radiol 1998;9(1 pt 1):81–83

Formichi M, Raybaud G, Benichou H, Ciosi G. Rupture of the external iliac artery during balloon angioplasty: endovascular treatment using a covered stent. J Endovasc Surg 1998;5(1):37–41

Hamdan MF, Maguire BG, Walker MA. Balloon-expandable stent deformation during deployment into the iliac artery: a procedural complication managed conservatively. Vascular 2012;20(4):233–235

Kufner S, Cassese S, Groha P, et al. Covered stents for endovascular repair of iatrogenic injuries of iliac and femoral arteries. Cardiovasc Revasc Med 2015;16(3):158–162

Molpus WM, McCowan TC, Eidt JF. External iliac artery rupture during angioplasty: control by balloon tamponade. South Med J 1991;84(9):1138–1139

Ozkan U, Oguzkurt L, Tercan F. Technique, complication, and long-term outcome for endovascular treatment of iliac artery occlusion. Cardiovasc Interv Radiol 2010;33(1):18–24

Park JK, Oh SJ, Shin JY. Delayed rupture of the iliac artery after percutaneous angioplasty. Ann Vasc Surg 2014;28(2):491.e1–e4

Redman A, Cope L, Uberoi R. Iliac artery injury following placement of the memotherm arterial stent. Cardiovasc Interv Radiol 2001;24(2):113–116

Reed H, Shandall A, Ruttley M. Iliac artery rupture during percutaneous angioplasty. Clin Radiol 1991;43(2):142–143

Sato K, Orihashi K, Hamanaka Y, Hirai S, Mitsui N, Chatani N. Treatment of iliac artery rupture during percutaneous transluminal angioplasty: a report of three cases. Hiroshima J Med Sci 2011;60(4):83–86

Scheinert D, Ludwig J, Steinkamp HJ, Schröder M, Balzer JO, Biamino G. Treatment of catheter-induced iliac artery injuries with self-expanding endografts. J Endovasc Ther 2000;7(3):213–220

Trehan V, Nigam A, Ramakrishnan S. Cardiovasc Interv Radiol 2007;30(1):108–110

Vorwerk D, Günther RW. Percutaneous interventions for treatment of iliac artery stenoses and occlusions. World J Surg 2001;25(3):319–326

Yeo KK, Rogers JH, Laird JR. Use of stent grafts and coils in vessel rupture and perforation. J Interv Cardiol 2008;21(1):86–99

Zollikofer CL, Salomonowitz E, Castaneda-Zuniga WR, Brühlmann WF, Amplatz K. The relation between arterial and balloon rupture in experimental angioplasty. AJR Am J Roentgenol 1985;144(4):777–779

Malplaced popliteal artery stent treated with crush stenting

Patient History

An 82-year-old woman with a long history of peripheral vascular disease presented with recurrence of rest pain in her left leg 4 weeks after in-situ vein bypass surgery. Clinically the patient was in a Rutherford IIa stage of acute limb ischemia. By interdisciplinary consensus it was de-

cided to salvage the bypass and the limb by locoregional thrombolysis.

Initial Treatment Received

Following retrograde puncture of the right common femoral artery (CFA) and insertion of 5F sheath, the left iliac artery was accessed using a Rösch inferior mesenteric (RIM)-shaped catheter (Cordis/Johnson & Johnson) over a 0.035-inch guidewire. The catheter was exchanged for a multipurpose catheter, which was used to intubate the occluded femoral vein bypass over the hydrophilic-coated wire (**Fig. 4.337a–c**). A bolus of 5 mg recombinant tissue plasminogen activator (rtPA) was injected into the proximal aspect of the bypass and locoregional low-dose thrombolysis was initiated with a dose of 1 mg of rtPA per hour. Following a bolus of 5,000 IU of heparin the patient was also continued on IV heparin 1,000 IU per hour. Twenty-four hours after initiation of thrombolysis, control angiography showed successful recanalization of the bypass (**Fig. 4.338a–c**); however, there was mid- to high-grade stenosis of the second popliteal arterial segment. It was decided to treat this lesion endovascularly to maximize outflow for the vein bypass.

Problems Encountered during Treatment

After placement of a hydrophilic-coated guidewire into the popliteal artery, a 45-mm-long 6F sheath was positioned in the left CFA. A 6 × 600-mm self-expanding stent (SES) was advanced over the wire into the target lesion and postdilated with a 6 × 60-mm balloon catheter. Following stent deployment the initial angiographic control showed "slow flow" in the stented segment

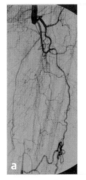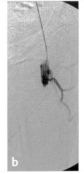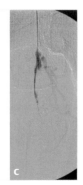

Fig. 4.337 **(a)** Acute occlusion of a femoral saphenous vein bypass. **(b)** Selective contrast injections in the CFA **(b)**. **(c)** Positioning of a multipurpose catheter in the proximal aspect of the bypass and application of a bolus of 5 mg rtPA.

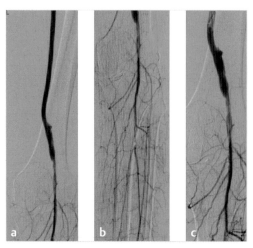

Fig. 4.338 (a–c) One day after initiation of long-term thrombolysis the vein bypass was fully patent. There was stenosis in the popliteal outflow vessel.

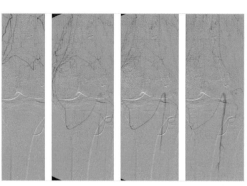

Fig. 4.340 RAO projection a few minutes after stent implantation shows functional occlusion of popliteal outflow. Note the distal wire position not following the course of the popliteal artery, but apparently located in a side branch.

(**Fig. 4.339**). Two minutes after implantation the second control in right anterior oblique (RAO) projection revealed total occlusion of the popliteal artery (**Fig. 4.340**). At this point the patient had already developed rest pain.

Imaging Plan

Selective angiography.

Resulting Complication

Stent occlusion. Due to a malpositioned guidewire the distal part of the stent had been implanted into a collateral of the popliteal artery (**Fig. 4.341**).

Possible Strategies for Complication Management

- Endovascular management with correction of guidewire position; passage of the malplaced

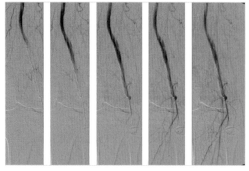

Fig. 4.339 First angiographic control after stent placement shows "slow flow."

stent outside the stent lumen; deployment of the second SES and angioplasty/crush stenting.
- Open surgical reconstruction, for example, infragenual bypass.

Final Complication Management

The malplaced stent was passed outside the stent struts using a Bern-shaped diagnostic catheter and a hydrophilic-coated guidewire (**Fig. 4.342**). The position of the intraluminal catheter distally to the stent in the popliteal artery was verified by direct contrast injection. A stiff, standard steel-core wire was used to bring a second longer SES (6 × 100 mm) into the target lesion. The device was postdilatated with a 6-mm balloon, which "crushed" the previously implanted stent (**Fig. 4.343**) and restored blood flow. Further long-term dilatation was able to achieve good patency with only mild residual stenosis (**Fig. 4.344**). The vein bypass and the new popliteal stent remained patent for at least 12 months, after which the patient was lost from follow-up.

Complication Analysis

Close review of the oblique images showed that the distal part of the guidewire had been positioned into a collateral artery, which coursed parallel to the popliteal artery in the posterior-anterior (PA) plane (**Fig. 4.345**). The distal end of the stent thus reached into the collateral and did not fully expand. The malplaced stent compromised flow and produced a functional occlusion. Because of the acute nature of the complication with instant onset of limb-threatening ischemia a prompt solution was needed. The minimally invasive endovascular approach with "crush stenting" was success-

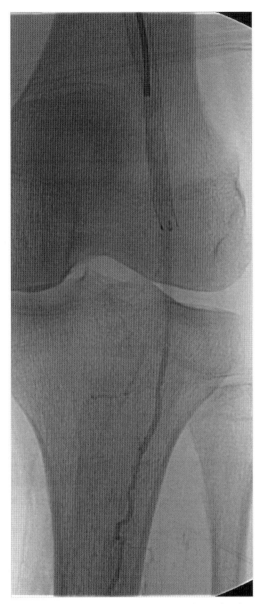

Fig. 4.341 Contrast injection directly into the popliteal artery confirms malpositioning of the distal stent, which is deployed inside a collateral artery.

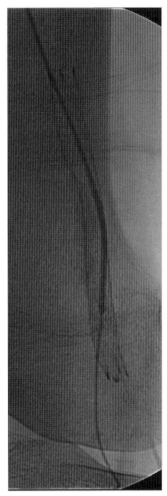

Fig. 4.342 Fluoroscopic image of the malplaced stent that has already been passed by a catheter and guidewire outside the stent lumen.

ful in restoring patency and completing the initial procedure.

J-shaped hydrophilic-coated guidewires are frequently used for peripheral interventions. They do have the tendency to run into side branches. In many cases the faulty position is obvious and easily visible in fluoroscopy. But sometimes, as in this case, the position appears correct in the working plane, especially, when the side branch "runs parallel" to the target vessel in a certain image projection. In order to rule out this pitfall, the working planes needs to be changed during the procedure. Only by doing that, looking at things from a different view/projection, can this complication be avoided. The correct catheter/ guidewire position can also be checked by selective contrast injections through the catheter once the target lesion has been recanalized.

A similar complication did occur a few weeks later in another institution although the above case had been personally communicated!

Prevention Strategies and Take-home Message

- Handle instruments with care. Always be familiar with the distal position of your guidewire.

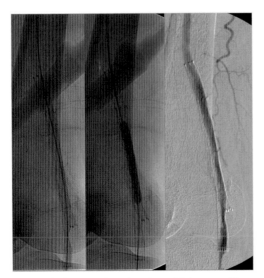

Fig. 4.343 Fluoroscopic and angiographic images of the popliteal artery after placement of a second stent and crush angioplasty.

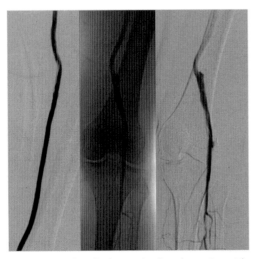

Fig. 4.344 Final result after popliteal crush stenting, with only mild residual stenosis.

- Change your angiographic plane during the procedure to make sure the guidewire position is correct in its entire course.
- Before stent placement check correct intraluminal catheter and wire position distally to the recanalized lesion, for example with injections through a Y-connector.
- Be aware that bizarre complications can occur even with experienced operators.

Further Reading

Cho YJ, Han SS, Lee SC. Guidewire malposition during central venous catheterization despite the use of ultrasound guidance. Korean J Anesthesiol 2013;64(5):469–471

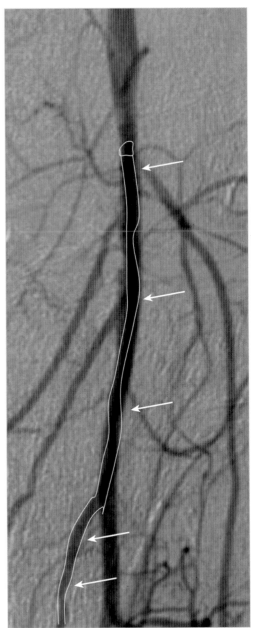

Fig. 4.345 Parallel course (*arrows*) of a collateral vessel to the popliteal artery in the PA plane—a dangerous pitfall.

Dawson DL, Terramani TT, Loberman Z, Lumsden AB, Lin PH. Simple technique to ensure coaxial guidewire positioning for placement of iliac limb of modular aortic endograft. J Interv Cardiol 2003;16(3):223–226

Vogel B, Strothmeyer A, Cebola R, Katus H, Blessing E. Crush implantation of a self-expanding interwoven stent over a subintimally recanalized standard stent in a TASC D lesion of the superficial femoral artery. Vasa 2012;41(6):458–462

Blind intraoperative subintimal stenting during thromboendarterectomy

Patient History

A 72-year-old man with subacute occlusion of both iliac arteries presented to the surgical department of a peripheral district hospital. The patient had a long history of peripheral vascular disease. In addition he was a heavy smoker and presented additional comorbidities like coronary heart disease, hypercholesterolemia, and diabetes mellitus.

Initial Treatment Received

Following bilateral surgical groin access, operative iliac thromboendarterectomy (TEA) was performed using Fogarty catheters and ring-stripper devices.

Problems Encountered during Treatment

Because no adequate flow could be established, balloon-expandable stents were implanted intraoperatively into both external iliac arteries. However, the procedure failed and patency was not restored. The patient was transported to a tertiary referral hospital for endovascular treatment.

Imaging Plan

Transbrachial angiography.

Resulting Complication

Digital subtraction angiography (DSA) via a left transbrachial route revealed an occlusion of the right external iliac artery (EIA) and a subtotal stenosis of the left EIA (**Fig. 4.346**). Apparently, stents had been implanted subintimally (**Fig. 4.347**).

Possible Strategies for Complication Management

- Endovascular recanalization and stenting.
- Open aortobifemoral bypass surgery.

Final Complication Management

Following placement of a 90-cm-long 6F sheath into the infrarenal aorta, the left EIA was recanalized using a 125-cm-long multipurpose catheter and a 0.035-inch hydrophilic-coated

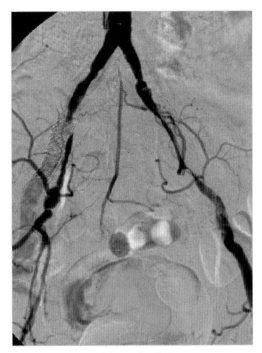

Fig. 4.346 DSA via a left transbrachial access route revealed occlusion of the right EIA and subtotal occlusion of the left EIA.

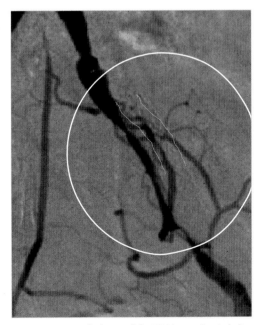

Fig. 4.347 Magnified view of the DSA image (*encircled*) shows a subintimally placed stent in the left EIA.

guidewire. Correct true-lumen catheter position was confirmed with direct contrast injections (**Fig. 4.348**). Two balloon-expandable stents were implanted intraluminally and patency was restored (**Fig. 4.349**). On the right the occlusion of the subintimally stented EIA could not be passed from the transbrachial approach (**Fig. 4.350**). Thus, the right common femoral artery (CFA) was punctured and a 6F sheath was inserted. Multiple attempts to reach the true vessel lumen of the right common iliac artery (CIA) from the retrograde approach failed. Then, a 6F re-entry catheter (Outback, Cordis/Johnson & Johnson) was used to create access to the true lumen of the CIA (**Fig. 4.351a–d**). Once this was achieved, a balloon-expandable stent was implanted and patency successfully restored. Computed tomography angiography (CTA) during follow-up showed the previously implanted stents in a subintimal position, crushed by the new correctly implanted stents (**Fig. 4.352**).

Complication Analysis

Following failed surgical TEA, stents had been implanted in the operating room with low-quality C-arm technology in a more or less "blind" fashion. Failed visualization of catheter and wire positions resulted in subintimal stent placement. This complication was managed endovascularly via a transbrachial approach and by additional stent placement in "crush-stenting" technique.

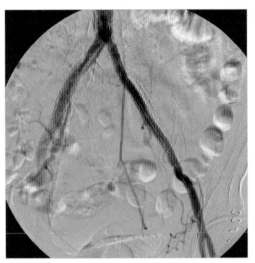

Fig. 4.349 Fully restored patency of the left iliac artery after additional stent placement.

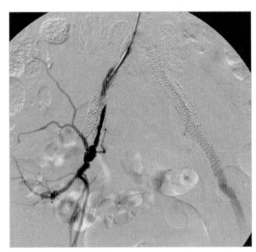

Fig. 4.350 Failed attempts to recanalize the right EIA from a transbrachial approach.

Prevention Strategies and Take-home Message

- Endovascular procedures for treatment of complex aortoiliac disease should be performed using state-of-the art angiographic equipment.
- An "endovascular first" approach should be considered for all aortoiliac lesions regardless of TASC (TransAtlantic Inter-Society Consensus) classification.
- Arterial occlusions due to subintimally placed stents can be corrected by endovascular means using modern technology (e.g., re-entry catheters, crush stenting) and alternative vascular access routes.

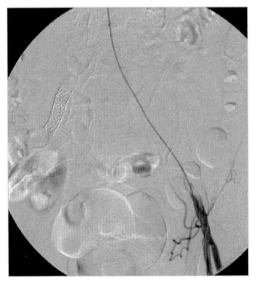

Fig. 4.348 Successful recanalization of the left EIA and documentation of intraluminal catheter position.

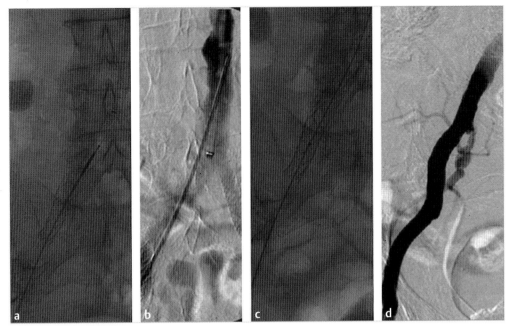

Fig. 4.351 (a) Retrograde recanalization of the right iliac artery using a re-entry device. **(b)** Documentation of correct intraluminal catheter position. **(c,d)** Fluoroscopic and angiographic result after additional stent placement.

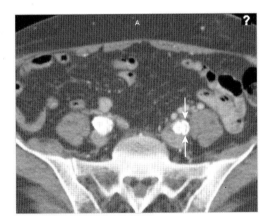

Fig. 4.352 CTA following endovascular bail-out procedure. Patent iliac arteries on both sides. Note the crushed subintimal stent (*arrows*) on the left.

Further Reading

De Donato G, Bosiers M, Setacci F, et al. 24-month data from the BRAVISSIMO: a large-scale prospective registry on iliac stenting for TASC A & B and TASC C & D lesions. Ann Vasc Surg 2015;29(4):738–750

Vogel B, Strothmeyer A, Cebola R, Katus H, Blessing E. Crush implantation of a self-expanding interwoven stent over a subintimally recanalized standard stent in a TASC D lesion of the superficial femoral artery. Vasa 2012;41(6):458–462

4.3.5 Special Procedures and Tools

Endovascular Abdominal and Thoracic Aneurysm Repair

Unexpected covering of a main renal artery during endovascular aneurysm repair

Patient History

A 62-year-old man with a 5.5-cm infrarenal aortic aneurysm was scheduled for interdisciplinary endovascular aneurysm repair (EVAR). Based on computed tomography (CT) scan the measurement for a standard aortobiiliacal prosthesis was performed. It was decided that the entire infrarenal neck should be covered by the covered part of the prosthesis in order to avoid the risk of type 1 endoleak. The angles for the angiographic planes during implantation, such as in the craniocaudal and the oblique plane, were measured; it was communicated that the origin of the right renal artery was some millimeters lower (caudal) than the contralateral one.

Initial Treatment Received

Following surgical cut-down of the left and right groin, the main body of the prosthesis was inserted from the right groin and angiographic control of final deployment of the suprarenal fixation was done via a pigtail catheter placed through the contralateral groin. When the main body was placed and deployed completely and catheterization of the contralateral limb was performed successfully, the contralateral limb was inserted and deployed. Final angiography after dilatating the two prosthesis components depicted a complete covering of the right renal artery without any contrast media filling (**Fig. 4.353**).

Problems Encountered during Treatment

Incidental, complete covering of the right renal artery by the cover of the endoprosthesis.

Imaging Plan

Fluoroscopy in order to depict the exact location of the cover and estimating the exact origin of the renal artery. Trying to achieve contrast media filling of the artery for further evaluation

Resulting Complication

Acute, iatrogenic occlusion of a main renal artery.

Possible Strategies for Complication Management

- Trying to perform a pulling maneuver of the prosthesis main body, after threading a guidewire from one groin to the other one and pulling carefully at both ends; this procedure is unlikely to be successful because the prosthesis of the hooks has already fixed the main body at the suprarenal aortic level.
- Endovascular treatment via ipsilateral retrograde approach using the existing access coming from the right or left groin to try to engage the renal artery; that is, with right internal mammary catheter in combination with a 0.014- or 0.018-inch guidewire. Once access is successful, a direct stenting procedure can be performed in order to achieve inflow in the artery again by pushing away the cover with the expanded stainless steal stent.
- Endovascular treatment via a transbrachial access, followed by the procedural steps as mentioned above.
- Immediate explant of the prosthesis by surgery (open conversion).

Final Complication Management

Endovascular treatment via a left transbrachial approach. Once a 6F 90-cm-long sheath was placed, catheterization of the right renal artery was successful with a 4F multipurpose catheter in combination with a 0.014-inch catheter (**Fig. 4.354**). Direct stent advancement failed and direct access to the renal artery beyond the cover failed except with the already placed 0.014-inch wire. Therefore, a second 0.014-inch wire was placed via the multipurpose catheter (buddy wire technique) in order to achieve more support for further procedural steps such as predilatation with

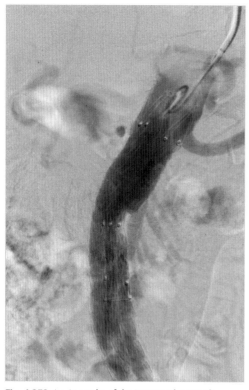

Fig. 4.353 Angiography of the juxtarenal aorta after placing a pigtail catheter from a transbrachial approach. Note, the left-side renal artery shows an uncompromised contrast media filling, whereas the right side is not enhanced.

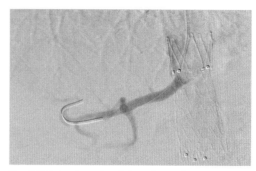

Fig. 4.354 Angiography of the right renal artery via a multipurpose catheter placed at the beginning of the prosthesis cover; note, a 0.014-inch wire is already placed in the renal artery.

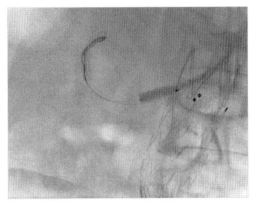

Fig. 4.355 Fluoroscopy during repeated predilatation with a 4 × 40-mm monorail balloon; a second 0.014-inch wire is already in place.

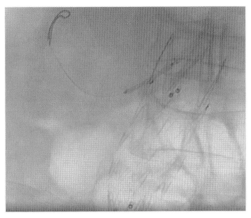

Fig. 4.357 Fluoroscopy showing the stent (6 × 18 mm) already in place centered at the renal ostium.

a 4 × 40-mm monorail balloon (**Fig. 4.355**). Stent placement failed once again. The ballooning procedure was repeated, and the sheath could then be advanced into the renal artery (**Fig. 4.356**). Then, the balloon-expandable stent was repositioned centrally toward the ostium, and the sheath was removed carefully, keeping the stent in a stable position (**Fig. 4.357**). Stent deployment was then performed (**Fig. 4.358**) and final angiography showed an unrestricted flow into the renal artery (**Fig. 4.359**).

Complication Analysis

Suspected uncontrolled and too-fast stent graft delivery or failure to interpret the final position of the covered part of the endoprosthesis resulted in incidental covering of a main renal artery by the prosthesis cover.

Prevention Strategies and Take-home Message

- Take your time for stent graft positioning and delivery.
- Try to handle systolic blood pressure at lower levels of around 90 to 100 mm Hg.
- Advise the patient to hold their breath for difficult procedural steps like positioning the prosthesis (or in case of general anesthesia, advise the anesthesiologist to hold patients' breath).
- Especially in difficult or complex anatomies, make an angiographic control before final prosthesis delivery to rule out that catheter or patient position has changed since the last run.
- In unclear situations, change angiographic projection in order to bring the marker (as in

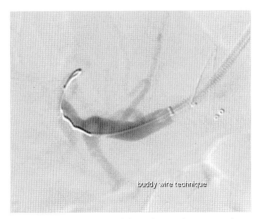

Fig. 4.356 Angiography of the right renal artery via the 6F sheath, which has already passed the prosthesis and entered the main renal artery.

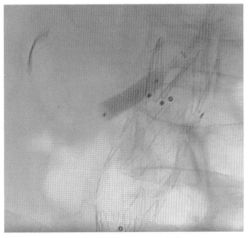

Fig. 4.358 Fluoroscopy of the inflated balloon–stent device at 8 atmospheres.

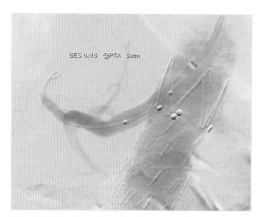

Fig. 4.359 Final angiography after stent deployment. Wire and deflated balloon are still in place.

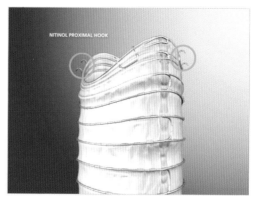

Fig. 4.360 "Fish mouth" design of the top end of the Aorfix graft with nitinol proximal hooks for infrarenal fixation.

the used device) into a horizontal line in order to determine and predict the final landing zone of the covered prosthesis part.

Further Reading

Adu J, Cheshire NJ, Riga CV, Hamady M, Bicknell CD. Strategies to tackle unrecognized bilateral renal artery occlusion after endovascular aneurysm repair. Ann Vasc Surg 2012;26(8):1127.e1–e7

Bracale UM, Giribono AM, Vitale G, Narese D, Santini G, Del Guercio L. Accidental coverage of both renal arteries during infrarenal aortic stent graft implantation: cause and treatment. Case Rep Vasc Med 2014;2014:710742

Hedayati N, Lin PH, Lumsden AB, Zhou W. Prolonged renal artery occlusion after endovascular aneurysm repair: endovascular rescue and renal function salvage. J Vasc Surg 2008;47(2):446–449

Hiramoto JS, Chang CK, Reilly LM, Schneider DB, Rapp JH, Chuter TA. Outcome of renal stenting for renal artery coverage during endovascular aortic aneurysm repair. J Vasc Surg 2009;49(5):1100–1106

Endoprosthesis migration during endovascular aneurysm repair— proximal type 1A endoleak management

Patient History

An abdominal aortic aneurysm (AAA) with a maximum diameter of 6.8 cm was detected in a 68-year-old man. Comorbidities included arterial hypertension, diabetes mellitus, and chronic obstructive pulmonary disease.

Initial Treatment Received

Endovascular abdominal aortic aneurysm repair. It was decided to use a flexible device due to neck angulation and flaring and in this context the Aorfix endograft (Lombard Medical) was selected as the most suitable device with those features. Aorfix is

an extremely flexible modular device composed of a circular nitinol frame covered by a woven polyester fabric. The top end of the Aorfix graft has a "fish mouth" for infrarenal fixation and requires accurate orientation of the graft (**Fig. 4.360**). Ideally the graft should be deployed with the troughs embracing the renal ostia and the anterior peak of the fish mouth positioned below the origin of the superior mesenteric origin (**Fig. 4.361**).

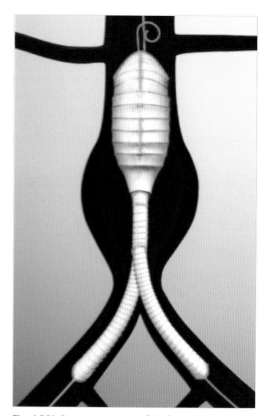

Fig. 4.361 Proper positioning of Aorfix endograft.

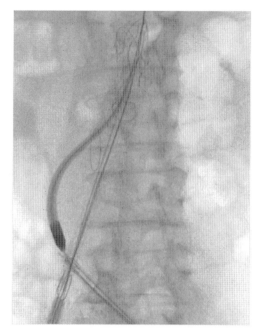

Fig. 4.362 Endograft twist during cannulation of the contralateral limb socket.

Problems Encountered during Treatment

During cannulation of the contralateral limb there was some endograft twist (**Fig. 4.362**) and, following endograft deployment, final angiography demonstrated caudal migration of the graft associated with a large proximal type 1A endoleak (**Fig. 4.363**).

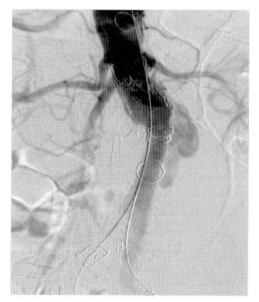

Fig. 4.363 Caudal migration of the graft associated with a large proximal type 1A endoleak.

Imaging Plan

Intraoperative digital subtraction angiography (DSA).

Resulting Complication

Type Ia endoleak.

Possible Strategies for Complication Management

- Balloon remodeling.
- Use of various extender cuffs.
- Bare stents (e.g., the giant Palmaz stent P4014 or P5014 [Cordis/Johnson & Johnson]).
- Obliteration of the lumen with coils, glue, thrombin, or other embolic agents, such as N-BCA (Trufill, Cordis) "glue" or Onyx (Ev3).
- Conversion to open repair (if endovascular approach fails).

Final Complication Management

The endoleak was fixed immediately with endovascular placement of an Aorfix proximal extender (cuff). The cuff is a short implant that has four pairs of barbs, a seam, and a fish mouth shape identical to the primary graft (**Figs. 4.364–4.367**).

Complication Analysis

Endograft twist during rigorous cannulation of the contralateral limb.

Prevention Strategies and Take-home Message

- Although relatively uncommon, significant endograft migration and/or twisting can occur during initial deployment.
- Never use excessive force during cannulation of the contralateral limb socket especially in flexible endografts like the Aorfix, as there is a high risk of pushing up and distorting the whole device.
- In order to keep proper orientation of the "fish mouth" proximal end of the endograft, always keep it in the field of view when alterations are made at the distal end of the endograft.
- Ensure that a member of the sterile team is holding the main delivery system and keeping it in place during cannulation of the contralateral limb socket!
- Always try endovascular techniques first for fixation of type 1 endoleaks.

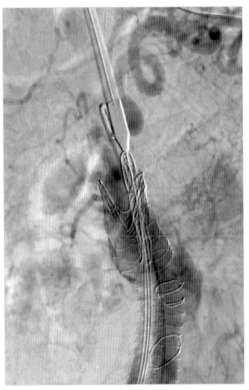

Fig. 4.364 Proper positioning of a 38-mm-long extender cuff before deployment.

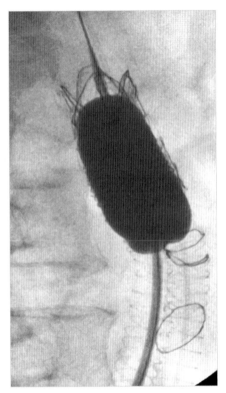

Fig. 4.366 Ballooning of the fully deployed extender cuff.

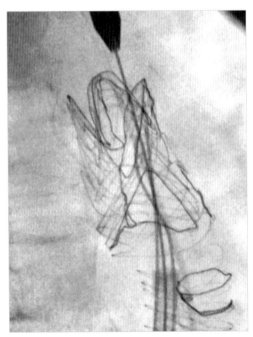

Fig. 4.365 Fully deployed extender cuff.

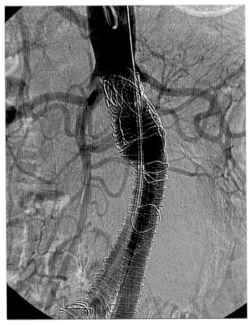

Fig. 4.367 Final intraoperative DSA demonstrates no type 1A endoleak.

Further Reading

Bastos Goncalves F, Hoeks SE, Teijink JA, et al. Risk factors for proximal neck complications after endovascular aneurysm repair using the endurant stentgraft. Eur J Vasc Endovasc Surg 2015;49(2):156–162

Bryce Y, Rogoff P, Romanelli D, Reichle R. Endovascular repair of abdominal aortic aneurysms: vascular anatomy, device selection, procedure, and procedure-specific complications. Radiographics 2015;35(2):593–615

Jayia P, Constantinou J, Morgan-Rowe L, Schroeder TV, Lonn L, Ivancev K. Are there fewer complications with third generation endografts in endovascular aneurysm repair? J Cardiovasc Surg (Torino) 2013;54(1):133–143

Valente T, Rossi G, Rea G, Pinto A, Romano L, Davies J, Scaglione M. Multidetector CT findings of complications of surgical and endovascular treatment of aortic aneurysms. Radiol Clin North Am 2014;52(5):961–989

Detachment and dislocation of iliac artery plaque into the abdominal aorta after thoracic endovascular aneurysm repair

Patient History

A 69-year-old woman, previously a smoker, with a history of hypertension, underwent investigation for an aneurysm of the descending thoracic aorta (TAA) with a maximum diameter of 61 mm extending 26 cm from D3 to D12. The TAA had been discovered 3 years previously and its maximum diameter had progressively increased (> 6 mm in the previous year). Multidetector computed tomography angiography (CTA) was performed to evaluate the morphology of the aorta and of the iliofemoral axis (**Fig. 4.368**).

Initial Treatment Received

Based on the CTA images and clinical signs, a multidisciplinary team decided in favor of an endovascular treatment with the insertion of two Zenith TX2 devices (Cook Medical). Via a percutaneous right common femoral artery (CFA) approach, a 5F calibrated pigtail catheter was inserted into the thoracic aorta for contrast medium injections. Surgical exposure of the left CFA was carried out. Due to high calcification in the femoroiliac vessels, a Zenith TX2 stent graft was selected because of the presence of a hydrophilic coating on its external surface. The morphology of the thoracic aorta, with a caliber of 34 mm in the proximal landing zone and 29 mm in the distal portion, suggested the insertion of two Zenith TX stent grafts, 38 mm and 40 mm in diameter, respectively. The first stent graft (38 × 186 mm)

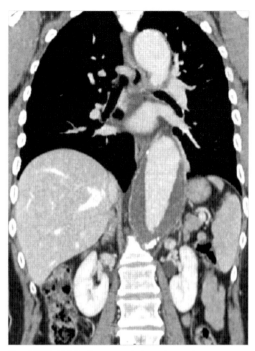

Fig. 4.368 CTA in the coronal plane shows the presence of an aneurysm of the descending thoracic aorta extending 26 cm from D3 to D12.

was released 25 mm distally to the origin of the left subclavian artery (LSA) while the second (40 × 126 mm), deployed at a lower level, landed in the abdominal aorta, just above the origin of the superior mesenteric artery (SMA), as the coeliac trunk was occluded. The two stent grafts were positioned with an overlap of > 5 cm to avoid misinsertion of the two components during the follow-up. A dilatation of the proximal and distal portions of the stent grafts, as well as of the overlapping area, was performed using a balloon catheter (Coda, Cook Medical).

Digital subtraction angiography (DSA) was done at the end of the procedure and it confirmed the complete exclusion of the aneurysm and regular blood flow within the abdominal aorta, the SMA, and the iliac and femoral arteries. Surgical reconstruction of the left CFA was performed, while the right femoral access was managed with manual compression. The postprocedure period was uneventful and 3 days later the patient was discharged in good clinical condition.

Problems Encountered during Treatment

At 1-month follow-up, a CTA showed the presence of some calcified material inside the abdominal

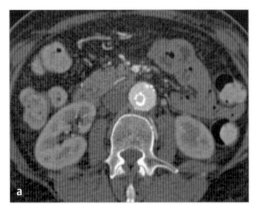
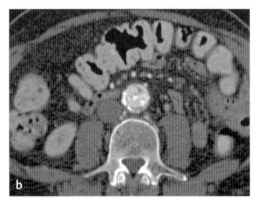

Fig. 4.369 CTA performed at 1-month follow-up showed complete exclusion of the aneurysm along the descending aorta. At the level of the abdominal aorta, below the origin of the renal arteries, some calcified material was spotted within the aortic lumen (a, b). The blood flow was regular.

aorta, below the origin of the renal arteries (Fig. 4.369a, b). The blood flow was normal within the two stent grafts and no endoleak was present. During a thorough analysis, complete absence of calcification was observed in the left common iliac artery (CIA) in a context of diffuse vasculopathy associated with multiple arterial calcifications.[1,2,3] The calcified material, which was floating in the abdominal aorta, was interpreted as calcified intima detached from the iliac arterial wall and was assumed to be secondary to the passage of the stent graft devices (Fig. 4.370a, b).

Imaging Plan

Not applicable.

Resulting Complication

No acute consequence, but potential risk of distal embolization.

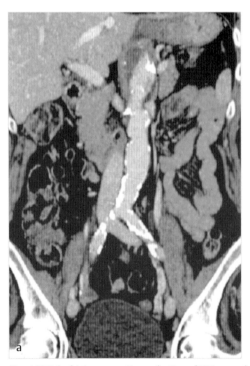
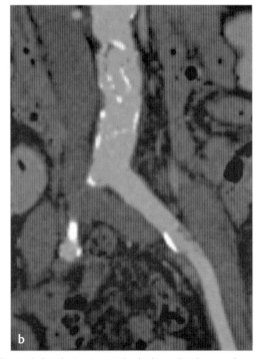

Fig. 4.370 (a, b) A comparative evaluation of CT images before and after the treatment clearly shows the absence of calcium along the arterial wall of the left CIA. Calcified material in the lower portion of the abdominal aorta is also visible.

Possible Strategies for Complication Management

- Conservative treatment with medical therapy (aspirin 100 mg/day).
- Endovascular treatment with the insertion of a stent graft below the origin of the renal arteries.
- Surgery (if above approaches fail).

Final Complication Management

As the patient was completely asymptomatic, a multidisciplinary (vascular surgeons, cardiothoracic surgeons, and interventional radiologists) discussion led to the decision to keep the patient on aspirin therapy and to perform CTA during the follow-up on a regular basis, every 6 months in the first year and then annually. At 4-year follow-up the patient was in good clinical condition without any symptoms, and the CTA showed no significant imaging modifications (**Fig. 4.371**). A progressive shrinkage of the thoracic aneurysm (from 61 mm to 40 mm maximum diameter) was also observed.

Complication Analysis

As a consequence of the large caliber of the thoracic aortic stent graft devices, with an outer diameter ranging from 20 to 26F, several complications at the level of the entry site have been reported, such as arterial rupture, arterial dissection, and arterial stenosis.[4,5] The complications described above were undoubtedly correlated with the high amount of calcium in the iliac arteries. The hydrophilic coating of the devices reduces

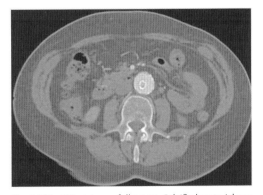

Fig. 4.371 CTA at 4-year follow-up. Calcified material can clearly be seen in the same place in the abdominal aorta. No modifications of aorta morphology can be observed and there is no alteration of the flow within the inner lumen.

friction during insertion but it can potentially increase the risk of plaque mobilization, as occurred in this case.

Prevention Strategies and Take-home Message

- Continuous fluoroscopic control of the insertion devices is mandatory because the hydrophilic coating reduces the resistance the operator is able to feel.

References

1. Heilmaier C, Koester A, Moysidis T, Weishaupt D, Kröger K. Abdominal aortic calcification and its distribution in normal-sized and aneurysmatic abdominal aortas. Vasa 2014;43(2):132–140
2. Chuang ML, Leslie RW, Massaro JM, et al. Distribution of abdominal aortic calcium by computed tomography: impact of analysis method on quantitative calcium score. Acad Radiol 2013;20(11):1422–1428
3. Hofmann Bowman MA, McNally EM. Genetic pathways of vascular calcification. Trends Cardiovasc Med 2012;22(4):93–98
4. Toggweiler S, Leipsic J, Binder RK, et al. Management of vascular access in transcatheter aortic valve replacement: part 2: Vascular complications. JACC Cardiovasc Interv 2013;6(8):767–776
5. Tsetis D. Endovascular treatment of complications of femoral arterial access. Cardiovasc Interv Radiol 2010;33(3):457–468

Endovascular aneurysm repair type 1 endoleak due to inadequate sealing at the proximal end

Patient History

In a 68-year-old man with a past medical history of hypertension and dyslipidemia, an abdominal aortic aneurysm (AAA) was diagnosed during a routine ultrasound examination of the abdomen. Multidetector computed tomography angiography (CTA) was undertaken to evaluate the morphology of the aorta and of the iliofemoral axis.

Transverse dimension of the AAA was 4.5 cm and longitudinal diameter was 8 cm; length and diameter of the aneurysmal neck were 29 mm and 34 mm, respectively. The patient was scheduled for endovascular aneurysm repair (EVAR).

Initial Treatment Received

Because of the tortuous course and small diameter of the iliac arteries an Ovation Prime

Abdominal Stent Graft System (TriVascular) was selected—a trimodular device designed with the aortic body delivered via a flexible, hydrophilic-coated, ultra–low-profile catheter (14F outer diameter). The aortic body is composed of a proximal bare nitinol stent for suprarenal fixation and a polytetrafluoroethylene (PTFE) graft. For proximal sealing and appropriate support to the aortic body legs into which the iliac limbs are deployed, the graft body contains a system of inflatable ring tubes. These tubes are filled with a liquid polymer that solidifies after being injected to inflate these rings. The radial force of the stents provides both fixation and sealing between the aortic body and the distal landing zone in the iliac vessels.

As the size of the stent graft device was small, two Prostar XLs (Abbott Vascular) were preimplanted at the level of both common femoral arteries (CFAs).

On the right side, the aortic main body was introduced over an extra-stiff guidewire (Lunderquist, Cook Medical). On the left side, a 5F pigtail catheter was positioned in the suprarenal aorta, to make contrast medium injections.

The aortic body section (29 × 80 mm diameter) was deployed and followed by polymer injection to provide an effective sealing. When the polymer hardened (20 min), contralateral (18 × 100 mm) and ipsilateral stent graft extensions (16 × 100 mm) were deployed.

The following digital subtraction angiography (DSA) showed an incomplete exclusion of the aneurysm due to an endoleak from the proximal (type 1A) attachment site (**Fig. 4.372a, b**).

Problems Encountered during Treatment

An endoleak is defined as persistent blood flow outside the graft and within an aneurysm sac. In this case, a type 1 endoleak occurred because of inadequate sealing at the proximal end of the endoprosthesis (type 1A).

Imaging Plan

Not applicable.

Resulting Complication

Type 1 endoleaks are known to be associated with high sac pressure, aneurysmal dilatation, and rupture of aneurysm; therefore, treatment at the time of diagnosis is recommended. Generally

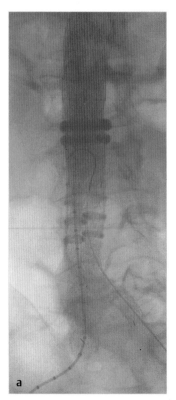

a

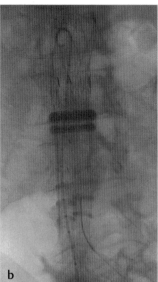

b

Fig. 4.372 **(a, b)** DSA showed an incomplete exclusion of the aneurysm due to an endoleak from the proximal (type 1A) attachment site.

speaking, a type 1 endoleak requires immediate surgical conversion due to the high risk of aneurysm dilatation and rupture.

Possible Strategies for Complication Management

- Endovascular treatment: proximal stent graft insertion, aneurysm sac embolization.
- Surgical conversion.

Final Complication Management

A proximal stent graft extension (32 mm diameter—Excluder, WL Gore & Associates) was deployed at the level of the aneurysmal neck, below the origin of the renal arteries and dilatated using a compliant balloon catheter (Coda, Cook Medical) (**Fig. 4.373**).

Subsequent angiogram showed persistence of blood flow into the aneurysmal sac.

As the patient was considered unfit for surgery, an endovascular attempt was made. Surgery was also considered difficult for the structural characteristics of the Ovation stent graft.

A microcatheter (2.7F Progreat, Terumo) was advanced into the space between the stent graft and the aortic wall (**Fig. 4.374**) and then the endoleak was treated with microcoil embolization and Onyx (Medtronic) liquid embolic system injection (**Fig. 4.375a, b**).

An angiogram was done at the end of the procedure and it confirmed the complete exclusion of the aneurysm.

At 1-year follow-up, the patient was in good clinical condition, without any symptoms, and at

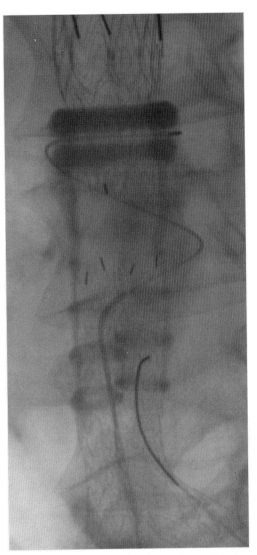

Fig. 4.374 A microcatheter (2.7F) was advanced into the space between the stent graft and the aortic wall.

3 years CTA showed no recurrence of type 1 endoleak or sac expansion (**Fig. 4.376**).

Complication Analysis

Type 1 endoleaks are caused by an inadequate seal at the proximal and distal ends of a stent graft. They result in a rupture of the aneurysm for the presence of persistent blood flow in the aneurysmal sac. Treatment at the time of diagnosis is recommended.

An early (periprocedural) endoleak is defined as one that is found on completion angiography immediately after EVAR. An early endoleak (peri-

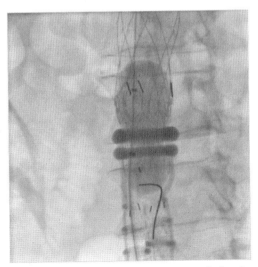

Fig. 4.373 Proximal stent graft extension was deployed at the level of the aneurysmal neck and then dilatated using a compliant balloon catheter.

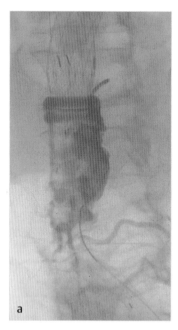

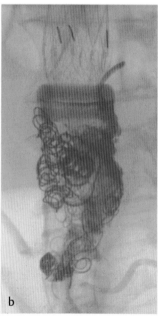

Fig. 4.375 (a, b) The endoleak was treated with microcoil embolization and Onyx.

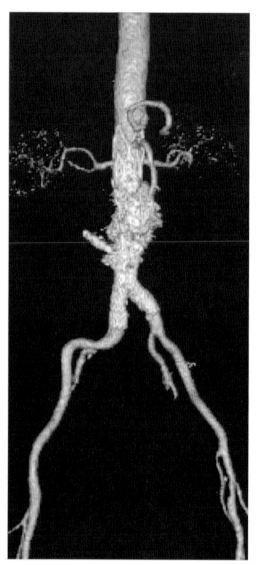

Fig. 4.376 Three-year CTA showed no recurrence of type 1 endoleak or sac expansion.

procedural) can be found when angiography is on the way to be completed immediately after EVAR. It is distinguished from a delayed endoleak that occurs during the follow-up. The prognosis of type 1 endoleaks is serious and surgical conversion or endovascular treatment are mandatory and urgent.

Prevention Strategies and Take-home Message

- Preoperative planning and patient selection are important to prevent type 1 endoleaks.
- Several morphologic risk factors have been reported to be risk factors for type 1 endoleaks, including a large aneurysm, and a heavily calcified, angulated and wide neck.
- Intraoperative factors, such as type of stent graft, stent graft oversizing, and residual uncovered landing zones, are reported to be causes of graft migration and type 1 endoleaks.

Further Reading

Chun JY, Morgan R. Transcatheter embolisation of type 1 endoleaks after endovascular aortic aneurysm repair with Onyx: when no other treatment option is feasible. Eur J Vasc Endovasc Surg 2013;45(2):141–144

Faries PL, Cadot H, Agarwal G, Kent KC, Hollier LH, Marin ML. Management of endoleak after endovascular aneurysm repair: cuffs, coils, and conversion. J Vasc Surg 2003;37(6):1155–1161

Ghouri M, Krajcer Z. Endoluminal abdominal aortic aneurysm repair: the latest advances in prevention of distal endograft migration and type 1 endoleak. Tex Heart Inst J 2010;37(1):19–24

Hobo R, Kievit J, Leurs LJ, Buth J; EUROSTAR collaborators. Influence of severe infrarenal aortic neck angulation on complications at the proximal neck following endovascular AAA repair: a EUROSTAR study. J Endovasc Ther 2007;14(1):1–11

Kim SM, Ra HD, Min SI, Jae HJ, Ha J, Min SK. Clinical significance of type 1 endoleak on completion angiography. Ann Surg Treat Res 2014;86(2):95–99

Venermo MA, Arko FR III, Salenius JP, Saarinen JP, Zvaigzne A, Zarins CK. EVAR may reduce the risk of aneurysm rupture despite persisting type 1a endoleaks. J Endovasc Ther 2011;18(5):676–682

Pressure gradient after stent graft repair of the descending thoracic aorta

Patient History

A 31-year-old man with history of a car accident and rupture of the thoracic descending aorta at the level of the isthmus underwent stent graft repair with a Relay stent graft (Bolton Medical). The procedure was technically uneventful and postprocedure imaging demonstrated exclusion of the traumatic injury.

Three years after the initial event he suffered of weakness, bilateral claudication (ankle-brachial index [ABI] 0.6), headache, and visual impairment.

He underwent a computed tomography angiography (CTA) that showed a filling defect within the lumen of the stent graft in the distal portion (**Fig. 4.377a–c**). This was correlated with thrombus formation or focal dissection.

The patient was admitted and clinical evaluation showed severe hypertension in the upper extremities (BP 180/110 mm Hg) and hypotension in the lower extremities (BP 108/70 mm Hg).

An endovascular reintervention was decided upon after multidisciplinary discussion.

Initial Treatment Received

CTA showed an anomalous flow within the stent graft, in the distal portion. Thrombus apposition or focal dissection was suspected.

A transesophageal echocardiogram (TEE) was also performed but final diagnosis was still unclear.

Problems Encountered during Treatment

This remains unclear.

Imaging Plan

An angiography was planned to evaluate the hemodynamic characteristics of the blood flow within the stent graft.

Resulting Complication

The presence of a pressure gradient between the upper and lower extremities should be correlated with flow impairment within the thoracic stent graft.

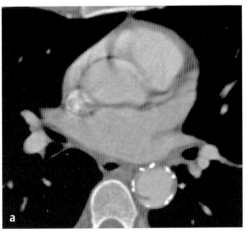
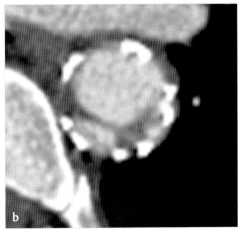

Fig. 4.377 (a–c) CTA images on the axial plan showed the presence of a filling defect within the stent graft. Above this area no alterations were evident. (*continued*)

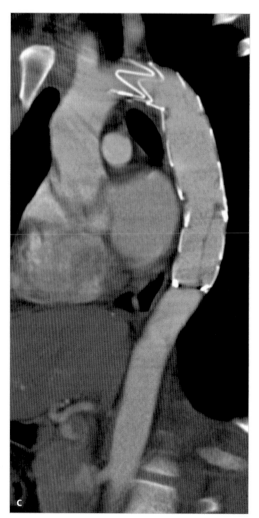

Fig. 4.377 (*continued*) **(a–c)** CTA images on the axial plan showed the presence of a filling defect within the stent graft. Above this area no alterations were evident.

Possible Strategies for Complication Management

- Wait and see.
- Medical therapy (anticoagulant).
- Endovascular treatment:[1]
  - angioplasty;
  - stenting (relining) with stent graft or bare stent;
  - a combination of the two above;
  - distal extension of the stent graft.
- Surgical conversion.[2]

Final Complication Management

Reintervention by implantation of a Valiant endograft (26 × 22 × 150 mm, Medtronic) inside the previous one. Digital subtraction angiography (DSA) after the insertion of the second stent graft showed a severe residual stenosis at the level of the diseased segment (**Fig. 4.378**). The stent graft was postdilatated using a Reliant aortic balloon (Medtronic) (**Fig. 4.379**). The second stent graft was deployed, extending around 2 cm below the previous one. DSA performed at the end of the procedure showed a good position of the stent graft without any alteration of the blood flow along all the descending aorta (**Fig. 4.380**).

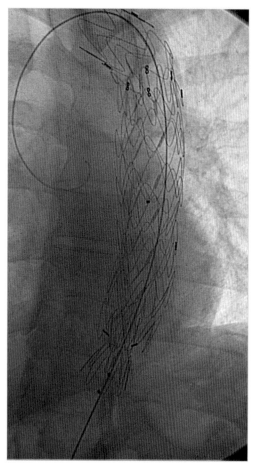

Fig. 4.378 Digital subtraction angiography (DSA) after the insertion of the second stent graft showed a severe residual stenosis at the level of the diseased segment.

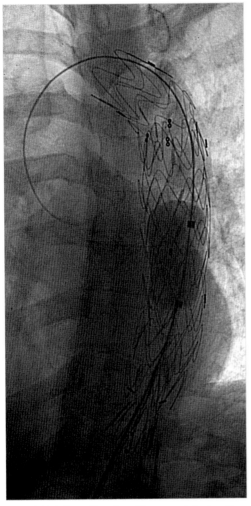

Fig. 4.379 Balloon dilatation of the second stent graft using a dedicated balloon.

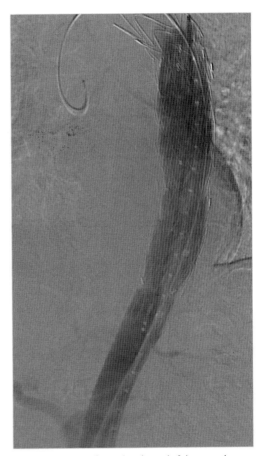

Fig. 4.380 DSA performed at the end of the procedure showed a good position of the stent graft without any alteration of the blood flow along all the descending aorta.

Complication Analysis

Late formation of thrombus/dissection at the edge of a thoracic stent graft is a rare complication.[2]

After stent graft deployment, a regular flow within the stent was observed at CTA performed 1 week after the procedure.

The absence of gradient pressure between upper and lower extremities at the end of the procedure was a clear sign of good management of the complication.

Prevention Strategies and Take-home Message

- This is a rare complication and difficult to predict. However, appropriate medical therapy is required after stent graft insertion, for example, ASA, dual antiplatelet therapy, or other anticoagulant.[3]
- Other cases with similar complications have been reported in the literature.

References

1. Khoynezhad A, Azizzadeh A, Donayre CE, et al; RESCUE investigators. Results of a multicenter, prospective trial of thoracic endovascular aortic repair for blunt thoracic aortic injury (RESCUE trial). J Vasc Surg 2013;57(4):899–890
2. Kumpati GS, Patel AN, Bull DA. Thrombosis of a descending thoracic aortic endovascular stent graft in a patient with factor V Leiden: case report. J Cardiothorac Surg 2014;9:47
3. Mirakhur A, Appoo JJ, Kent W, Herget EJ, Wong JK. Delayed intimal blowout after endovascular repair of aortic dissection. J Vasc Interv Radiol 2013;24(10):1471–1475

Stent graft migration during endovascular aneurysm repair resulting in incidental covering of the renal arteries

Patient History

A 67-year-old man, heavy smoker (> 30 cigarettes/day) with hypertension, chronic kidney disease (creatinine 4.6 mg/dL), and previous endovascular treatment for thoracic aortic aneurysm. He suffered an abdominal aortic aneurysm (AAA) that increased in caliber during the last year (> 1 cm/y) up to 56 × 50 mm.

A computed tomography (CT) scan, performed without contrast media due to renal insufficiency, confirmed the suggested findings (**Fig. 4.381**). After a multidisciplinary discussion an endovascular intervention was planned.

Initial Treatment Received

The procedure was performed under local anesthesia with bilateral surgical cut-down of the common femoral arteries (CFAs). Through the left femoral access the main body of the aortic

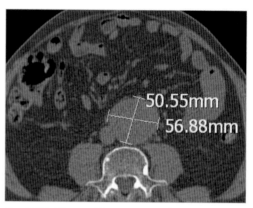

Fig. 4.381 CT scan without injection of contrast media: axial view shows that the aneurysm sac is 56 × 50 mm in diameter.

endoprothesis (Excluder—26 × 14 × 140 mm, WL Gore & Associates) was inserted and deployed just at the bottom of the renal arteries origin. The landing zone was decided on the basis of the first aortography, which confirmed the presence of the AAA (**Fig. 4.382a, b**). One of the procedural goals was to use the lowest amount possible of contrast media.

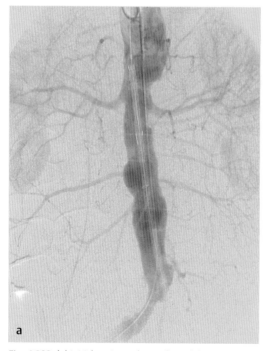
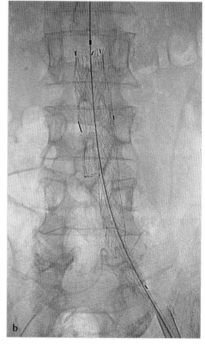

Fig. 4.382 **(a)** Initial angiography confirmed the presence of the AAA. **(b)** The renal arteries were localized immediately.

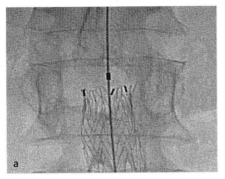 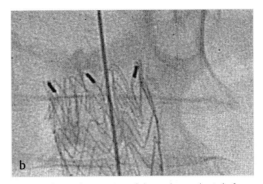

Fig. 4.383 **(a)** Comparative evaluation of unsubtracted images shows the position of the endoprosthesis before introduction of the contralateral sheath through the right femoral access **(b)** and after. In this image the upper edge of the endoprosthesis is located above the inferior aspect of L1, covering both renal arteries.

Problems Encountered during Treatment

Immediately after insertion of the contralateral introducer a change was observed in the position of the upper edge of the endoprosthesis, which was now above the inferior aspect of L1 (**Fig. 4.383a, b**).

A stent graft migration had occurred with subsequent occlusion of the origin of the renal arteries.

Imaging Plan

Proceed with fluoroscopy and if necessary contrast-enhanced angiography.

Resulting Complication

Both renal arteries were occluded in a patient with chronic renal insufficiency.

Possible Strategies for Complication Management

- Endovascular treatment by pulling down the endoprothesis with an aortic balloon or a guidewire loop.
- Renal stenting.
- Surgical conversion (if endovascular approaches fail).

Final Complication Management

From the right femoral access a standard hydrophilic guidewire (0.035-inch Terumo) was inserted and directed into the left common iliac artery

(CIA) with a Simmons 1 catheter. The guidewire was snared with a snare loop (30 mm) and pulled out from the femoral access. The two extremities of the guidewire were pulled down in order to replace the stent graft in the correct position, below the renal arteries. An angiogram showed the correct position of the endoprosthesis below the renal arteries with a regular flow (**Fig. 4.384a, b**).

To restore a normal morphology of the stent graft and its iliac limbs, a balloon angioplasty (33 mm) was used. The contralateral limb was then inserted (**Fig 4.385a–c**).

Final angiography showed an endograft with crossed limbs ("ballerina" configuration). No endoleaks were detected (**Fig. 4.386**). Follow-up CT exam performed 4 years later showed further decrease of the aneurysm sac dimensions and normal shape of the endoprosthesis (**Fig. 4.387**).

Complication Analysis

The endoprosthesis's accidental dislodgement upwards might have occurred during the insertion of the introducer sheath through the right femoral access. This could be the consequence of an incomplete adhesion of the stent graft to the aortic wall.

Prevention Strategies and Take-home Message

- Such a complication is quite a rare event.[1,2] To prevent it, other authors have investigated the change in the position of the renal arteries during the respiratory cycle.[3]

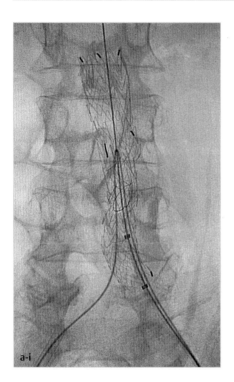
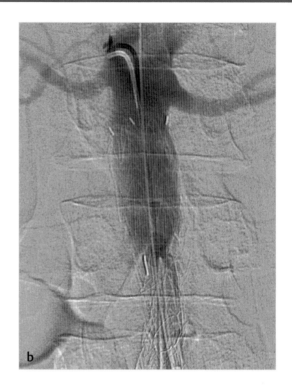
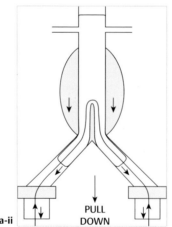

Fig. 4.384 (a-i, a-ii) Through the right femoral access a standard hydrophilic guidewire was inserted and directed into the left CIA with a Simmons 1 catheter. The guidewire was snared with a snare loop (30 mm) and pulled out from the femoral access. The two extremities of the guidewire were pulled down in order to replace the stent graft in the correct position, below the renal arteries. **(b)** A subsequent angiogram showing patency of both renal arteries.

- We suggest dilatating the main body of the stent graft immediately after its deployment. Then the procedure can be completed with insertion of the contralateral limb in the standard fashion.
- The rescue maneuver described above is not easy to perform and cannot be used with all

endoprostheses. The great risk is aortic wall damage.
- When this technique cannot be applied, bilateral renal stenting should be selected and if not applicable a surgical conversion should be performed.

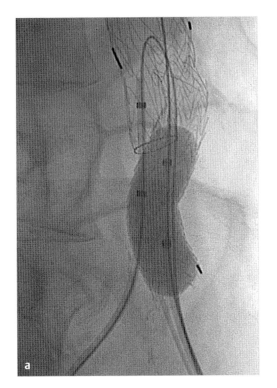
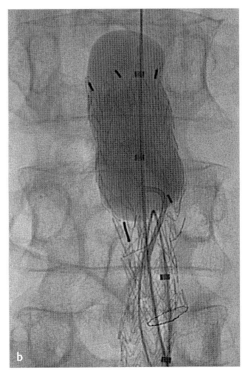
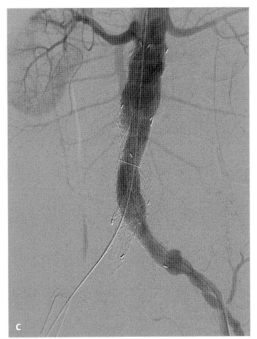

Fig. 4.385 (a, b) A 33-mm balloon was inflated to reshape the endoprosthesis which was morphologically altered during the "pulling down" maneuver. (c) After dilatation the right branch (14 mm) was correctly deployed.

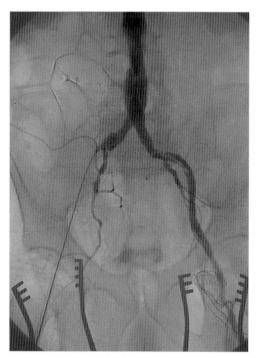

Fig. 4.386 Final angiography showed the endoprosthesis normal shape with a crossed limbs configuration with no evidence of endoleaks.

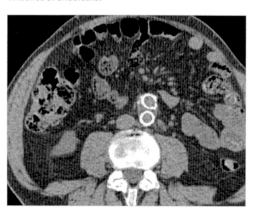

Fig. 4.387 Follow-up CT exam performed 4 years later showed further decrease of the aneurysm sac dimensions and normal shape of the endoprosthesis.

References

1. Adu J, Cheshire NJ, Riga CV, Hamady M, Bicknell CD. Strategies to tackle unrecognized bilateral renal artery occlusion after endovascular aneurysm repair. Ann Vasc Surg 2012;26(8):1127.e1–e7

2. McWilliams RG, Fisher RK, Lawrence-Brown M. Renal artery rescue after EVAR. J Endovasc Ther 2013;20(3):295–297

3. Scavée V, Banice R, Parisel A, et al. Influence of respiratory cycle on proximal renal artery motion: an angiographic study in patients undergoing endovascular aneurysm repair. Acta Chir Belg 2012;112(1):65–68

Sizing failure during endovascular aneurysm repair

Patient History

An 86-year-old man with an incidental 10-cm infrarenal abdominal aortic aneurysm (AAA) was scheduled for semielective conventional endovascular aneurysm repair (EVAR).

Initial Treatment Received

The computed tomography angiography (CTA) was reviewed and a percutaneous aortobiiliac EVAR was planned. Zenith (Cook Medical) devices were chosen. The main body was to be 32 × 140 mm with bilateral 24 × 90-mm iliac extensions.

Problems Encountered during Treatment

When the main body of the graft was placed via the right common femoral artery (CFA) the delivery system was found to be too short (Fig. 4.388).

Imaging Plan

Further angiographic evaluation.

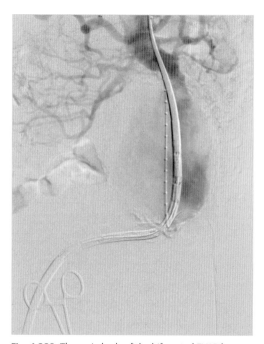

Fig. 4.388 The main body of the bifurcated EVAR has been delivered via the right CFA. Even with the delivery system advanced maximally in the groin access site the proximal end of the graft is seen to lie at the level of the middle of the aneurysm.

Resulting Complication

Inability to deliver the stent graft to the infrarenal landing zone with inadequate exclusion of the aneurysm.

Possible Strategies for Complication Management

- Place the stent where it is and build cranially.
- Place a thoracic stent proximally and then place the main body, continuing the EVAR as normal.
- Convert from percutaneous access to a cutdown on the right (the main body delivery side) and place an iliac conduit.
- Convert to open surgery if the patient is fit.

Final Complication Management

An off-the-shelf 34-mm thoracic stent (Zenith) was placed proximally (**Fig. 4.389**), thus allowing distal deployment of the bifurcated main body and 24-mm limb extensions. Balloon molding was performed in the usual manner. Initial postprocedure angiogram demonstrated a proximal type 1 endoleak that was excluded with a 38-mm Zenith cuff (**Fig. 4.390**).

Complication Analysis

Though rare, delivery systems for EVAR can be too short. This is something that should be considered in tall patients or in patients with excessively elongated/ectatic iliacs.

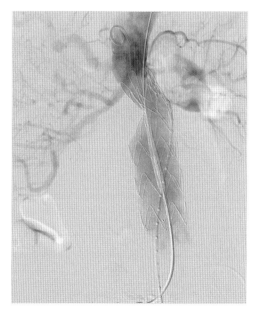

Fig. 4.389 34-mm thoracic stent placed proximally within the infrarenal aneurysm.

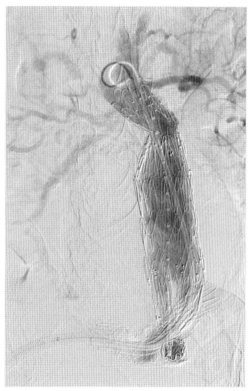

Fig. 4.390 Final angiogram demonstrating satisfactory occlusion of the proximal type 1 endoleak with a 38-mm cuff.

Prevention Strategies and Take-home Message

- Having off-the-shelf devices available can be of benefit for unforeseen circumstances.

Further Reading

Jordan WD Jr, Moore WM Jr, Melton JG, Brown OW, Carpenter JP; Endologix investigators. Secure fixation following EVAR with the Powerlink XL System in wide aortic necks: results of a prospective, multicenter trial. J Vasc Surg 2009;50(5):979–986

Access-related thrombosis after total percutaneous aortic repair

Patient History

A 63-year-old woman presented with an ultrasound diagnosis of an abdominal aortic aneurysm. Abdominal computed tomography angiography (CTA) was performed, which demonstrated a focal eccentric infrarenal abdominal aortic aneurysm (AAA) (**Fig. 4.391**).

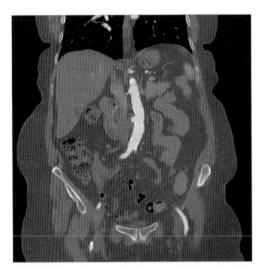

Fig. 4.391 CTA showing a focal eccentric infrarenal AAA.

Initial Treatment Received

The patient underwent a percutaneous endovascular repair of the focal AAA. A right common femoral artery (CFA) access was performed using a micropuncture kit under ultrasound guidance. After access was obtained, two suture-mediated ProGlide (Abbott Vascular) closure devices were inserted to perform a planned "preclose" closure at the end of the case due to the large-sized access required for the placement of the abdominal aortic stent graft. A diagnostic abdominal aortic angiogram was performed (**Fig. 4.392**). A 0.035-inch Super Stiff Amplatz wire (Boston Scientific) was inserted into the abdominal aorta. A 12 × 41-mm balloon-expandable stent graft was manually mounted on an 18 × 60-mm angioplasty balloon. A 12F sheath was inserted in the right groin. The stent and was inserted and deployed at the site of the focal eccentric AAA followed by an angiogram (**Fig. 4.393**). The closure devices were applied in the right groin. There were no complications at the time of the procedure.

Problems Encountered after Treatment

One week after the initial procedure, the patient presented with acute right leg pain on walking up one flight of stairs with progressive worsening. The patient was brought to the Emergency Department for further assessment.

Imaging Plan

CTA.

Resulting Complication

There was an occlusion of the right external iliac artery (EIA) at its origin on the right CFA

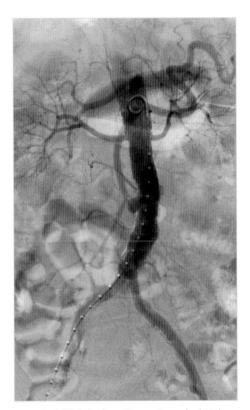

Fig. 4.392 Digital subtraction angiography (DSA) imaging of the eccentric focal AAA.

(**Fig. 4.394**). There was a puncture site or access-related thrombosis.

Possible Strategies for Complication Management

- Endovascular treatment via contralateral left CFA percutaneous access over the aortic bifurcation with thrombolysis and angioplasty.
- CFA-to-CFA bypass graft placement.

Final Complication Management

Endovascular treatment via left CFA access was performed. A 6F Balkin sheath (Cook Medical) was placed over the aortic bifurcation and a diagnostic angiogram was performed (**Fig. 4.395**). Pulse spray thrombolysis was performed with 10 mg of intra-arterial recombinant tissue plasminogen activator (rtPA). Post-thrombolysis there was recanalization with severe stenosis in the distal right EIA at the site of the previous suture-mediated closure device placement (**Fig. 4.396**). A 7 × 40-mm angioplasty was performed with significant improvement and minimal (less than 20%) residual stenosis (**Fig. 4.397**). After manual compression hemostasis was obtained in the left groin.

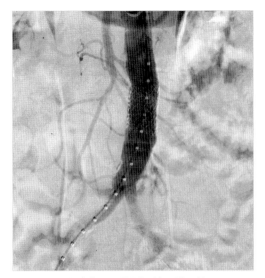

Fig. 4.393 DSA following EVAR with a 12 × 41-mm balloon-expandable stent graft.

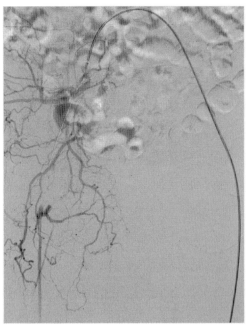

Fig. 4.395 Selective angiogram of the right iliac axis after sheath placement from the contralateral groin.

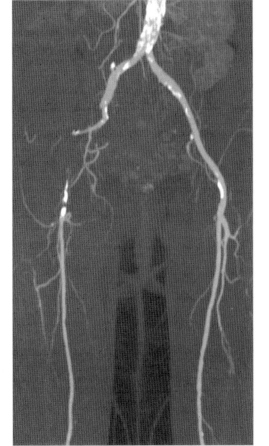

Fig. 4.394 CTA maximum intensity projection (MIP) imaging showing an occlusion of the right EIA.

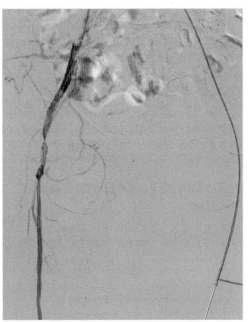

Fig. 4.396 Post-thrombolysis recanalization with severe stenosis in the distal right EIA at the site of the previous suture-mediated closure device placement.

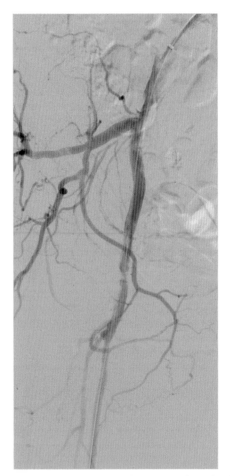

Fig. 4.397 A 7 × 40-mm angioplasty was performed with significant improvement and minimal residual stenosis.

Complication Analysis

In this case, there was an access-related thrombosis of the right EIA secondary to placement of a large sheath for aortic stent graft placement, which was corrected with thrombolysis and angioplasty.

Prevention Strategies and Take-home Message

- There should be aggressive heparinization at the time of placement of large intra-arterial vascular sheaths.
- There should be sufficient flushing after placement of large vascular sheaths to prevent access-related vessel thrombosis.
- There should be close monitoring of patients post–complex endovascular procedures with early intervention if there are any access-related stenoses.

Further Reading

Mathisen SR, Zimmermann E, Markström U, Mattsson K, Larzon T. Complication rate of the fascia closure technique in endovascular aneurysm repair. J Endovasc Ther 2012; 19(3):392–396

Ye P, Chen Y, Zeng Q, He X, Li Y, Zhao J. Long-term follow-up of the femoral artery after total percutaneous endovascular aortic repair with preclose technique using a vascular closure device. Nan Fang Yi Ke Da Xue Xue Bao 2014;34(5):747–750

Limb occlusion 4 months after successful endovascular aneurysm repair

Patient History

An 80-year-old man presented with an infrarenal abdominal aortic aneurysm (AAA) on external ultrasound. Abdominal computed tomography angiography (CTA) was performed and confirmed the findings (**Fig. 4.398**).

Initial Treatment Received

The patient underwent a percutaneous endovascular repair of the infrarenal AAA. A bilateral common femoral artery (CFA) access was performed using a micropuncture kit under ultrasound

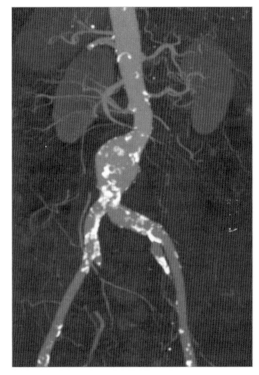

Fig. 4.398 CTA showing an infrarenal abdominal aortic aneurysm.

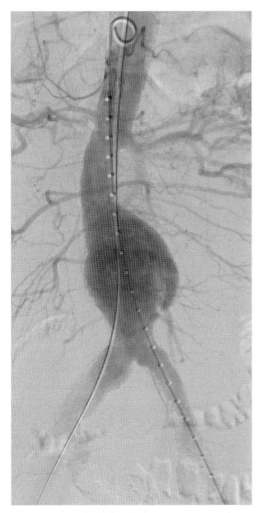

Fig. 4.399 Procedural digital subtraction angiography (DSA) imaging of the AAA.

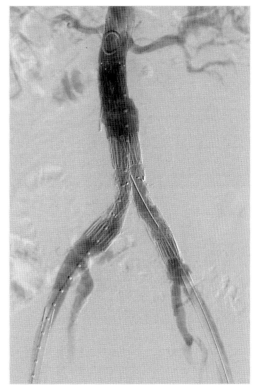

Fig. 4.400 Postinterventional DSA showing the excluded aneurysm following endovascular aneurysm repair (EVAR).

guidance. After access was obtained two suture-mediated ProGlide closure devices (Abbott Vascular) were inserted to perform a planned "preclose" closure at the end of the case due to the large-sized access required for the placement of the abdominal aortic stent graft in both groins. A diagnostic abdominal aortic angiogram was performed (Fig. 4.399). A 0.035-inch × 300-cm-long Lunderquist wire (Cook Medical) was inserted into the abdominal aorta through the right groin access. An 18F sequential dilatation was performed in the right groin at 2F increments. The main body measuring 24 × 58 mm was inserted through the right groin through an 18F sheath. The main body was deployed below the origin of both renal arteries. The contralateral gate was cannulated and a 16 × 60-mm contralateral limb was placed. An ipsilateral 16 × 48-mm limb was placed followed by compliant balloon dilatation at all the landing zones and junctions. An abdominal aortic angiogram demonstrated no evidence of a type 1 or type 3 endoleak (Fig. 4.400). The closure devices were completed in both groins. There were no complications at the time of the procedure.

Problems Encountered after Treatment

Four months after the initial procedure, the patient presented with acute right leg pain on walking for less than one block on a flat surface. A duplex arterial ultrasound was performed.

Imaging Plan

CTA.

Resulting Complication

There was an occlusion of the right limb of the abdominal aortic endograft (Figs. 4.401 and 4.402). The right CFA and access site were patent.

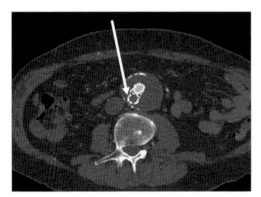

Fig. 4.401 CTA image of the occlusion of the right limb of the abdominal aortic endograft (*arrow*).

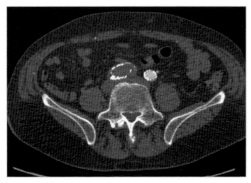

Fig. 4.402 CTA image of the occlusion of the right limb of the abdominal aortic endograft.

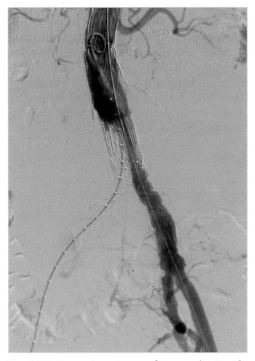

Fig. 4.403 Diagnostic angiogram after recanalization of the occlusion.

Possible Strategies for Complication Management

- Endovascular treatment via ipsilateral percutaneous vascular access.
- CFA-to-CFA bypass graft placement.

Final Complication Management

Endovascular treatment via a bilateral CFA ultrasound guided access. A 6F vascular sheath was inserted. Using an angled 40-cm, 5F Kumpe catheter and 0.035-inch × 145-cm-long Rosen wire, cannulation through the occlusion into the main body of the abdominal aortic endograft was performed. After access was obtained two suture-mediated ProGlide closure devices (Abbott Vascular) were inserted to perform a planned "preclose" closure at the end of the case due to the large-sized access required for the placement stent graft placement in both groins. A diagnostic angiogram was performed (**Fig. 4.403**). Pulse spray thrombolysis was performed with 10 mg of intra-arterial recombinant tissue plasminogen activator (rtPA). Post-thrombolysis bilateral 12 × 60-mm balloon-expandable stents were placed (**Fig. 4.404**), followed by a extension endograft

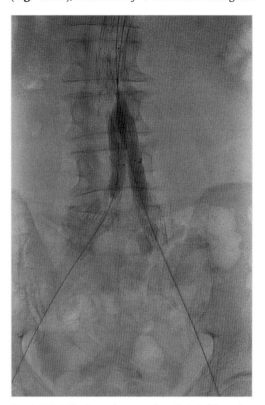

Fig. 4.404 Following pulse spray thrombolysis bilateral balloon-expandable stents were placed.

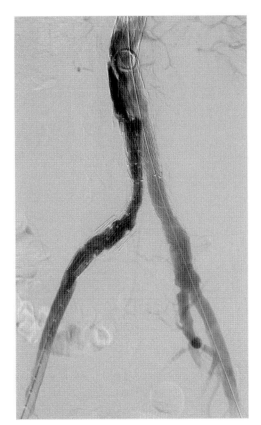

Fig. 4.405 Final angiogram following extension endograft limb in the right EIA.

limb in the right external iliac artery (EIA) (**Fig. 4.405**). The closure devices were completed in both groins. There were no complications at the time of the procedure.

Complication Analysis

In this case there was delayed thrombosis of the right limb of the abdominal aortic endograft, suggesting this was not an access-related thrombosis.

Prevention Strategies and Take-home Message

- There should be aggressive heparinization at the time of placement of large intra-arterial vascular sheaths.
- There should be aggressive flushing after placement of large vascular sheaths to prevent access-related vessel thrombosis.
- There should be close monitoring of patients post–complex endovascular procedures with

consideration of early intervention if there are any access-related stenosis.
- Limb occlusion will occur in abdominal aortic endografts even with ideal anatomy and optimal procedure technique.

Further Reading

Conway AM, Modarai B, Taylor PR, et al. Stent graft limb deployment in the external iliac artery increases the risk of limb occlusion following endovascular AAA repair. J Endovasc Ther 2012;19(1):79–85

Coulston J, Baigent A, Selvachandran H, Jones S, Torella F, Fisher R. The impact of endovascular aneurysm repair on aortoiliac tortuosity and its use as a predictor of iliac limb complications. J Vasc Surg 2014;60(3):585–589

Lau YF, Senaratne J, Ghatwary T. Re. "Endograft limb occlusion in EVAR: iliac tortuosity quantified by three different indices on the basis of pre-operative CTA." Eur J Vasc Endovasc Surg 2014;48(6):711–712

Mantas GK, Antonopoulos CN, Sfyroeras GS, et al. Factors predisposing to endograft limb occlusion after endovascular aortic repair. Eur J Vasc Endovasc Surg 2015;49(1):39–41

O'Neill S, Collins A, Harkin D. Limb occlusion after endovascular repair of an abdominal aortic aneurysm: beware the narrow distal aorta. Ir J Med Sci 2012;181(3):373–376

Rancic Z. Commentary on: "Endograft limb occlusion in EVAR: iliac tortuosity quantified by three different indices on the basis of preoperative CTA." Eur J Vasc Endovasc Surg 2014;48(5):534–535

Ronsivalle S, Faresin F, Franz F, et al. A new management for limb graft occlusion after endovascular aneurysm repair adding a Vollmar ring stripper: the unclogging technique. Ann Vasc Surg 2013;27(8):1216–1222

Taudorf M, Jensen LP, Vogt KC, Grønvall J, Schroeder TV, Lönn L. Endograft limb occlusion in EVAR: iliac tortuosity quantified by three different indices on the basis of preoperative CTA. Eur J Vasc Endovasc Surg 2014;48(5):527–533

Taudorf M, Schroeder TV, Lönn L. Response to letter to the editor: "Re: Endograft limb occlusion in EVAR: iliac tortuosity quantified by three different indices on the basis of pre-operative CTA." Eur J Vasc Endovasc Surg 2014;48(6):712

Van Zeggeren L, Bastos Gonçalves F, Van Herwaarden JA, et al. Incidence and treatment results of Endurant endograft occlusion. J Vasc Surg 2013;57(5):1246–1254

Wu MS, Boyle JR. Strategies that minimize the risk of iliac limb occlusion after EVAR. J Endovasc Ther 2012;19(1):86–87

When everything is going too smoothly: limb malplacement in an easy endovascular aneurysm repair (EVAR) case

Patient History

A 64-year-old patient with a 4-cm aneurysm of the left common iliac artery (CIA) was referred for vascular surgery for endovascular aneurysm repair (EVAR). Due to the proximity of the aneurysm to the aortic bifurcation it was decided to implant a bifurcated endoprosthesis.

Initial Treatment Received

The procedure was performed under general anesthesia. Following surgical exposure of the femoral arteries and retrograde sheath placement, the left internal iliac artery (IIA) was cannulated and embolized with coils. Digital subtraction angiography (DSA) was performed using a pigtail catheter inserted from the right groin (**Fig. 4.406**). Before the main body of the prosthesis was implanted the pigtail catheter was pulled back and positioned into the right iliac artery. After implantation of the main body the guidewire was advanced and both wire and catheter seemed to easily pass into the limb socket as seen in posterior-anterior fluoroscopy view (**Fig. 4.407**). The hydrophylic-coated wire was exchanged for a stiff guide wire and the contralateral limb was implanted from the right side (**Fig. 4.408**).

Problems Encountered during Treatment

Control angiography from the left side now showed that the limb had not been implanted into the socket, but that the wire had passed the prosthesis outside and ventral to the main body. The aneurysm was not excluded, the stent was malplaced into the aneurysm sack (**Fig. 4.409**).

Imaging Plan

Further angiographic evaluation.

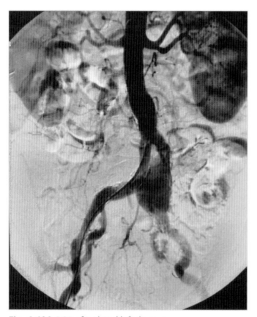

Fig. 4.406 DSA of isolated left iliac aneurysm.

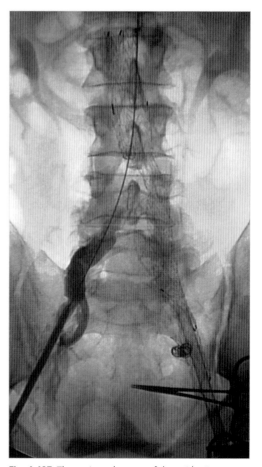

Fig. 4.407 The projected course of the guidewire seemed to pass into the limb socket.

Resulting Complication

Limb malplacement, lack of aneurysm exclusion.

Possible Strategies for Complication Management

- Endovascular management by intraluminal recannulation of the limb socket and implantation of a second graft limb.
- Surgical conversion with open aneurysm repair.

Final Complication Management

First, cannulating the limb socket was tried from the right side using a diagnostic catheter over a hydrophilic-coated guidewire. However, this was not possible due to the fully expanded malplaced limb, which obstructed the ostium. Then, a guidewire was advanced from the left side through the socket in an antegrade fashion using a Rösch in-

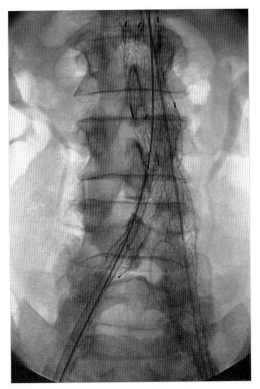

Fig. 4.408 Fully expanded, but malplaced limb.

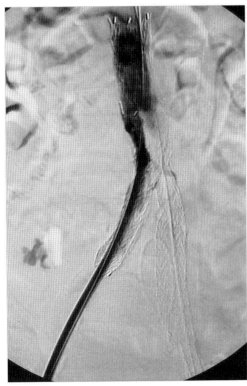

Fig. 4.409 Failure of aneurysm exclusion, contrast medium injected through a long sheath inserted into the aneurysm from the right groin.

ferior mesenteric (RIM) catheter (Cordis/Johnson & Johnson) (**Fig. 4.410**). The wire was caught with a snare and pulled through the sheath in the right groin (**Fig. 4.411**). After the wire had been exchanged for a stiff steel guide (Back-Up Meier, Boston Scientific), a second contralateral limb was implanted (**Fig. 4.412**). The prosthesis was expanded using a semicompliant balloon and the malplaced limb was "crushed" as shown in postinterventional computed tomography angiography (CTA) (**Fig. 4.413**).

Complication Analysis

What started as an easy case of EVAR ended in a serious complication with the potential need for surgical conversion. The critical error in this case was that the operator had forgotten to test the correct intraluminal wire position by rotating a pigtail catheter in the proximal aspect of the prosthesis before implantation of the limb. Because the aorta was not aneurysmatic the guidewire took a straight course, which projected over the limb socket and looked correct.

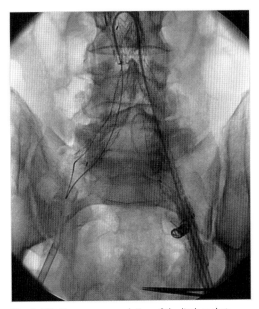

Fig. 4.410 Crossover cannulation of the limb socket using a hook-shaped RIM catheter

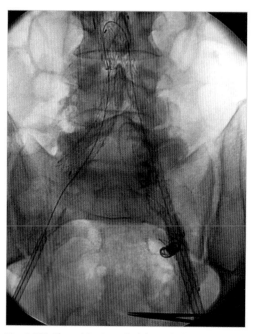

Fig. 4.411 The guidewire pulled through the sheath in the right groin.

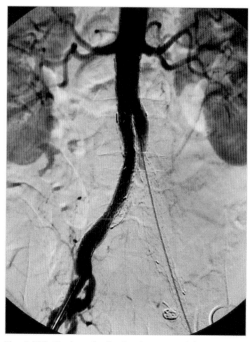

Fig. 4.412 Final result after implantation of the second limb and "crush stenting" of the malplaced device.

Prevention Strategies and Take-home Message

- Always follow a strict protocol of implantation steps, even in seemingly simple cases. These steps should include use of at least two different angiographic planes after cannulation of the limb socket and a pigtail rotation test.
- Have a variety of spare limbs available as bail-out tools for complicated cases.

Further Reading

Bryce Y, Rogoff P, Romanelli D, Reichle R. Endovascular repair of abdominal aortic aneurysms: vascular anatomy, device selection, procedure, and procedure-specific complications. Radiographics 2015;35(2):593–615

Törnqvist P, Dias N, Sonesson B, Kristmundsson T, Resch T. Intraoperative cone beam computed tomography can help avoid reinterventions and reduce CT follow up after infrarenal EVAR. Eur J Vasc Endovasc Surg 2015;49(4):390–395

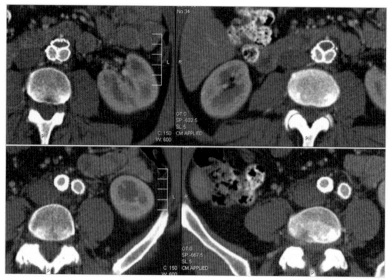

Fig. 4.413 CTA shows the "crushed" malplaced stent ventral to both now adequately perfused limbs.

Supra-aortic Stenting

When a hydrophilic 0.035-inch guidewire is lost

Patient History

A 55-year-old man with severe neurological problems related to a basilar artery stenosis, refractory to optimized medical treatment, was scheduled for direct stenting.

Initial Treatment Received

Direct stenting with a 3 × 11-mm drug-eluting stent (DES) was performed under general anesthesia; the final angiographic control presented an acceptable technical result (**Fig. 4.414**).

Problems Encountered during Treatment

After completion of the procedure, the long 6F guiding sheath was removed down to the groin, while a 0.035-inch guidewire was reinserted. The plan was to leave it in place during sheath removal and vascular closure device–specific sheath insertion. Suddenly, it was noticed that the wire had disappeared into the sheath (**Fig. 4.415**) and flushed into the external iliac artery. Any at-

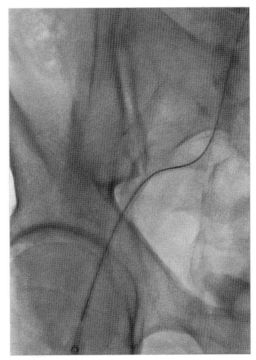

Fig. 4.415 Fluoroscopy image shows the 0.035-inch wire initially placed prior to sheath removal as an exchange wire, had disappeared into the sheath.

tempts to snare the stiff end of the wire at the end of the sheath in the external iliac artery (EIA) failed (**Fig. 4.416**).

Imaging Plan

Fluoroscopy.

Resulting Complication

There was dislodgement of a hydrophilic wire into the body.

Possible Strategies for Complication Management

- Insert a larger lumen sheath for better steerability of the wire into the sheath opening.
- Try to snare the distal soft angle-tip of the wire with a snare.

Final Complication Management

Endovascular treatment with snaring the distal soft angle-tip (**Fig. 4.417**) for final guidewire removal.

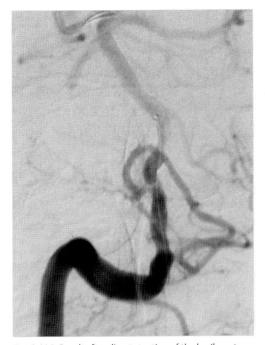

Fig. 4.414 Result after direct stenting of the basilar artery.

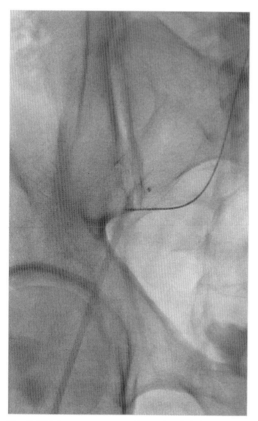

Fig. 4.416 Attempts to snare the stiff end of the wire at the end of the sheath in the EIA failed.

Complication Analysis

Suspected uncontrolled advancement of the hydrophilic guidewire during sheath removal; additional permanent flush of the sheath via the side port might have transported the hydrophilic-coated wire into the body.

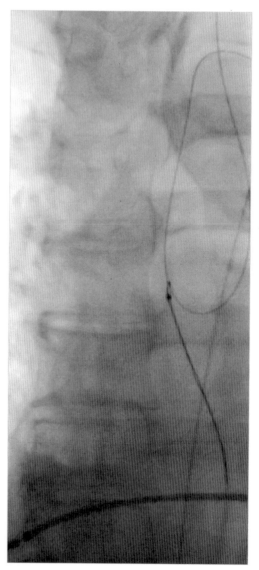

Fig. 4.417 Endovascular treatment with snaring the distal soft angle-tip at the level of the right atrium for final guidewire removal.

Prevention Strategies and Take-home Message

- Guidewire advancement should be constantly controlled under fluoroscopy, especially when using hydrophilic-coated wires!
- Be aware of the wire length in order not to lose you wire in the body!

Further Reading

Barbiero G, Cognolato D, Polverosi R, Guarise A. Percutaneous retrieval of a radiolucent foreign body from an EVAR device by combining different image modalities. Cardiovasc Interv Radiol 2009;32(4):785–788

Sheth R, Someshwar V, Warawdekar G. Percutaneous retrieval of misplaced intravascular foreign objects with the Dormia basket: an effective solution. Cardiovasc Interv Radiol 2007;30(1):48–53

Embolization Procedures

Displacement of microcoils during side-branch embolization prior to endovascular aneurysm repair

Patient History

A 72-year-old man was planned for abdominal endovascular aneurysm repair (EVAR). In the preinterventional computed tomography (CT) imaging a large lumen patent inferior mesenteric artery (IMA) was detected.

Initial Treatment Received

The patient was scheduled for coil embolization of the IMA via a retrograde groin access prior to EVAR in order to decrease the risk of type 2 endoleak. Catheterization of the IMA origin was performed with an 0.038-inch 5F renal double-curve (RDC) catheter. A 2.7F microcatheter was placed coaxially via the diagnostic catheter and positioned into the mid-part of the IMA trunk. Under fluoroscopic guidance an 0.018-inch complex helical coil (6 × 6 mm) was delivered into the IMA trunk with a dedicated coil-pusher wire.

Problems Encountered after Treatment

Immediately after placement there was dislocation of the coil into the trifurcation of the superior rectal artery, left colic artery, and sigmoid arteries, probably due to high blood pressure and insufficient coil attachment to the vessel wall (**Fig. 4.418**)!

Imaging Plan

Angiography.

Resulting Complication

No acute consequences, but potential of distal vessel occlusion and development of bowel ischemia.

Possible Strategies for Complication Management

- Conservative treatment; for example, heparinization/anticoagulation.
- Endovascular treatment via 5F RDC (guiding) catheter that is already in place:
- Snaring the coil with small-diameter snares.
  - Snaring the coil with a stent retriever (usually used for clot removal during stroke management).
- Surgery (if an endovascular approach fails).

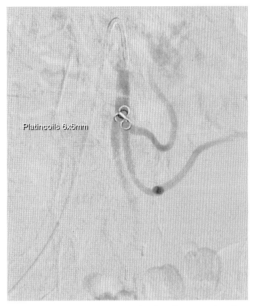

Fig. 4.418 Selective angiography already presenting the dislodged 0.018-inch pushable platinum microcoil.

Final Complication Management

Endovascular treatment via the catheter that was still in place. Positioning of a multisnare with diameter ranging from 20 to 30 mm. The coil was captured by rotating the snare around the foreign body until it could be fixed and removed safely (**Figs. 4.419** and **4.420**). The initial procedure was then completed by placement of a 5F guiding sheath 1 cm distally of the origin of the IMA. A

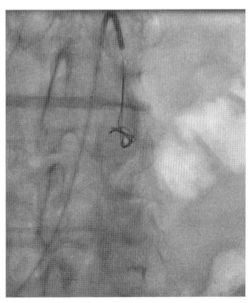

Fig. 4.419 Fluoroscopic view with snare already placed around the coil.

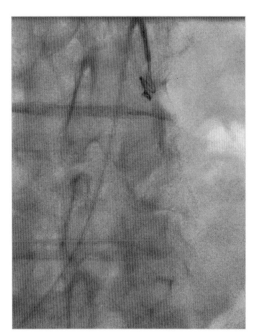

Fig. 4.420 Engagement of the coil was possible by rotating the open snare around the coil. The originally placed 5F RDC catheter was still in place and was used a guide catheter during the snaring procedure.

6-mm Amplatzer Vascular Plug II (St. Jude Medical) was placed successfully (**Fig. 4.421**).

Complication Analysis

Improper selection of coil size and length in regard to vessel diameter, blood pressure, and flow, resulting in immediate coil dislodgement.

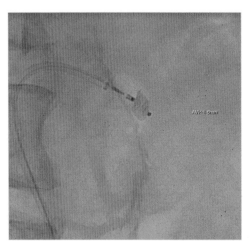

Fig. 4.421 A 5F guide sheath was placed over a soft angle-tip Terumo wire in the origin of the IMA. An Amplatzer Vascular Plug II (6 mm) was successfully placed and anchored in the proximal part of the IMA, allowing flow in all bowel arteries via Riolan's anastomosis.

Prevention Strategies and Take-home Message

- Evaluate exact size of target vessels before coil embolization; for example, by noninvasive imaging, with adequate sizing of embolization material.
- If the risk of potential coil dislodgement is high, devices with higher radial force for controlled placement in the target vessel like detachable coils or plugs should be used if possible!
- Use of scaffolding technique with placement of a high radial force coil followed by packing with multiple coils into the resulting scaffold.
- Use of the anchoring technique with deployment of the distal part of the coil into a noncritical side branch.
- Always have different snare sizes available for foreign body retrieval!
- Use plugs instead of coils, if possible.

Coil dislocation during patient preparation for further selective internal radiation therapy

Patient History

A 56-year-old man with bilobar colorectal liver metastases, whose disease progressed on first- and second-line chemotherapy agents, was planned for selective internal radiation therapy (SIRT). Preprocedural computed tomography (CT) angiogram demonstrated conventional hepatic, right gastric and gastroduodenal artery (GDA) anatomy. A calcified plaque was noted at the origin of the GDA.

Initial Treatment

SIRT procedure 1. The initial treatment plan was to embolize the GDA, right gastric artery (RGA), and any gastric or duodenal branches thought to be at risk. The coeliac trunk was accessed using a 5F Simmons 1 catheter. Accessing the GDA with a 2.7F microcatheter proved difficult despite attempts being made with multiple 0.014-inch wires. Ultimately a 5F Rösch inferior mesenteric (RIM) catheter (Cordis/Johnson & Johnson) was anchored in the GDA origin and a coaxial microcatheter placed through this (**Fig. 4.422**). Two 6 × 30-mm detachable coils were placed in the GDA for occlusion. A subsequent angiogram demonstrated satisfactory deployment.

SIRT procedure 2. To be performed 8 days later, delivery of 60% of yttrium dose to the right hepatic arterial territory and 40% of the dose to the left hepatic arterial territory.

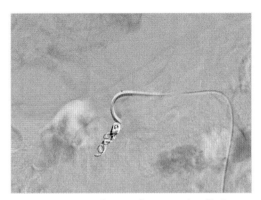

Fig. 4.422 5F RIM catheter in the GDA with coil ball.

Problems Encountered during Treatment

The microcatheter was withdrawn into the 5F catheter. However, on removing the RIM from the GDA origin, the end of a coil was flicked into the left hepatic artery (**Fig. 4.423**).

Imaging Plan

Angiography.
   Radionuclide imaging.

Resulting Complication

No acute consequences. However, the presence of a coil extending from the left hepatic artery, across the common hepatic artery proper into the GDA, could ultimately result in occlusion of any or all of these vessels.

Possible Strategies for Complication Management

- Occlude the entire left hepatic artery and ultimately deliver the full SIRT dose via the right hepatic artery.
- Attempt endovascular removal of the displaced coil.
- Abandon the procedure, rendering the patient unable to undergo SIRT, bearing in mind that occlusion of hepatic arterial flow in most cases is unlikely to cause liver dysfunction in its own right given the portal venous supply.

Final Complication Management

A 5F Destination sheath (Terumo) was placed in the common hepatic artery. A 5F C2 catheter was placed selectively in the artery and then a 2.7 microcatheter placed coaxially. The microwire was advanced into the left hepatic artery to attempt endovascular snare retrieval. Immediately the wire accessed the right gastric artery. Given that this vessel was to be embolized as part of the planned SIRT, the opportunity was taken to deploy two 3 × 3.3-cm coils with resultant satisfactory occlusion (**Fig. 4.424**). Subsequently the microwire was directed to the left hepatic segmental branch in which the end of the displaced coil ball was located. Attempts to guide a snare catheter over the wire proved fruitless due to the stiffness of this catheter. Instead, the microcatheter was advanced to this position, the microwire removed and replaced with a 7-mm 0.018-inch gooseneck snare. The coil was captured using the standard snaring technique. It

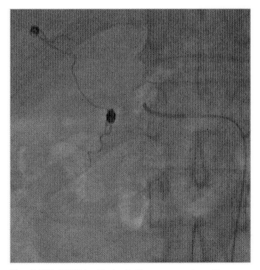

Fig. 4.423 5F RIM catheter in the common hepatic artery. Displaced coil spanning the left hepatic artery, common hepatic artery, and GDA.

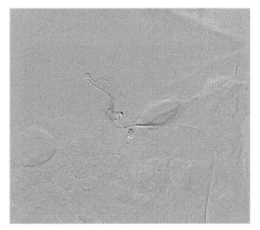

Fig. 4.424 While attempting to access the left hepatic artery the microcatheter immediately accessed the RGA. The opportunity was taken to place coils in the origin of the RGA. A 2.7F microcatheter, 5F C2 catheter, and 5F Destination sheath were all identified originating from the common hepatic artery.

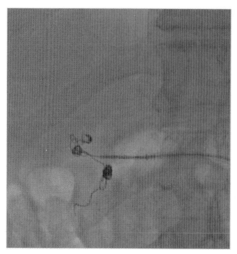

Fig. 4.425 The coil was snared. Coil and microcatheter were withdrawn into the 5F C2 catheter and removed from the arterial sheath.

was retrieved into the microcatheter, which was removed through the 5F C2 catheter (**Fig. 4.425**).

At the end of the procedure both GDA and RGA were occluded and the patient was sent for preliminary radionuclide imaging (**Fig. 4.426**).

Complication Analysis

Coil dislodgement occurred despite only minimal adjacent catheter activity.

Prevention Strategies and Take-home Message

- Care must be taken when removing catheters post–coil deployment regardless of the perceived stability of the coil scaffold.

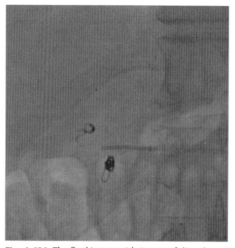

Fig. 4.426 The final image with "successful" coil deployment in the RGA and GDA.

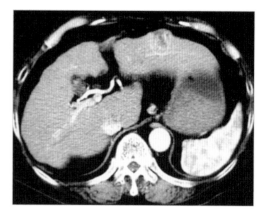

Fig. 4.427 Abdominal computed tomography (CT) showed an inhomogeneously enhanced tumor on the anterior surface of the lateral segment.

- If presented with an opportunity to coil a target vessel during SIRT, take it! In this case, the RGA was inadvertently accessed while trying to retrieve the dislodged coil, however this vessel was coiled anyway.

Gastric ulcer after chemoembolization for hepatocellular carcinoma treatment

Patient History

An 80-year-old man with cirrhosis type C was referred for chemoembolization of hepatocellular carcinoma (HCC) in the left lobe (**Fig. 4.427**).

Initial Treatment Received

Lipiodol chemoembolization was selectively performed from a possible tumor-feeding artery originating from the left hepatic artery (**Figs. 4.428** and **4.429**).

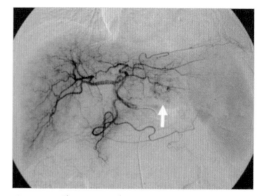

Fig. 4.428 The common hepatic arteriogram showed a tumor stain in segment III (*arrow*).

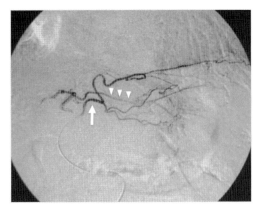

Fig. 4.429 A microcatheter was advanced into the possible tumor-feeding artery (*arrow*). However, this artery originating proximally to the umbilical point was revealed as the accessory left gastric artery. Note the overlapped course of the segment II artery (*arrowheads*) as the true tumor-feeder artery.

Problems Encountered after Treatment

Soon after chemoembolization the patient complained of severe epigastralgia.

Imaging Plan

Gastroscopy.
    Re-assessment of the celiac and hepatic arteriograms.

Resulting Complication

On the next day, gastroscopy revealed a large gastric ulcer (**Fig. 4.430**).

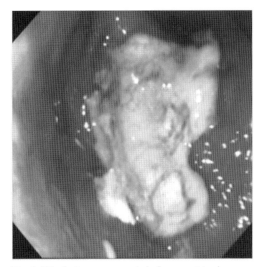

Fig. 4.430 Gastroscopy revealed a huge gastric ulcer.

Possible Strategies for Complication Management

Gastroprotective treatment.

Final Complication Management

The ulcer was healed conservatively with gastroprotective agents. Chemoembolization was performed again to treat the true tumor after 2 weeks.

Complication Analysis

The microcatheter was inserted into the accessory left gastric artery, and the gastric mucosal stain mimicked the tumor stain. As a result, inadvertent embolization induced the gastric ischemia.

Prevention Strategies and Take-home Message

- When chemoembolization is performed for tumors in the lateral segment, the existence of the accessory left gastric artery should be recognized to avoid inadvertent embolization.
- The reported incidence of the accessory left gastric artery is 3–21%, and it always originates from the left hepatic artery proximal to the umbilical point.
- Gastric mucosal stain in the territory of the accessory left gastric artery may mimic the tumor stain in the lateral segment.

Further Reading

Huang CM, Chen QY, Lin JX, et al. Short-term clinical implications of the accessory left hepatic artery in patients undergoing radical gastrectomy for gastric cancer. PLoS One 2013;8(5):e64300. doi:10.1371/journal.pone.0064300

Ishigami K, Yoshimitsu K, Irie H, et al. Accessory left gastric artery from left hepatic artery shown on MDCT and conventional angiography: correlation with CT hepatic arteriography. AJR Am J Roentgenol 2006;187(4):1002–1009

Liver abscess after chemoembolization for hepatocellular carcinoma treatment

Patient History

A 72-year-old man with cirrhosis type C, Child-Pugh class B, was referred for chemoembolization of hepatocellular carcinoma (HCC) in the right lobe.

Initial Treatment Received

Angiography revealed a large tumor stain with arteriovenous (AV) shunt in the right lobe (**Fig. 4.431**). Embolization was performed using large gelatin sponge particles alone to avoid the

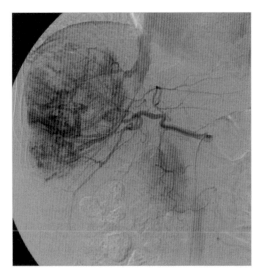

Fig. 4.431 The common hepatic arteriogram showed a hypervascular tumor stain with AV shunt.

pulmonary embolism or chemical lung damage via the AV shunt (**Fig. 4.432**).

Problems Encountered after Treatment

Five days after embolization, the patient presented with fever > 38°C, leukocytosis (34,200/mm³), and elevated C-reactive protein level (12.0 mg/dL). The blood culture was positive for *E. coli*.

Imaging Plan

Abdominal ultrasound.

Abdominal contrast-enhanced computed tomography (CT).

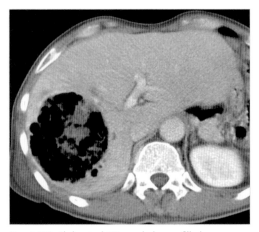

Fig. 4.433 Abdominal CT revealed a gas-filled mass, indicating liver abscess formation.

Resulting Complication

Liver abscess was developed following significant tumor necrosis induced by embolization (**Fig. 4.433**).

Possible Strategies for Complication Management

- Antibiotics.
- Percutaneous abscess drainage.
- Surgical resection.

Final Complication Management

Percutaneous abscess drainage was performed (**Fig. 4.434**). After 1 month, although the patient's

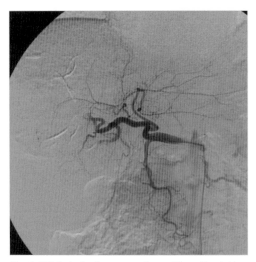

Fig. 4.432 Embolization was performed from the right hepatic artery with gelatin sponge alone.

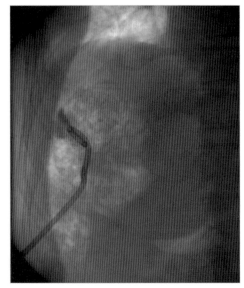

Fig. 4.434 A 12F pigtail drainage tube was percutaneously inserted into the gas-filled lesion.

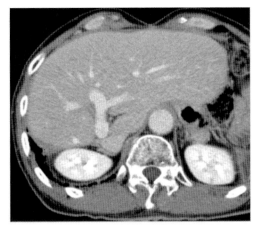

Fig. 4.435 Abdominal CT showed no tumor recurrence at follow-up 1 year 6 months after the right hepatectomy.

condition improved, right hepatectomy was performed as a definitive therapy (**Fig. 4.435**).

Complication Analysis

Colonization of the extensive large tumor necrosis by embolization was induced by *E. coli*. The patient had no history of biliary reconstructive surgery.

Prevention Strategies and Take-home Message

- The risk of liver abscess after embolization or chemoembolization is low in general with an incidence of 0.2–2%.
- Symptoms are similar to postembolization syndrome (fever, nausea and vomiting, and abdominal pain). However, if these symptoms appear or persist for 5 days after procedure, abscess formation should be suspected.
- Management includes antibiotics, drainage, and surgery, although the preventive role of prophylactic antibiotics remains uncertain.
- Prior biliary reconstructive surgery is a known risk for abscess formation.

Further Reading

Brown DB, Geschwind JF, Soulen MC, Millward SF, Sacks D. Society of Interventional Radiology Position Statement on Chemoembolization of Hepatic Malignancies. J Vasc Interv Radiol 2006;17(2 Pt 1):217–223

Coil migration during embolization for treatment of type 2 endoleak after hybrid thoracic endovascular repair

Patient History

A 66-year-old woman with aortic dissection had undergone hybrid thoracic endovascular repair (TEVAR) with total arch replacement. She was referred for embolization of type 2 endoleak due to incomplete ligation of the right brachiocephalic artery.

Initial Treatment Received

Coil embolization of the right brachiocephalic artery 15 mm in diameter was performed via the right brachial approach.

Problems Encountered after Treatment

Because of the large arterial size, oversized detachable microcoils up to 20 mm in loop diameter were used to make a dense coil frame. Subsequently, 8-mm-loop pushable fibered microcoils were deployed by forceful saline flush for tight filling inside the frame. However, the last microcoil dislocated out proximally and migrated into the right common carotid artery (**Fig. 4.436**).

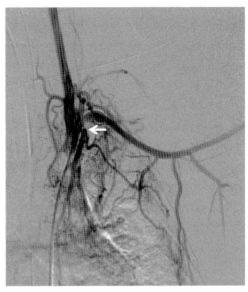

Fig. 4.436 During embolization of the right brachiocephalic artery, the last microcoil migrated proximally (*arrow*). Immediately, the operator's hand compressed the neck.

Imaging Plan

Close fluoroscopy monitoring of the migrated microcoil.

Resulting Complication

The patient presented with no symptoms, although there was a risk of cerebral thromboembolism.

Possible Strategies for Complication Management

- Immediate manual compression of the affected side of the neck to prevent further coil migration (as the effect is uncertain).
- Full heparinization to avoid thrombus formation around the fibered microcoils.
- Insertion of a balloon catheter beyond the microcoil to prevent further migration.
- Removal of the microcoil using a retrieval catheter device.
- Surgical removal (if endovascular approach fails).

Final Complication Management

Directly following the coil migration, the operator manually compressed the right side of the neck. Under full heparinization, a 4-mm-loop microsnare catheter was carefully advanced beyond the migrated microcoil via the same guiding catheter (**Fig. 4.437**). By pulling back and rotating the loop

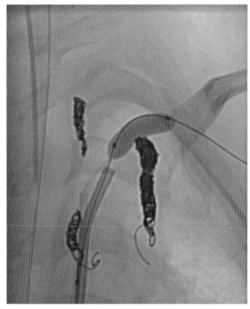

Fig. 4.438 The microcoil was captured in the microsnare loop and pulled down to the right subclavian artery.

snare, the proximal end of microcoil was successfully captured and retrieved (**Figs. 4.438** and **4.439**).

Complication Analysis

The delivery microcatheter was unstable inside the wide brachiocephalic artery. Then the microcatheter was kicked back due to the forceful saline flush during deployment of the last microcoil.

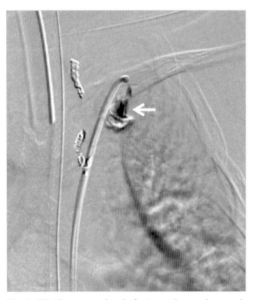

Fig. 4.437 The proximal end of microcoil moved upward to the right common carotid artery, while the distal end remained in the coil mass. The microsnare loop was inserted beyond the migrated microcoil to catch the proximal end (*arrow*).

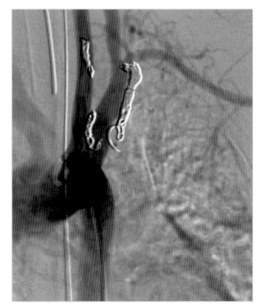

Fig. 4.439 The microcoil was successfully retrieved.

The microcoil was prone to being directed to the common carotid artery affected by the retrograde blood flow of the right subclavian artery.

Prevention Strategies and Take-home Message

- Saline flush technique is not suitable for the delivery of pushable microcoils in critical vascular territories; for example, supra-aortic vessels.
- Coil-push technique is preferable to deliver pushable microcoils, or detachable coils can be alternatively used, when the microcatheter is unstable in the target vessel.
- Proper selection of coil size is also important to avoid migration.
- Retrieval devices should always be kept in stock.

Displacement of a microcoil during internal iliac artery occlusion prior to endovascular aneurysm repair

Patient History

A 76-year-old man was planned for abdominal endovascular aneurysm repair (EVAR). In the preinterventional computed tomography (CT) imaging an enlarged common iliac artery (CIA) diameter was depicted. Therefore, it was planned to cover the origin of the internal iliac artery (IIA), ending the stent graft in the ipsilateral left external iliac artery (EIA). It was planned to exclude the IIA with plug occlusion.

Initial Treatment

The patient was scheduled for plug embolization of the IIA via a retrograde groin access (crossover approach) prior to EVAR in order to decrease the risk of type 2 endoleak. Catheterization of the IIA origin was performed with a 4F 0.038-inch Bern (Cordis) catheter. The initial plan of plug placement was abandoned due to the impossibility of placing a guiding catheter or a large guiding sheath into the IIA. Therefore, the Bern catheter was used coaxially in a 6F 45-cm sheath, placed crossover and fixed by an 0.014-inch wire threaded out through both sheaths (4F sheath placed in the left groin) in order to fix the crossover sheath during manipulation while the iliac arteries were elongated (**Figs. 4.440** and **4.441**). Under fluoroscopic guidance a 0.035-inch complex helical MReye coil (15 × 8 m; Cook Medical) was delivered into the IIA with a 0.035-inch hydrophilic-coated wire.

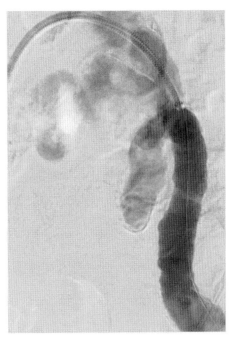

Fig. 4.440 Selective angiography via the 0.014-inch guidewire-fixed 6F sheath.

Problems Encountered during Treatment

Immediately after placement there was dislocation of one coil end into the CIA, probably due to an uncontrolled coil-pushing maneuver (**Fig. 4.442**)!

Imaging Plan

Angiography.

Resulting Complication

No acute consequences, but potential risk of thrombus formation around the coil in the CIA.

Possible Strategies for Complication Management

- Conservative treatment; for example, heparinization/anticoagulation.
- Endovascular treatment via 4F Bern (guiding catheter), which is already in place:
- Snaring the coil with small-diameter snares.
- Surgery (if an endovascular approach fails).

Final Complication Management

Endovascular treatment via the catheter, which was still in place. Positioning of a multisnare with ranging diameter from 20 to 30 mm. The coil was captured by rotating the snare around the foreign body at the level of the IIA until it could be fixed and

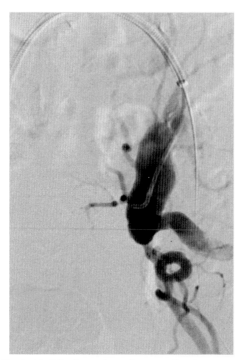

Fig. 4.441 Selective angiography presenting the 4F Bern catheter securely placed in the IIA in front of the bifurcation in the main anterior and posterior branch.

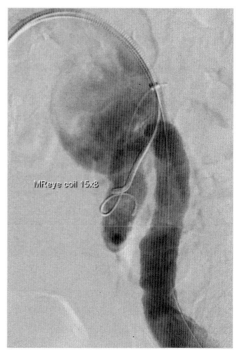

Fig. 4.442 Selective angiography showing the protrusion of one coil end into the CIA, whereas the other end is still in the IIA.

removed safely (**Fig. 4.443**). The initial procedure was then completed by placement of four smaller-diameter MReye coils (10 × 8 m; **Fig. 4.444**).

Complication Analysis

Improper selection of coil size in relation to vessel diameter; catheter instability; and fast coil pushing, resulting in immediate coil dislodgement.

Prevention Strategies and Take-home Message

- Evaluate exact size of target vessels before coil embolization, for example, by noninvasive imaging, with adequate sizing of embolization material.
- If the risk of potential coil dislodgement is high, devices with higher radial force for controlled placement in the target vessel like detachable coils or plugs should be used if possible!
- Use of scaffolding technique with placement of a high-radial-force coil followed by packing with multiple coils into the resulting scaffold.
- Use anchoring technique with deployment of the distal part of the coil into a noncritical side branch.
- Use guide catheters or guide sheath with larger diameter in order to achieve a safer guide

position and stability resistant to coil forces during placement.
- Always have different snare sizes available for foreign body retrieval!

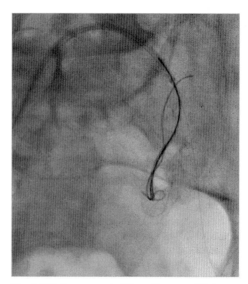

Fig. 4.443 Engagement of the coil was possible by rotating the open snare around the coil. The originally placed 4F Bern catheter was still in place and was used a guide catheter during the snaring procedure.

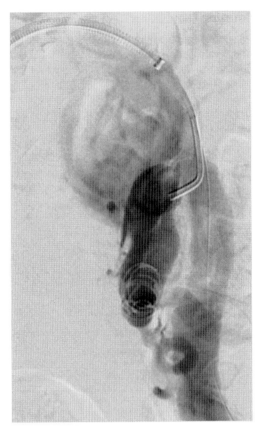

Fig. 4.444 Final angiography after placement of four 0.035-inch pushable platinum microcoils.

Further Reading

Barbiero G, Cognolato D, Polverosi R, Guarise A. Percutaneous retrieval of a radiolucent foreign body from an EVAR device by combining different image modalities. Cardiovasc Interv Radiol 2009;32(4):785–788

Sheth R, Someshwar V, Warawdekar G. Percutaneous retrieval of misplaced intravascular foreign objects with the Dormia basket: an effective solution. Cardiovasc Interv Radiol 2007;30(1):48–53

Mechanical Thrombectomy, Fibrinolysis, and Atherectomy

Interaction between open-cell superficial femoral artery stent and atherectomy device

Patient History

An 80-year-old man was scheduled for treatment of in-stent restenosis (ISR) 6 months after the index procedure. For initial superficial femoral artery (SFA) treatment, two self-expanding stents (SESs—6 × 60 mm and 6 × 40 mm) had been im-planted in an overlapping manner in the proximal part of the SFA. Color duplex ultrasound depicted high-grade ISR. Therefore, the patient was scheduled for reintervention.

Initial Treatment Received

After successful and uncomplicated antegrade puncture of the right common femoral artery (CFA), successful recanalization of the high-grade stenosis was performed using a 0.014-inch hydrophilic-coated wire in combination with a 4F angle-tip end-hole catheter (**Fig. 4.445**). Atherectomy for ISR treatment was begun with a Silver-Hawk LS device (Ev3) (**Fig. 4.446**). Although use of this technique is "off-label" it was regarded as

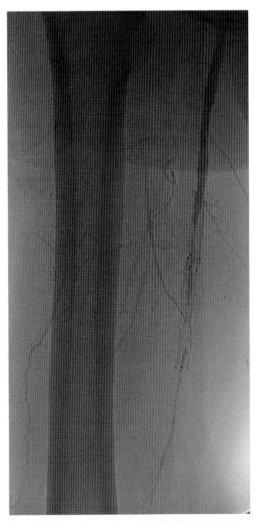

Fig. 4.445 Unsubtracted angiography showing severe intimal hyperplasia resulting in high-grade ISR of the stented and unstented SFA.

a potentially suitable treatment modality due to the high level of intimal hyperplasia.

Problems Encountered during Treatment

After some initially successful runs with the atherectomy device, there was an interaction with the stent struts. The atherectomy device became entangled with the distal aspect of the stent (**Fig. 4.447**). It was possible to pull back the atherectomy device with some force; however, this resulted in infolding of the distal stent into the proximal stent (**Fig. 4.448**). It was impossible to remove the atherectomy device without dislocating more of the stent.

Imaging Plan

Magnified angiography and fluoroscopy for further evaluation (i.e., determination of the exact location of stent elongation and looking for the zone of stent engagement).

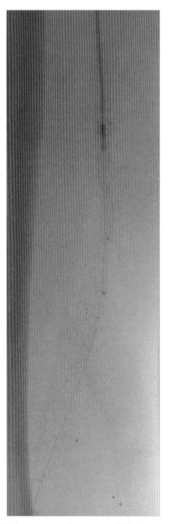

Fig. 4.446 Fluoroscopy after successful lesion crossing with a 0.014-inch guidewire. The atherectomy device was already in place.

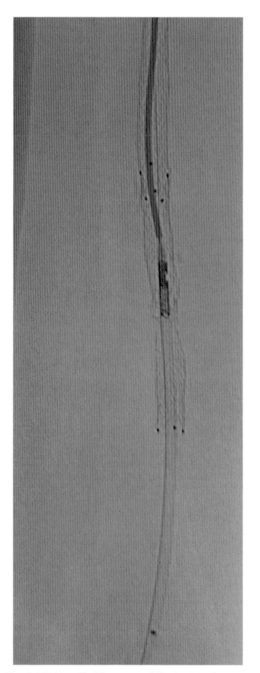

Fig. 4.447 Magnified fluoroscopy following initially successful runs of the atherectomy device shortly before interaction between the device and stent struts.

Resulting Complication

Interaction between the atherectomy device and an SES resulted in stent engagement and disruption of parts of the stent.

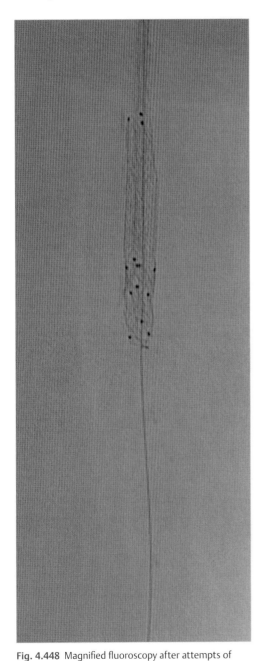

Fig. 4.448 Magnified fluoroscopy after attempts of atherectomy device retrieval. The engagement of the struts and the mechanical parts of the catheter resulted in stent dislocation and destruction of stent strut architecture. It was impossible to remove the atherectomy device.

Possible Strategies for Complication Management

- Forceful removal of the atherectomy device, taking into account that severe damage to the SFA and embolization of stent strut particles could occur.
- Surgical removal and vascular reconstruction.

Final Complication Management

The vascular surgeon was informed and asked to undertake open repair. After surgical cut-down to the groin, the atherectomy device was forcefully removed (**Fig. 4.449**). Then an SES (6 × 200 mm)

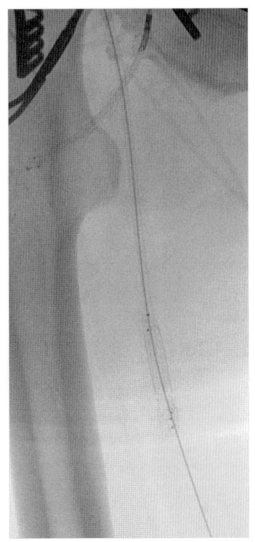

Fig. 4.449 Fluoroscopy following forceful removal of the atherectomy device after surgical cut-down.

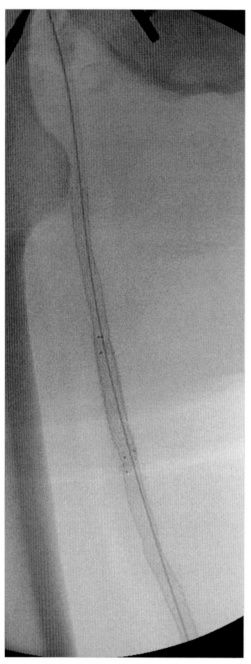

Fig. 4.450 Magnified fluoroscopy after additional stent placement (6 × 200 mm) in order to treat the previously affected vessel area and the stenosed SFA distally.

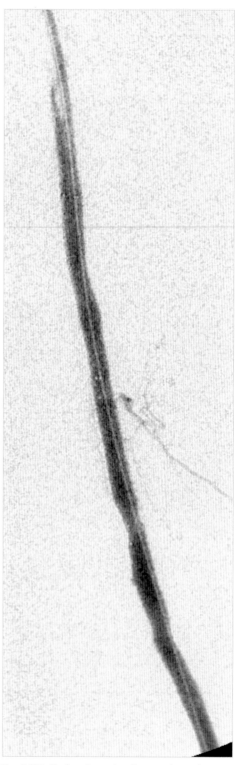

was implanted to cover the stented area and the stenosed SFA distally (**Fig. 4.450**). The final angiography showed a patent SFA without any signs of residual stenosis (**Fig. 4.451**).

Fig. 4.451 Final angiography after stenting and percutaneous transluminal angioplasty (6 mm) of the treated proximal and mid-part of the SFA.

Complication Analysis

Off-label use of an atherectomy for treatment of in-stent restenosis 6 months after the index stenting procedure resulted in stent disruption and dislocation.

Prevention Strategies and Take-home Message

• Handle instruments with care and according to instructions for use; keep restrictions for application (off-label use) in mind!

Further Reading

Cook JR, Haery C, Montoya A. Potential contribution of open-cell stent design to balloon entrapment and review of techniques to recover. J Invasive Cardiol 2011;23(8):E183–E187

Kim JH, Jang WJ, Ahn KJ, et al. Successful retrieval of intravascular stent remnants with a combination of rotational atherectomy and a gooseneck snare. Korean Circ J 2012;42(7): 492–496

Kimura M, Shiraishi J, Kohno Y. Successful retrieval of an entrapped Rotablator burr using 5 Fr guiding catheter. Catheter Cardiovasc Interv 2011;78(4):558–564

Li Y, Honye J, Takayama T, Yokoyama S, Saito S. A potential complication of directional coronary atherectomy for in-stent restenosis. Tex Heart Inst J 2005;32(1):108–109

Sakakura K, Ako J, Momomura S. Successful removal of an entrapped rotablation burr by extracting drive shaft sheath followed by balloon dilatation. Catheter Cardiovasc Interv 2011;78(4):567–570

Thromboembolism resistant to long-term fibrinolysis therapy

Patient History

A 74-year-old man suffered from sudden onset of a painfully limited walking distance without rest pain. He was admitted to the hospital for further diagnostics and treatment. The patient's history reported surgical repair of an infrarenal abdominal aneurysm with an aortobiiliacal prosthesis a few years before. Therefore, instead of a crossover approach for endovascular treatment the patient was scheduled for diagnostic antegrade angiography of the right limb; pulses of both femoral arteries were palpable.

Initial Treatment Received

Following antegrade puncture of the right groin with sheath insertion (6F), diagnostic angiography was performed. Thromboembolic occlusion of the distal popliteal artery involving the anterior tibial artery, the peroneal trunk, and the origin of both the peroneal artery and the posterior tibial artery was detected (**Fig. 4.452**). With interdisciplinary consensus, local fibrinolysis via a 4F angle-tip end-hole catheter was begun for 24 hours with admission of 1 mg recombinant tissue plasminogen activator (rtPA) per hour. Control angiography after 24 hours showed a short-distance thromboembolus in the distal part of the popliteal artery, while the peroneal and tibial posterior arteries were patent. The anterior tibial artery was still occluded (**Fig. 4.453**). A decision was made

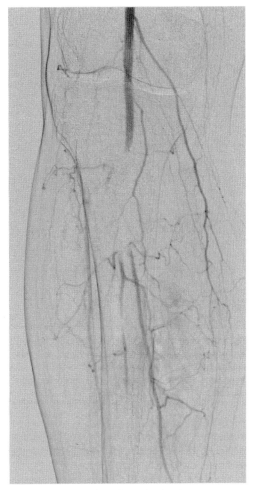

Fig. 4.452 Diagnostic angiography showing thromboembolic occlusion of distal popliteal artery involving the anterior tibial artery, the peroneal trunk, and the origin of both the peroneal artery and the posterior tibial artery.

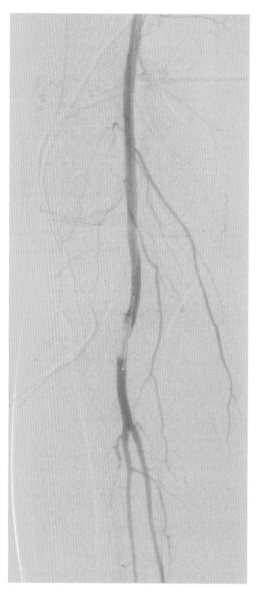

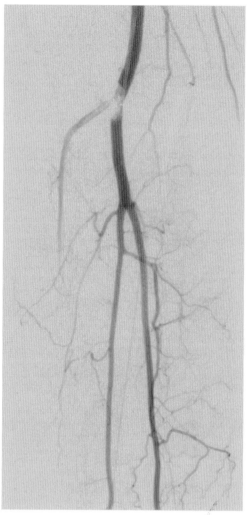

Fig. 4.454 After a total dose of 48 mg rtPA over 48 hours, the thromboembolic material was still visible at the same location, but the anterior tibial artery was partially open.

Fig. 4.453 Control angiography after 24 hours showed a short-distance thromboembolus in the distal part of the popliteal artery. The peroneal and tibial posterior arteries were patent, whereas the anterior tibial artery was still occluded.

to continue local fibrinolyisis therapy for another 24 hours. After a total dose of 48 mg of rtPA over 48 hours, the thromboembolic material was still visible at the same location; however, the anterior tibial artery was partially open (**Fig. 4.454**).

Problems Encountered during Treatment

Remaining thromboembolic material below the knee resistant to 48-hour long-term fibrinolysis therapy.

Imaging Plan

Careful image interpretation of last angiography to plan any further treatment.

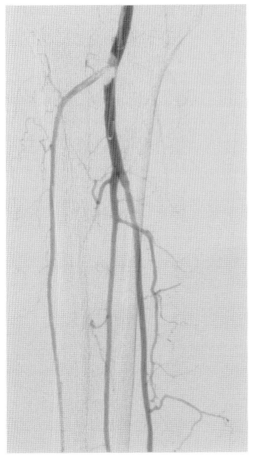

Fig. 4.455 Angiography showing the 6F catheter in place, before advancing it towards the embolus over the wire.

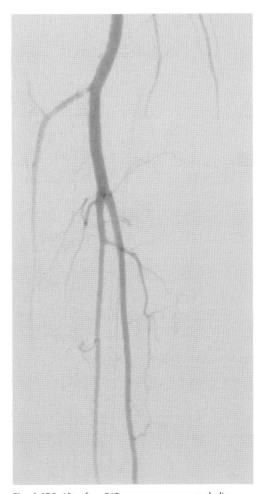

Fig. 4.456 After four PAT maneuvers some embolic material remains in the proximal anterior tibial artery.

Resulting Complication

So far no real complications appeared (apart from the initial thromboembolic event).

Possible Strategies for Complication Management

- Continuation of low-dose fibrinolysis.
- Further endovascular therapy; for example, percutaneous aspiration thrombectomy (PAT).
- Surgical thrombembolectomy.

Final Complication Management

PAT using a large lumen guide catheter (6F Envoy, 0.070-inch × 90 cm, angle-tip, Johnson & Johnson). Five PAT maneuvers are very necessary to remove the entire clot material (**Figs. 4.455–4.457**). For removal of embolic material from the anterior tibial artery, the Envoy catheter was steered over an 0.035-inch hydrophilic-coated wire into its origin. Spasm was treated with 0.2 mg intra-arterial nitroglycerin. The final angiography showed a sufficient three-vessel run-off (**Fig. 4.458**). The removed debris looked like old white clot material (**Fig. 4.459**). The groin was closed successfully with a 6F Angio-Seal (St. Jude Medical) closure device.

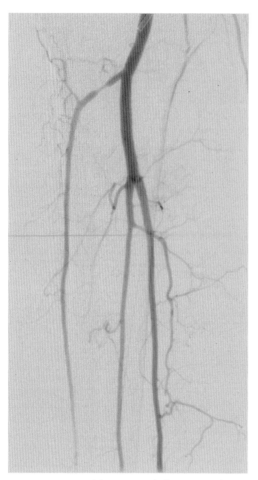

Fig. 4.457 Spasm of the anterior tibial artery is visible after successful fifth PAT maneuver.

Complication Analysis

No real complications occurred. This case should highlight that in the case of local fibrinolyisis failure, PAT is a suitable alternative for successful endovascular treatment.

Prevention Strategies and Take-home Message

- PAT is an easy and effective treatment option for endovascular management of thromboembolic complications.
- Large inner lumen catheters and dedicated PAT devices should be kept in stock.

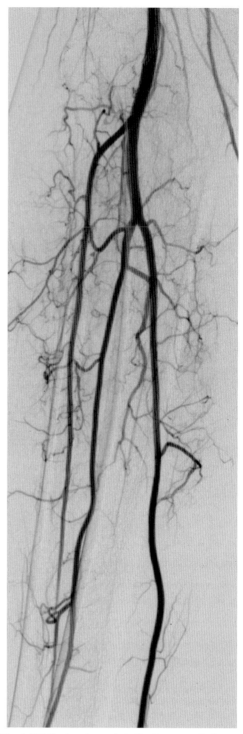

Fig. 4.458 Final angiography indicating no residual emboli.

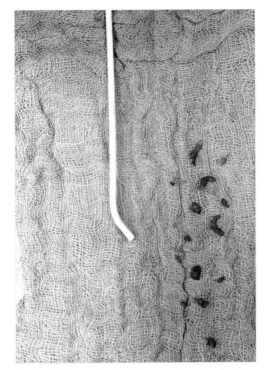

Fig. 4.459 Removed embolic fragments next to the 6F large lumen guide catheter that was used for PAT.

Further Reading

Brossmann J, Mueller-Huelsbeck S, Heller M. Percutaneous thrombectomy and mechanical thrombolysis. Rofo 1998;169(4):344–354

Daly B, Patel M, Prasad A. The use of the Trellis-6 thrombectomy device in the management of acute limb ischemia due to native vessel occlusion: challenges, tips, and limitations. Catheter Cardiovasc Interv 2013;81(1):142–147

Dorros G, Jamnadas P, Lewin RF, Sachdev N. Percutaneous aspiration of a thromboembolus. Cathet Cardiovasc Diagn 1989;17(4):202–206

Turnipseed WD, Starck EE, McDermott JC, et al. Percutaneous aspiration thromboembolectomy (PAT): an alternative to surgical balloon techniques for clot retrieval. J Vasc Surg 1986;3(3):437–441

False superficial femoral artery aneurysm postlysis

Patient History

A 78-year-old obese woman with atrial fibrillation and peripheral vascular disease presented with acute limb ischemia of her left leg due to segmental femoropopliteal thromboembolism. Clinical stage of acute limb ischemia was Ruther-

ford IIa; locoregional long-term thrombolysis was planned as the primary treatment strategy.

Initial Treatment Received

Following retrograde puncture of the right common femoral artery (CFA) and placement of a standard 5F sheath the left femoral artery was cannulated with a 4F multipurpose catheter over a J-shaped 0.035-inch hydrophilic-coated guidewire. The guidewire easily entered the thrombus and the catheter was positioned into the proximal aspect of the left CFA. Locoregional low-dose thrombolysis was initiated with a bolus of 5 mg recombinant tissue plasminogen activator (rtPA), followed by application of 1 mg rtPA per hour. Additionally, heparin was administered intravenously (20,000 IU/24 h; 1,000 IU/h).

Problems Encountered during Treatment

One day after initiation of lysis the patient complained about thigh pain in her left leg. There was mild to moderate swelling.

Imaging Plan

Computed tomography angiography (CTA).

Resulting Complication

CT showed only mild swelling of the left thigh in comparison to the right side. There was a 2 × 1-cm pseudoaneurysm of the proximal superficial femoral artery (SFA) (**Fig. 4.460**).

Possible Strategies for Complication Management

- Leave as it is, abort lysis, wait and see.
- Endovascular management (e.g., stent graft placement, embolization).
- Transcutaneous ultrasound-guided thrombin injection.
- Surgical repair (if other approaches fail).

Final Complication Management

The patient was transferred back to the Interventional Radiology Department for selective angiography. Contrast injections through the catheter in place confirmed an oval-shaped pseudoaneurysm at the base of a collateral of the SFA (**Fig. 4.461**). The aneurysm was intubated with a 4F (5-mm) diagnostic catheter and was filled with

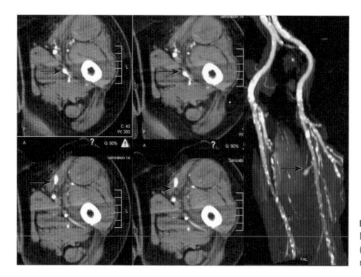

Fig. 4.460 Axial CT images at the level of the femoral pseudoaneurysm (*red arrows*) and corresponding MIP-reconstruction.

conventional pushable 0.035-inch platinum coils (6-mm MReye embolization coils, Cook Medical) (**Fig. 4.462**). After coil embolization there was near total occlusion of the aneurysm (**Fig. 4.463**). Since complete revascularization of the SFA had been achieved, locoregional thrombolysis was stopped. A total dose of 30 mg rtPA had been applied.

Complication Analysis

Bleeding complications during locoregional thrombolysis are not uncommon. In this case

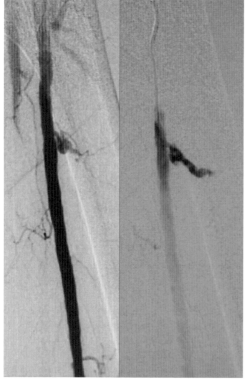

Fig. 4.461 Contrast injections through the catheter in place confirmed the false aneurysm at the base of a collateral of the superficial femoral artery.

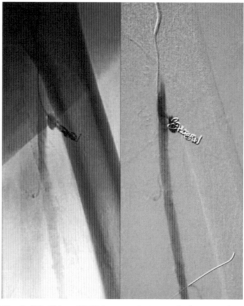

Fig. 4.462 DA and DSA images during embolization of the aneurysm using pushable platin coils.

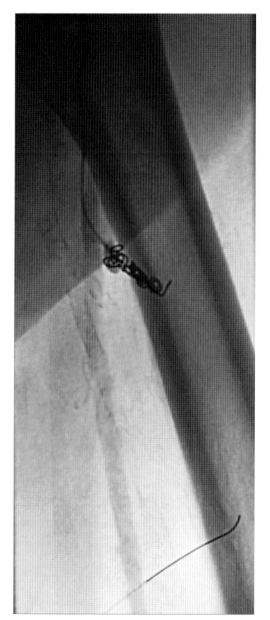

Fig. 4.463 Digital angiography image showing the coiled pseudoaneurysm.

it can be assumed that iatrogenic injury to the collateral with the J-shaped hydrophilic-coated guidewire from cannulation of the occlusion was responsible for development of the pseudoaneurysm. Endovascular management with coil embolization was successful. It is important that in patients scheduled for thrombolysis all instruments (puncture needles, guidewires etc.) are handled with extreme care to prevent vessel injury and subsequent bleeding complications.

Prevention Strategies and Take-home Message

- Be prepared to deal with bleeding complications in patients treated with thrombolysis.
- Avoid multiple punctures.
- Carefully steer hydrophilic-coated guidewires under fluoroscopy to prevent injury to collateral arteries, especially when locoregional thrombolysis is planned.

Further Reading

Abisi S, Chick C, Williams I, Hill S, Gordon A. Endovascular coil embolization for large femoral false aneurysms: two case reports. Vasc Endovasc Surg 2006;40(5):414–417

DerDerian T, Hingorani A, Gallagher J, Ascher E. Use of duplex guided stent graft placement to prevent bleeding from previously thrombosed pseudo-aneurysms during thrombolytic therapy for acute popliteal artery occlusion. Vascular 2014;22(4):302–305

Imsand D, Hayoz D. Current treatment options of femoral pseudoaneurysms. Vasa 2007;36(2):91–95

Kobeiter H, Lapeyre M, Becquemin JP, Mathieu D, Melliere D, Desgranges P. Percutaneous coil embolization of postcatheterization arterial femoral pseudoaneurysms. J Vasc Surg 2002;36(1):127–131

Korn P, Khilnani NM, Fellers JC, et al. Thrombolysis for native arterial occlusions of the lower extremities: clinical outcome and cost. J Vasc Surg 2001;33(6):1148–1157

Lichtenberg M, Käunicke M, Hailer B. Percutaneous mechanical thrombectomy for treatment of acute femoropopliteal bypass occlusion. Vasc Health Risk Manag 2012;8:283–289

Miura T, Soga Y, Nobuyoshi M. Iatrogenic peroneal artery pseudoaneurysm treated by transluminal coil embolization. Cardiovasc Interv Ther 2013;28(1):128–130

Si TG, Guo Z, Hao XS. Can catheter-directed thrombolysis be applied to acute lower extremity artery embolism after recent cerebral embolism from atrial fibrillation? Clin Radiol 2008;63(10):1136–1141

Swischuk JL, Fox PF, Young K, et al. Transcatheter intraarterial infusion of rt-PA for acute lower limb ischemia: results and complications. J Vasc Interv Radiol 2001;12(4):423–430

Tam M, Ahnood D, Tanqueray A, Wang W, Salter M. Endovascular treatment of a superficial femoral artery aneurysm using an Amplatzer Vascular Plug. Diagn Interv Radiol 2013;19(6):516–517.

Venous Interventions
Arteriovenous Fistula

Problems encountered during percutaneous exchange of a permanent hemodialysis catheter

Patient History

A 79-year-old patient on chronic hemodialysis (HD) with a left permanent (tunneled) HD catheter was referred to the Interventional Radiology Unit due to catheter dysfunction, prolonged HD time, and difficulty in aspiration.

Initial Treatment Received

Chronic HD catheter placement.

Problems Encountered during Treatment

Unremarkable procedure reports.

Imaging Plan

Initial contrast injection under fluoroscopy revealed that the catheter had a split-tip configuration. Although both tips were in an intravascular position, with no extravasation, the catheter tips were clearly malpositioned (in a high superior vena cava [SVC] location) and maloriented (i.e., abutting the SVC wall) (**Fig. 4.464a**).

Resulting Complication

The HD catheter was surgically exposed under local anesthesia in the neck region, near the access site and a stiff hydrophilic guidewire (Radiofocus, Terumo) was inserted in one of the lumens.

An HD catheter removal and exchange to a new one over a guidewire was attempted.

After removing the old catheter and introducing the new one through a peel-away sheath, it was impossible to advance the catheter past the left innominate vein–SVC junction (**Fig. 4.464b**).

The catheter was removed again over the wire and a 9F vascular sheath was introduced. Venography performed via the sheath revealed a tight stenosis in the left innominate vein (LIV), along with a contrast filling defect consistent with thrombus formation (**Fig. 4.465**).

Possible Strategies for Complication Management

- Balloon angioplasty of the stenotic region with regular or high-pressure balloon.
- Balloon angioplasty of the stenotic region with bail-out stenting.
- Direct stenting of the stenotic region.
- Catheterizing of the contralateral internal jugular vein (IJV) for catheter placement.

Final Complication Management

Balloon angioplasty of the stenotic lesion was performed using a high-pressure 12 × 40 mm balloon (Atlas, Bard PV) and catheter reinsertion was attempted. The catheter still could not pass into the SVC and another angioplasty with the same balloon followed in the LIV–SVC junction. It was then possible to introduce the HD catheter and complete the procedure (**Fig. 4.466a–c**).

Complication Analysis

HD catheter tip malpositioning and malorientation resulted in catheter malfunction, but also caused stenosis and thrombus formation in the LIV–SVC region.

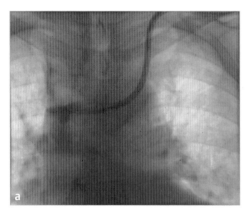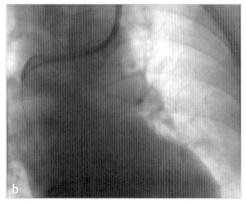

Fig. 4.464 Contrast injected through one of the lumens of hemodialysis catheter, with no evidence of extravasation. Notice the catheter-tip malpositioning and malorientation **(a)**. Inability to advance the new hemodialysis catheter into the SVC **(b)**.

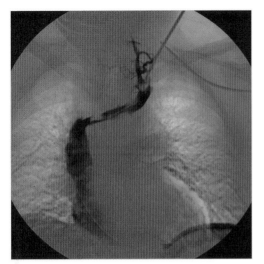

Fig. 4.465 Venography revealing high-grade stenosis of the LIV, with possible thrombus formation. The metal tunneler is also being used to create a subcutaneous tunnel.

Prevention Strategies and Take-home Message

- For patients with chronic renal insufficiency dependent on HD catheters, catheter tip malposition and malorientation is never trivial!
- Apart from causing inadequate HD, catheter malpositioning can cause venous stenoses, further decreasing catheter flow and/or creating blood recirculation.
- Balloon angioplasty is an effective method for dilatation of venous stenoses and stenting is usually not required, especially with the advent of high-pressure balloons.
- The number of patients on permanent HD catheters should be as few as possible as serious complications can occur.

Perforation during cutting-balloon angioplasty of a central vein stenosis in a patient with failing dialysis fistula

Patient History

A 74-year-old patient on chronic hemodialysis (HD) with a failing arteriovenous fistula (AVF) in his left arm was referred to the Interventional Radiology for endovascular therapy.

Initial Treatment Received

Native forearm AVF with an anastomosis to the left cephalic vein.

Problems Encountered during Treatment

High venous pressures during dialysis indicated central venous stenosis.

Imaging Plan

Antegrade puncture of the proximal AVF with angiographic assessment of central venous outflow revealed a subtotal stenosis of the cephalic vein close to the junction of the subclavian vein (**Fig. 4.467**).

Resulting Complication

After placement of a 6F sheath into the proximal aspect of the fistula, the stenosis was easily recanalized using a diagnostic catheter and a 0.035-inch hydrophilic guidewire. Angioplasty with a 6 × 40-mm standard percutaneous transluminal angioplasty (PTA) balloon left a high-grade residual stenosis (**Figs. 4.468** and **4.469**). After

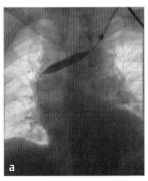
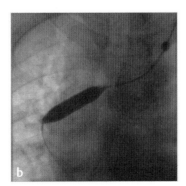
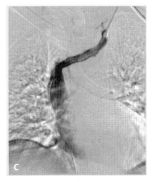

Fig. 4.466 Percutaneous transluminal angioplasty (PTA) of the LIV **(a)** and LIV–SVC **(b)** junction with a 12 × 40 mm balloon, leading to a good final result **(c)**.

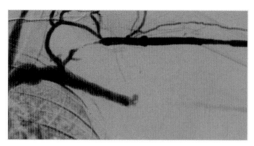

Fig. 4.467 Subtotal stenosis of the cephalic vein close to the junction of the subclavian vein.

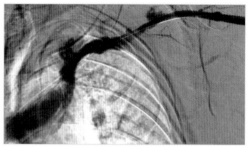

Fig. 4.470 Initial control angiography after CBA revealed contrast medium extravasation indicating vessel perforation.

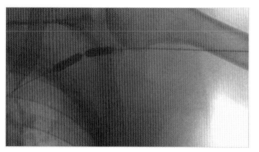

Fig. 4.468 Angioplasty with a 6 × 40-mm standard PTA balloon. Note the indentation of the balloon.

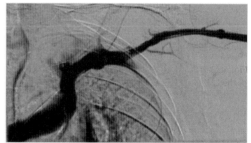

Fig. 4.471 Following balloon tamponade, control angiography showed no signs of persistent bleeding.

Final Complication Management

The perforation site was occluded by inflating a standard balloon (6 × 40 mm) and leaving it in place for 10 minutes. Meanwhile, heparinization was reversed using venous protamine. Control angiography showed no signs of persistent bleeding (**Fig. 4.471**). Ultrasound did not show relevant hematoma formation.

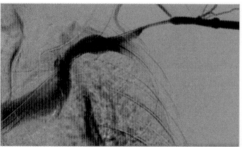

Fig. 4.469 Following standard balloon angioplasty there was a high-grade residual stenosis.

Complication Analysis

There was significant high-grade residual stenosis in a severely chronically diseased outflow vein. Cutting-balloon angioplasty perforated the vessel. Endovascular management with balloon tamponade was successfully used to manage the complication.

changing the guidewire to a 0.014-inch wire, a 6 × 20-mm cutting balloon was used to dilatate the residual stenosis. Initial control angiography revealed contrast medium extravasation, indicating vessel perforation (**Fig. 4.470**).

Possible Strategies for Complication Management

- Balloon tamponade of the rupture site.
- Stent graft implantation.
- Embolization of the entire cephalic vein.
- Surgery (if endovascular approach fails).

Prevention Strategies and Take-home Message

- Avoid cutting balloons in central venous locations because of the potential risk of vessel perforation.
- When using cutting balloons they should primarily be undersized to avoid vessel perforation.

Further Reading

Backer M, Zangan S. Delayed presentation of rupture after venous angioplasty. Semin Interv Radiol 2007;24(3): 324–326

Beathard GA. Management of complications of endovascular dialysis access procedures. Semin Dial 2003;16(4): 309–313

Bittl JA. Venous rupture during percutaneous treatment of hemodialysis fistulas and grafts. Catheter Cardiovasc Interv 2009;74(7):1097–1101

Dale JD, Dolmatch BL, Duch JM, Winder R, Davidson IJ. Expanded polytetrafluoroethylene-covered stent treatment of angioplasty-related extravasation during hemodialysis access intervention: technical and 180-day patency. J Vasc Interv Radiol 2010;21(3):322–326

Murakami R, Tajima H, Kumita S. Cutting balloon-associated hemodialysis fistula rupture after failed standard balloon angioplasty. Kidney Int 2006;70(5):825

Rundback JH, Leonardo RF, Poplausky MR, Rozenblit G. Venous rupture complicating hemodialysis access angioplasty: percutaneous treatment and outcomes in seven patients. AJR Am J Roentgenol 1998;171(4):1081–1084

Shemesh D, Goldin I, Zaghal I, Berelowitz D, Verstandig AG, Olsha O. Stent graft treatment for hemodialysis access aneurysms. J Vasc Surg 2011;54(4):1088–1094

Valentin CN, Zangan SM. Axillary vein rupture after angioplasty. Semin Interv Radiol 2009;26(3):276–278

Webb KM, Cull DL, Carsten CG III, Johnson BL, Taylor SM. Outcome of the use of stent grafts to salvage failed arteriovenous accesses. Ann Vasc Surg 2010;24(1):34–38

Weng MJ, Chen MC, Liang HL, Pan HB. Treatment of hemodialysis vascular access rupture irresponsive to prolonged balloon tamponade: retrospective evaluation of the effectiveness of N-butyl cyanoacrylate seal-off technique. Korean J Radiol 2013;14(1):70–80

Venous access—loss of fistula

Patient History

A 68-year-old woman with chronic renal failure on hemodialysis (HD) with a brachial artery to cephalic vein fistula created after failure of the left arm fistulae (at radial artery and at brachial artery) in the past. The dialysis team reported poor venous pressures and an unsatisfactory dialysis attempt.

A right internal jugular permacath was inserted and the patient referred for investigation and possible correction of the arteriovenous fistula (AVF).

Initial Treatment Received

Angiography was performed after manual examination of the dialysis fistula site and evidence of adequate arterial flow. A 5F Kumpe catheter was inserted into the venous side of the fistula just beyond the arterial anastomosis. Without an arterial tourniquet, contrast refluxed into the distal artery and no stenosis was seen at the arte-

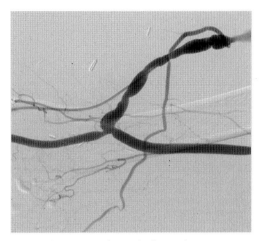

Fig. 4.472 Unstenosed arterial inflow and severe venous stenosis in the cephalic vein at the junction of the proximal and middle thirds shown in digital subtraction angiography (DSA).

rial inflow (**Fig. 4.472**). However, a severe venous stenosis was identified in the cephalic vein at the junction of the proximal and middle thirds and a further string of even more severe stenoses at the distal end of the cephalic vein as it entered the clavipectoral fascia to terminate in the subclavian vein (**Fig. 4.473**).

The radiologist decided to use a 6-mm high-pressure balloon to dilatate the most distal stenosis before attempting to clear the more proximal stenosis. The angioplasty image with the balloon inflated revealed a size discrepancy of the balloon (**Fig. 4.474**).

Problems Encountered during Treatment

The patient complained loudly of pain in the right arm during and immediately after the first angio-

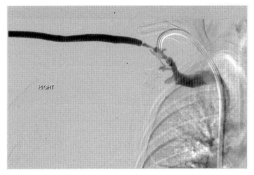

Fig. 4.473 Severe stenoses at the distal end of the cephalic vein as shown in DSA.

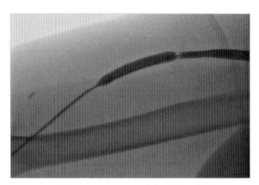

Fig. 4.474 Fluoroscopic image of the inflated balloon in the proximal venous stenosis showing a size discrepancy of the balloon.

plasty and was given sedation with fentanyl and midazolam with good effect. However, angiography revealed a localized rupture of the vein at the angioplasty site (**Fig. 4.475**).

The same angioplasty balloon was then advanced to perform angioplasty of the distal portion of the cephalic vein and junction with the subclavian vein. Angiography post angioplasty showed a single residual stenosis (**Fig. 4.476**).

Further angiography from lower in the cephalic vein now showed an extensive extravasation had occurred during occlusion of the outflow vein during the second series of angioplasties (**Figs. 4.477** and **4.478**).

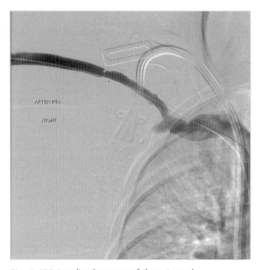

Fig. 4.475 Localized rupture of the vein at the angioplasty site.

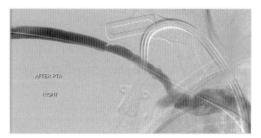

Fig. 4.476 Angiography post angioplasty showed a single residual stenosis.

Possible Strategies for Complication Management

- Further long-term angioplasty with a 100-mm-long balloon of smaller diameter.
- An alternative may be a long series of covered stents but this would have restricted dialysis access.
- Surgical repair.

Final Complication Management.

A series of long inflations with a long balloon catheter resulted in complete loss of the dialysis fistula. This patient is now dependent on central venous access for dialysis.

Complication Analysis

Dialysis fistula veins become relatively thick-walled in response to arterial pressure. The wall is thickened by collagen that stretches until it reaches its burst point, then ruptures.

Angioplasty of veins should begin at the outflow and work back to the inflow. Not doing this was the first error. The second error was attempting to overdilatate the vein with a high-pressure balloon with a further stenosis obstructing outflow.

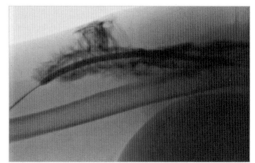

Fig. 4.477 Extensive contrast extravasation at the proximal angioplasty site occurred during occlusion of the outflow vein.

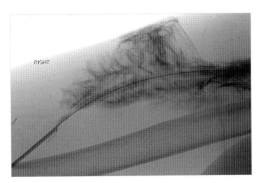

Fig. 4.478 Massive extravasation at the proximal angioplasty site and total loss of AVF function.

Prevention Strategies and Take-home Message

- Care must be taken to prevent overdilatation of dialysis fistula veins.
- In a very severe stenosis a smaller-diameter cutting balloon may be helpful prior to a larger-diameter conventional angioplasty.

Further Reading

Backer M, Zangan S. Delayed presentation of rupture after venous angioplasty. Semin Interv Radiol 2007;24(3): 324–326

Beathard GA. Management of complications of endovascular dialysis access procedures. Semin Dial 2003;16(4): 309–313

Bittl JA. Venous rupture during percutaneous treatment of hemodialysis fistulas and grafts. Catheter Cardiovasc Interv 2009;74(7):1097–1101

Dale JD, Dolmatch BL, Duch JM, Winder R, Davidson IJ. Expanded polytetrafluoroethylene-covered stent treatment of angioplasty-related extravasation during hemodialysis access intervention: technical and 180-day patency. J Vasc Interv Radiol 2010;21(3):322–326

Murakami R, Tajima H, Kumita S. Cutting balloon-associated hemodialysis fistula rupture after failed standard balloon angioplasty. Kidney Int 2006;70(5):825

Rundback JH, Leonardo RF, Poplausky MR, Rozenblit G. Venous rupture complicating hemodialysis access angioplasty: percutaneous treatment and outcomes in seven patients. AJR Am J Roentgenol 1998;171(4):1081–1084

Shemesh D, Goldin I, Zaghal I, Berelowitz D, Verstandig AG, Olsha O. Stent graft treatment for hemodialysis access aneurysms. J Vasc Surg 2011;54(4):1088–1094

Valentin CN, Zangan SM. Axillary vein rupture after angioplasty. Semin Interv Radiol 2009;26(3):276–278

Webb KM, Cull DL, Carsten CG III, Johnson BL, Taylor SM. Outcome of the use of stent grafts to salvage failed arteriovenous accesses. Ann Vasc Surg 2010;24(1):34–38

Weng MJ, Chen MC, Liang HL, Pan HB. Treatment of hemodialysis vascular access rupture irresponsive to prolonged balloon tamponade: retrospective evaluation of the effectiveness of N-butyl cyanoacrylate seal-off technique. Korean J Radiol 2013;14(1):70–80

Transjugular Intrahepatic Portosystemic Shunt

Portal vein dissection during transjugular intrahepatic portosystemic shunt (TIPS)

Patient History

An obese 62-year-old woman with nonalcoholic steatohepatitis (NASH) cirrhosis and recurrent right hepatic hydrothorax was referred for a TIPS to control the pleural effusion.

Initial Treatment Received

Prior ultrasound demonstrated a patent large-diameter portal vein with hepatofugal flow.

The patient underwent a percutaneous puncture of the right internal jugular vein (IJV) using a Haskal TIPS set (Cook Medical) and the right hepatic vein was accessed as usual. Prior to the access to the portal vein, the intrahepatic bile ducts were punctured and contrast injected into these ducts. Finally, access to the portal vein was obtained but the wire guide would not advance down the portal vein to the splenic or mesenteric veins.

Problems Encountered during Treatment

Portal angiography (**Fig. 4.479**) showed a catheter in the region of the portal vein but the vein was incompletely opacified with a long filling defect. Partially subtracted contrast was noted in the hepatic ducts and main bile duct.

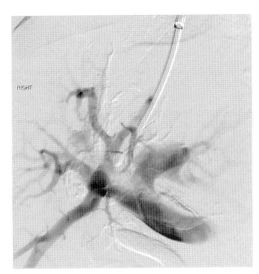

Fig. 4.479 Portogram.

Imaging Plan

The procedure was performed in a biplane Angiography/Interventional Suite with access to ultrasound.

Resulting Complication

Dissection and or partial thrombus of the portal vein. Previous bile duct puncture with Colapinto needle.

Possible Strategies for Complication Management

- Stop the procedure and wait for the dissection to resolve over a few weeks then repeat the TIPS.
- Withdraw the catheter until free flow of blood was obtained and gently advance a guidewire.
- Attempt subintimal recanalization of the dissection.

Final Complication Management

While it was not urgent that this patient had a TIPS, there was no guarantee that the dissection would not extend and rupture or cause thrombosis of the portal vein. Subintimal dissection would possibly cause a fatal rupture of the portal system. There is little time for emergency surgery after portal vein rupture in the peritoneal cavity.

The catheter was gently withdrawn until free flow of blood was obtained. Then a Terumo Glidewire was gently advanced into the lumen of the portal vein. Once a good position was obtained, the TIPS catheters were advanced and a Gore Viatorr stent graft inserted (**Figs. 4.480**). Following stent implantation, successful TIPS creation with patent flow was documented with DSA (**Fig. 4.481**). During follow-up several years later, colored Doppler ultrasound showed long-term patency of the shunt (**Fig. 4.482**).

Complication Analysis

An unrecognized puncture of the portal vein in a region unsupported by the liver may be fatal. Dissection is not usually associated with morbidity as long as the lumen of the portal vein can be re-entered. A focal area of rupture may be covered by a longer than usual Gore Viatorr graft as long as the portal vein is sized to the graft (usually not).

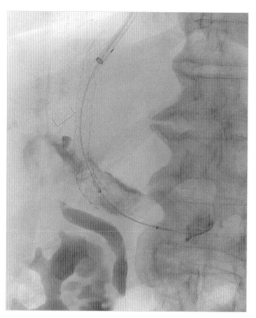

Fig. 4.480 Late image after portogram and stent graft placed. Note the extravasated contrast and the contrast in the main bile duct and duodenum.

Prevention Strategies and Take-home Message

- This complication looks worse than it is and it can be simply managed by basic angiographic techniques.
- Dissection is caused by advancing the stiff catheters and needles into the portal vein when there is inadequate guidewire support.

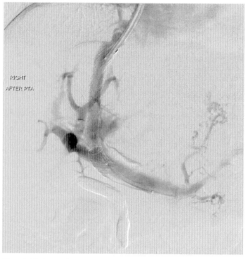

RIGHT
AFTER PTA

Fig. 4.481 Final result.

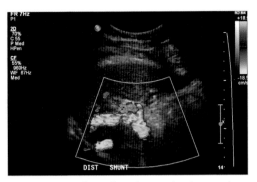

Fig. 4.482 Several years later the Doppler ultrasound showed that the shunt was still patent.

Further Reading

Paoli V, Durieux-Courbière M, Dumortier J, Pilleul F. Portal dissection during TIPS placement. J Radiol 2007;88(5 pt 1): 687–688. [In French]

Petit P, Lazar I, Chagnaud C, Moulin G, Castellani P, Bartoli JM. Iatrogenic dissection of the portal vein during TIPS procedure. Eur Radiol 2000;10(6):930–934

Liver laceration during transjugular intrahepatic portosystemic shunt (TIPS)

Patient History

A 44-year-old male with alcoholic cirrhosis and atrophy of the right lobe of the liver was to undergo a TIPS procedure because of recurrent ascites and variceal bleeding.

Initial Treatment Received

The patient underwent a percutaneous puncture of the right internal jugular vein (IJV) using a Haskal TIPS set (Cook Medical) and the right hepatic vein was accessed to perform a wedged injection (**Fig. 4.483**) to identify the position of the portal vein.

Problems Encountered during Treatment

The angiography shows a focal dense collection of contrast (**Fig. 4.484**) with later extravasation into the subhepatic space (**Fig. 4.485**). The portal vein was poorly opacified.

Imaging Plan

The procedure was performed in a biplane Angiography/Interventional Suite with access to ultrasound.

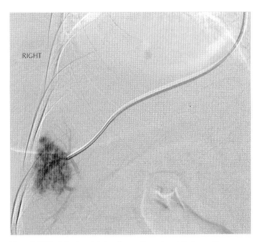

Fig. 4.483 Wedged injection of contrast in hepatic venule.

Resulting Complication

Extravasation of contrast into an intrahepatic hematoma and rupture of the liver capsule with extravasation.

Possible Strategies for Complication Management

- No treatment is generally required as the intrahepatic venous pressure is low.
- Observation while the TIPS proceeds, to confirm the hematoma does not enlarge.
- Use carbon dioxide angiography to prevent this complication.
- Avoid a wedge hepatic vein injection.

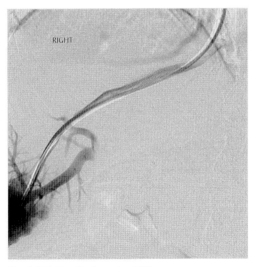

Fig. 4.484 Portal vein contrast filling.

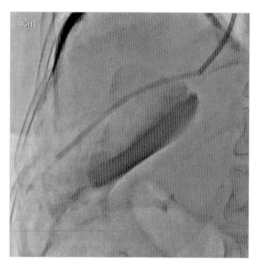

Fig. 4.485 Extravasation into subhepatic space.

- In cases of increasing or extracapsular hemorrhage the vein may be coiled or occluded with gelfoam pledgets (**Fig. 4.486**).

Final Complication Management

After embolization of the vein, the TIPS procedure was completed without further incident and no treatment was required.

Complication Analysis

A forceful injection with a wedged catheter position is designed to force contrast retrograde across the hepatic sinusoids to the portal vein. There is always a risk of intrahepatic hematoma

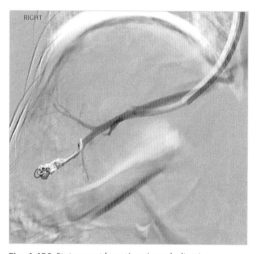

Fig. 4.486 Status post hepatic vein embolization.

or even rupture of the capsule of the liver with further bleeding.

Prevention Strategies and Take-home Message

- The relative positions of the left hepatic vein and left branch of the portal vein are known from prior cross-sectional imaging and wedged hepatic venography is no longer essential.
- In variant anatomy, the position of the portal vein can be marked with fiducials if necessary.
- Consider carbon dioxide angiography if wedged injections are necessary.

Further Reading

Kanterman RY. Hepatic laceration from wedged hepatic venography before transjugular intrahepatic portosystemic shunt placement: one survivor. J Vasc Interv Radiol 1996;7(5):776–777

Krajina A, Hulek P, Ferko A, Nozicka J. Extrahepatic portal venous laceration in TIPS treated with stent graft placement. Hepatogastroenterology 1997;44(15):667–670

Leong S, Kok HK, Govender P, Torreggiani W. Reducing risk of transjugular intrahepatic portosystemic shunt using ultrasound guided single needle pass. World J Gastroenterol 2013;19(22):3528–3530

Owen RJ, Rose JD. Endovascular treatment of a portal vein tear during TIPS. Cardiovasc Interv Radiol 2000;23(3):230–232

Semba CP, Saperstein L, Nyman U, Dake MD. Hepatic laceration from wedged venography performed before transjugular intrahepatic portosystemic shunt placement. J Vasc Interv Radiol 1996;7(1):143–146

Theuerkauf I, Strunk H, Brensing KA, Schild HH, Pfeifer U. Infarction and laceration of liver parenchyma caused by wedged CO_2 venography before TIPS insertion. Cardiovasc Interv Radiol 2001;24(1):64–67

Pericardial hemorrhage during transjugular intrahepatic portosystemic shunt (TIPS)

Patient History

A 51-year-old man with cirrhosis (Child-Pugh class B) secondary to heavy alcohol abuse and a history of mild clotting abnormalities presented with severe hematemesis following failed endoscopic banding. An emergency TIPS was requested during the hematemesis.

Initial Treatment Received

The patient underwent a percutaneous puncture of the right internal jugular vein (IJV) using a Haskal TIPS set (Cook Medical) and the right hepatic vein was accessed to perform a wedged injection to identify the position of the portal vein.

Problems Encountered during Treatment

The angiography (**Fig. 4.487**) shows a good opacification of the right branch of the portal vein from a superior branch of the middle hepatic vein. Subsequently it proved very difficult to advance the Colapinto needle and sheath into the vein and during manipulation the anesthetist noted a problem with falling blood pressure and rising venous pressure.

Imaging Plan

The procedure was performed in a biplane Angiography/Interventional Suite with access to ultrasound. The radiologist performed a transthoracic cardiac ultrasound and observed the presence of a pericardial tamponade from acute hemorrhage.

Resulting Complication

Perforation of the right ventricle with pericardial hemorrhage and tamponade.

Possible Strategies for Complication Management

- Prior to emergency TIPS a management plan for the patient should be in place in case of complications.
- A pericardial drain to relieve the tamponade and stabilize the patient.
- Right atrial angiography to identify the area of perforation.
- Notification of cardiac surgery and the referring unit.

- Continuation of the TIPS if the patient's condition permits.

Final Complication Management

The management plan in place was palliation in the event of failure of the TIPS to control bleeding. Under ultrasound guidance an 8F pigtail drain was inserted into the pericardial sac via the subziphoid region (**Fig. 4.488**). Aspiration of about 100 mL of fresh blood resulted in stabilization of the patient. The site of the bleeding was not seen but this is not unusual.

Consultation with cardiac surgery was performed in the Angio Suite and in view of the general condition of the patient and the management plan no acute cardiac surgery was recommended.

Even though the patient was continuing to have hematemesis they were now more stable and the radiologist proceeded with the TIPS.

However, shortly afterwards the patient had a further large hematemesis and died.

Complication Analysis

It is easy to puncture the wall of the right ventricle with more rigid catheters and even some long vascular sheaths have resulted in cardiac tamponade. In this case the perforation was in the inferior wall of the right ventricle close to the tricuspid valve at a point where the wall of the ventricle was only 3 mm thick.

Pressure on the right atrium and ventricle is more likely when the Colapinto needle and sheath are directed more horizontally. This is more likely in small-volume livers.

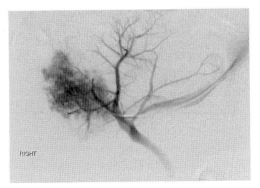

Fig. 4.487 Wedged injection of contrast in hepatic venule with portal vein filling.

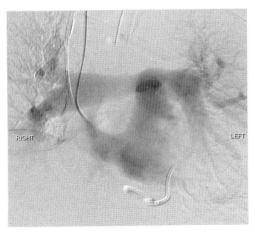

Fig. 4.488 Atrial venogram. Note the drain in the pericardium.

Prevention Strategies and Take-home Message

- Be careful of how much pressure is placed on the cardiac chambers during TIPS.
- Try to take a more vertical path from the middle hepatic vein to the portal vein.
- In very ill patients the radiologist needs specialist support—usually an intensivist or anesthetist.

Further Reading

Bala TM, Panda M. Cardiac perforation and tamponade: a potentially fatal complication during transjugular intrahepatic portosystemic shunt placement. South Med J 2006;99(9):1000–1002

Bañares R, Casado M, Rodríguez-Láiz JM, et al. Urgent transjugular intrahepatic portosystemic shunt for control of acute variceal bleeding. Am J Gastroenterol 1998;93(1):75–79

McCowan TC, Hummel MM, Schmucker T, Goertzen TC, Culp WC, Habbe TG. Cardiac perforation and tamponade during transjugular intrahepatic portosystemic shunt placement. Cardiovasc Interv Radiol 2000;23(4):298–300

Prahlow JA, O'Bryant TJ, Barnard JJ. Cardiac perforation due to Wallstent embolization: a fatal complication of the transjugular intrahepatic portosystemic shunt procedure. Radiology 199;205(1):170–172

4.4 Rejected Cases

Do not touch: arteriovenous malformation, not acute bleeding

Patient History

A 33-year-old man presented to the Emergency Department following a road traffic accident complaining of abdominal and lower back pain. Primary and secondary surveys performed by the trauma team demonstrated only a slight tachycardia (heart rate 112 bpm), normotensive self-ventilating, alert, and orientated patient. The patient had a tender abdomen and thoracolumbar junction. The cervical spine was cleared with plain radiography. There was no documented loss of consciousness and a trauma protocol computed tomography (CT) thorax, abdomen, and pelvis was performed.

Initial Treatment Received

The CT scan demonstrated abnormal arterial enhancement within the right lumbar musculature spanning L3 and L4 (4.2 cm craniocaudal dimension) (**Figs. 4.489–4.491**).

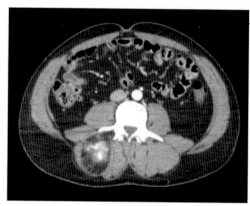

Fig. 4.489 Trauma protocol CT, axial slice at L4 level demonstrating an avidly enhancing lesion in the right lumbar musculature. Note the surrounding fat.

Problems Encountered during Treatment

No complication but the Emergency Department consultant approaches you asking to embolize an acute arterial bleed he has seen on the CT.

Possible Strategies for Complication Management

- Review the patient clinically yourself.
- Carry out additional imaging if unsure such as duplex and or magnetic resonance imaging (MRI) to further assess the lesion.

Final Complication Management

Symptomatic pain management and outpatient MRI follow-up.

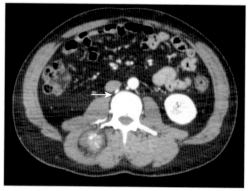

Fig. 4.490 Trauma protocol CT, axial slice at L3 level demonstrating hypertrophy of the right L3 lumbar artery (*arrow*).

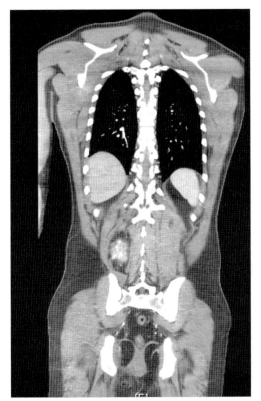

Fig. 4.491 Coronal reformats of the same CT study demonstrating the craniocaudal extent of the abnormality.

Complication Analysis

This is not an acute arterial hemorrhage. Note the hypertrophied lumbar and serpiginous dilated internal vasculature (**Fig. 4.490**). The lesion is surrounded by fat, as opposed to obliterating the fat plane. Features are in keeping with a vascular anomaly/arteriovenous malformation.

Prevention Strategies and Take-home Message

- Treat the patient not the imaging. While this patient was reported as having thoracolumbar tenderness, clinical examination by the IR consultant concluded that this tenderness was remote from the site of this lesion. With the exception of a mildly elevated heart rate there was nothing else to suggest active arterial hemorrhage in this patient.

Further Reading

Corr P, Royston D. Paravertebral arteriovenous malformation supplied by branches of the iliac arteries. Interv Neuroradiol 2003;9(4):379–381.

Do not touch: anterior spinal artery

Patient History

A 67-year-old man was planned for endovascular aneurysm repair (EVAR) procedure with branches supplying the right renal artery and main left-side renal artery. The endograft was planned aortouniiliac due to an occlusion of the right common iliac artery. In addition to contrast enhanced computed tomography (CT) (**Fig. 4.492**), conventional angiography was scheduled in order to determine the relevance of the left-side upper accessory renal artery, which should be coiled during this procedure for preparing branched EVAR.

Initial Treatment Received

Diagnostic angiography (**Fig. 4.493**) evaluating and coiling the left upper accessory renal artery.

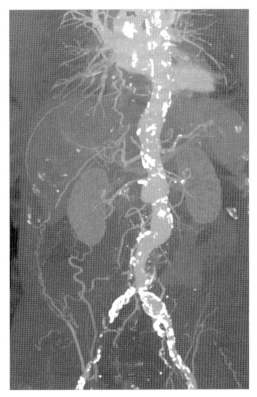

Fig. 4.492 Maximum intensity projection (MIP) reconstruction of contrast-enhanced CT scan showing aortic anatomy indicating a renal supply close to the sealing zone for EVAR. In addition, two renal arteries supply the left kidney.

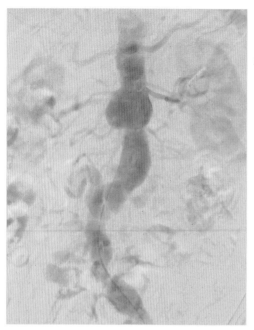

Fig. 4.493 Angiography proving CT findings. Selective angiography of the upper accessory artery should determine the exact volume of kidney supply prior to planned coiling.

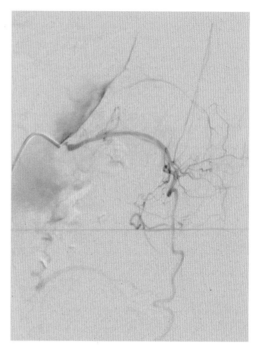

Fig. 4.494 Selective angiography of the third lumbar artery showing the opacification of the anterior spinal artery in a lateral projection.

Problems Encountered during Treatment

During accidental catheterization of the lumbar artery (L1) close to the origin of the suspect renal arteries, angiography depicted that this artery feeds the anterior spinal artery (ASA) (**Figs. 4.494–4.496**).

Imaging Plan

Fluoroscopy of the right groin including the external iliac artery.

Resulting Complication

No complication but there was further careful evaluation of obtained angiograms.

Possible Strategies for Complication Management

- In order to avoid spinal cord ischemia, EVAR should be evaluated carefully. Even though a reduction of flow feeding the anterior spinal artery after EVAR is rare (0.21%), it should be avoided.

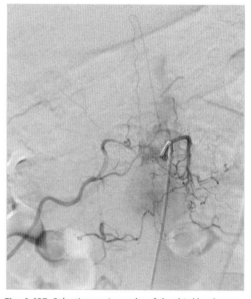

Fig. 4.495 Selective angiography of the third lumbar artery showing the opacification of the anterior spinal artery in an anteroposterior projection.

Final Complication Management

EVAR was not carried out due to the risk of spinal cord ischemia.

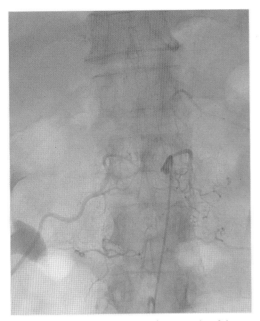

Fig. 4.496 Selective unsubtracted angiography of the third lumbar artery showing the opacification of the anterior spinal artery in a lateral projection.

Complication Analysis

Apparently, no complication occurred.

Prevention Strategies and Take-home Message

- Carefully evaluate angiograms for EVAR planning.
- In the case of a visible spinal cord supply, check whether this territory can be saved from covering, otherwise abandon the procedure.

Further Reading

Berg P, Kaufmann D, Van Marrewijk CJ, Buth J. Spinal cord ischemia after stent graft treatment for infrarenal abdominal aortic aneurysms. Analysis of the Eurostar database. Eur J Vasc Endovasc Surg 2001;22(4):342–347

4.5 Pseudocomplications

Falsely suspected vessel perforation during renal artery stent placement

Patient History

An 83-year-old man suffering from therapy-refractory hypertension and elevated serum creatinine levels was scheduled for renal artery stent placement. Moderate renal artery stenosis

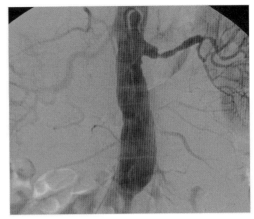

Fig. 4.497 Angiography via RDC catheter showing a moderate stenosis located at the proximal third of the left renal artery trunk.

on the left side was diagnosed by color duplex ultrasound.

Initial Treatment Received

Renal artery stent placement was performed via right-side femoral access. Catheterization of the left renal artery was performed using a 6F 45-cm-long sheath and a renal double-curve (RDC) 5F catheter in combination with a 0.014-inch guidewire (nonhydrophylic tip; **Fig. 4.497**). A 5 ×18-mm stent was deployed (inflation pressure 8 atmospheres [atm]). Opacification during angiographic control was not good (**Fig. 4.498**). A 4F diagnostic catheter was placed in the renal artery trunk, whereas the guidewire remained in a proper position. The angiogram was interpreted as showing contrast media extravasation (**Fig. 4.499**).

Problems Encountered during Treatment

Suspected perforation of the distal renal artery trunk immediately behind the distal stent end.

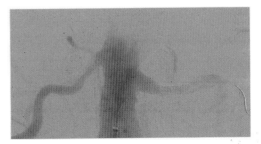

Fig. 4.498 First angiographic control after direct stent placement (5 ×18 mm at 8 atm for 10 s).

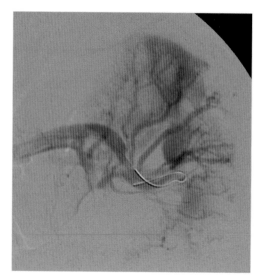

Fig. 4.499 Second control angiography after placing a 4F diagnostic catheter in the left renal artery keeping the 0.014-inch wire in place. Contrast extravasation was suspected at the distal third of the left renal artery, just behind the placed stent.

Imaging Plan

Careful interpretation of last angiography; repeated angiography.

Resulting Complication

Interpretation of DSA images led to diagnosis of vessel perforation.

Possible Strategies for Complication Management

- Long-term percutaneous transluminal angioplasty (PTA) at the level of suspected vessel injury in order to seal the bleeding.
- If the attempt at long-term PTA fails, additional placement of a self-expanding or balloon-expandable covered stent should be performed to achieve hemostasis.
- Embolization for failed control of bleeding with above means.

Final Complication Management

Repeated long-term PTA, which seemed without success, followed by additional placement of a balloon-expandable covered stent (**Figs. 4.500** and **4.501**). Even the latter stent seemed without effect and further bleeding was assumed as seen on repeated control angiograms (**Fig. 4.502**). Finally, the entire renal artery was coiled in order to stop suspected bleeding (**Fig. 4.503**).

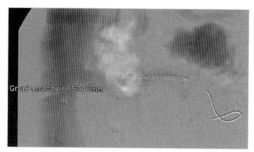

Fig. 4.500 Fluoroscopy before covered stent placement (Graftmaster 5 × 18 mm, Abbott Vascular).

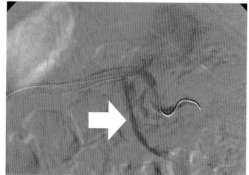

Fig. 4.501 Angiography after covered stent placement still presumably showing contrast extravasation (*arrow*).

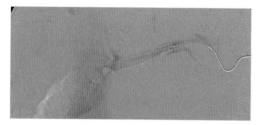

Fig. 4.502 Even additional, repeated long-term PTA could not control the assumed contrast extravasation.

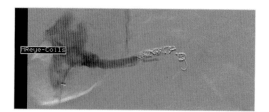

Fig. 4.503 Final angiography after placement of several 0.035-inch fibered coils. The assumed bleeding is no longer visible which was interpreted as successful complication management.

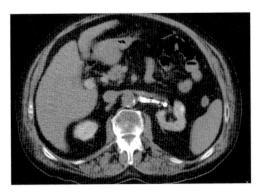

Fig. 4.504 Native control CT at the level of the main renal artery. No signs of blood and contrast extravasation are visible.

Complication Analysis

Vessel perforation was suspected during renal artery stenting. A common treatment algorithm was started in order to control and to stop the bleeding, finally ending in renal artery coiling, in order to prevent increasing retroperitoneal hematoma. It has to be noted that the patient did not show any clinical signs of blood loss and retroperitoneal bleeding such as hypovolemia and/or flank pain. Accordingly, the control computed tomography (CT) after the procedure did not show any contrast extravasation in the peri- and/or pararenal space (**Figs. 4.504** and **4.505**).

Retrospective analysis of the initial angiogram before stent placement already showed an artifact, which looked like contrast extravasation (see **Fig. 4.500**). Based on this artifact, which was falsely interpreted as vessel perforation with contrast extravasation, the above-mentioned cascade of vessel perforation treatment started, ending in the total loss of the left kidney.

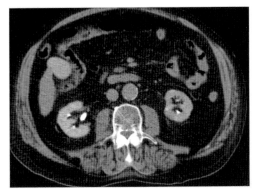

Fig. 4.505 Native control CT below the level of the main renal artery. No signs of blood and contrast extravasation are visible.

Prevention Strategies and Take-home Message

- Interpret images carefully. Take your time and be aware of artifacts.
- Beware of the pitfalls of the digital subtraction technique.
- Monitor the patient's condition and behavior closely during diagnostic and interventional procedures; control vital parameters and interview the patient referring to potential complaints.
- Ask for a second opinion, especially if vital parameters and patient's current condition are inconspicuous.

Superficial femoral artery pseudorupture during hydrophilic guidewire manipulation

Patient History

A 65-year-old man suffering from lifestyle-limiting claudication was scheduled for superficial femoral artery plain old balloon angioplasty (SFA POBA) (**Fig. 4.506**).

Initial Treatment Received

After successful contralateral retrograde groin access (common femoral artery) a 45-cm-long

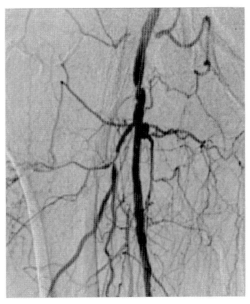

Fig. 4.506 Angiography of a severely stenosed proximal SFA before guidewire manipulation.

6F sheath was positioned in the right external iliac artery. The SFA was passed with a diagnostic catheter (multipurpose, 4F) and a hydrophylic 0.035-inch guidewire. During lesion passage only mild resistance was felt. The catheter was further advanced and contrast medium was injected.

Problems Encountered during Treatment

Selective contrast injection showed massive contrast filling "outside" of the SFA, presumably consistent with vessel rupture (**Fig. 4.507**).

Imaging Plan

Angiography.

Resulting Complication

Iatrogenic fistula with inadvertent cannulation of the femoral vein. Contrast filling of deep muscular veins and competent valves appearing like an extensive arterial injury.

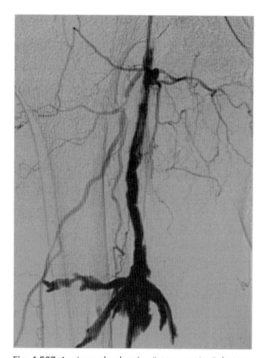

Fig. 4.507 Angiography showing "extravasation" during contrast injection. In fact the catheter had entered the femoral vein through an AV fistula in the groin. No arterial rupture was present.

Possible Strategies for Complication Management

- Do nothing.
- Long-term percutaneous transluminal angioplasty (PTA) in the groin or stent graft to close the AV fistula (AVF).
- Surgery.

Final Complication Management

The patient was without any symptoms (no pain, no limb swelling). After pulling back the catheter into the iliac artery, contrast injection did not show persistence of AVF. No arterial rupture was present.

Complication Analysis

The image of the selective angiography was interpreted by the resident performing the intervention as a huge arterial rupture. However, no serious complication was present.

Prevention Strategies and Take-home Message

- Handle instruments with care—advance them under fluoroscopic control, especially when manipulating with hydrophylic-coated guidewires, which are prone to penetrating the vessel wall.
- Be aware of the patient's condition and behavior during diagnostic and interventional procedures; control vital parameters and interview the patient referring to potential complaints.
- Ask for a second opinion, especially if vital parameters and patient's current condition is inconspicuous.
- Correlate angiographic images with clinical symptoms.

Further Reading

Shetty R, Lotun K. Treatment of an iatrogenic femoral artery pseudoaneurysm with concomitant arteriovenous fistula with percutaneous implantation of an Amplatzer vascular plug. Catheter Cardiovasc Interv 2013;81(1):E53–E57

Vena cava stent single strut fracture and dislocation

Patient History

Three years earlier a 55-year-old man received an inferior vena cava (IVC) stent (Günther Tulip,

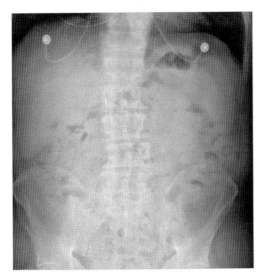

Fig. 4.508 X-ray of the abdomen indicating the position of the IVC stent at the right level; note a single stent strut distant from the stent dislodged to a position suspected beyond the IVC.

Cook Medical) due to repeated pulmonary embolism related to lower limb thrombosis.

Initial Treatment Received

Successful transjugular placement of a permanent cava filter at the juxtarenal level of the renal veins was performed.

Problems Encountered during Treatment

No problems occurred during filter placement. Follow-up computed tomography (CT) for restaging (colorectal cancer) showed a single stent strut fracture with strut dislocation into the right renal vein (**Figs. 4.508** and **4.509**).

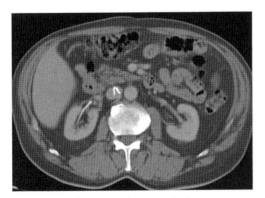

Fig. 4.509 Axial CT image showing a single stent strut from the IVC stent into the right renal vein.

Imaging Plan

Careful image interpretation of CT scans. Additional color duplex ultrasound.

Resulting Complication

Single stent strut fracture with strut dislocation into the right renal vein.

Possible Strategies for Complication Management

- Transjugular retrieval of both the cava stent and the stent strut using a snare.
- Leave everything as it is, depending on patient's condition.

Final Complication Management.

The patient was offered endovascular filter and strut removal; however, the patient rejected any further manipulation due to his underlying disease.

Complication Analysis

Stent strut fracture and dislodgement of the strut into the right renal vein. A stent fracture in this position is unpredictable. This event might be related to permanent movement (compression forces in axial and lateral projection) during inspiration and expiration.

Prevention Strategies and Take-home Message

- The editors know of no strategies to prevent a stent strut fracture of an IVC stent.
- IVC strut fracture occurs in fewer than 5% of cases, and embolization has been reported as a rare complication of strut fracture.

Further Reading

Ganguli S, Tham JC, Komlos F, Rabkin DJ. Fracture and migration of a suprarenal inferior vena cava filter in a pregnant patient. J Vasc Interv Radiol 2006;17:1707–1711

Kalva SP, Chlapoutaki C, Wicky S, Greenfield AJ, Waltman AC, Athanasoulis CA. Suprarenal inferior vena cava filters: a 20-year single-center experience. J Vasc Interv Radiol 2008;19(7):1041–1047

Kinney TB. Update on inferior vena cava filters. J Vasc Interv Radiol 2003;14(4):425–440

Rogers NA, Nguyen L, Minniefield NE, Jessen ME, de Lemos JA. Fracture and embolization of an inferior vena cava filter strut leading to cardiac tamponade. Circulation 2009;119(18): 2535–2536

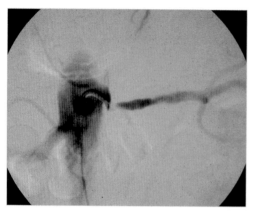

Fig. 4.510 Selective diagnostic angiogram of the left kidney showing a high-grade ostial stenosis.

Fracture of renal artery stent during short-term follow-up

Patient History

A 52-year-old man suffering from increased serum creatinine levels and therapy-refractory hypertension was treated 3 months earlier with a ostial renal artery stent for treatment of severe renal artery stenosis (**Figs. 4.510** and **4.511**). During color duplex ultrasound, a moderate in-stent restenosis (ISR) was depicted.

Initial Treatment Received

Technical successful ostial renal artery stent placement was performed via a transbrachial access route (balloon-expandable stent, 6 × 18 mm). Via groin access, stent placement was not possible, therefore a transbrachial access route was chosen in order to complete the procedure.

Problems Encountered during Treatment

No problems occurred during treatment. ISR detected at 3-month follow-up.

Imaging Plan

Angiography for treatment of ISR (**Fig. 4.512**).

Resulting Complication

Diagnostic angiography and fluoroscopy depicted a multiple stent strut fracture (**Fig. 4.513**).

Possible Strategies for Complication Management

- The editors know of no strategy to avoid stent fracture after renal artery stenting.
- Identification of a mobile kidney (in the current case not evaluated).

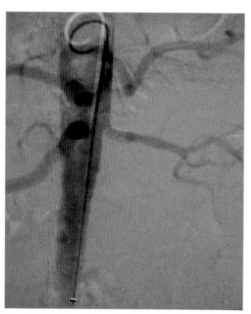

Fig. 4.511 Final angiography via pigtail catheter after technical successful stent placement from a transbrachial approach.

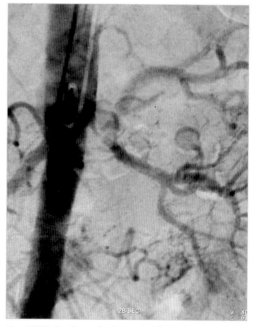

Fig. 4.512 Angiography 3 months after index procedure showing a moderate ISR.

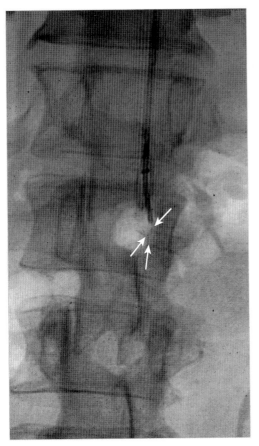

Fig. 4.513 Fluoroscopy showing the stent fracture of the aorta-protruding stent part (*arrows*).

Fig. 4.514 Fluoroscopy after successful crossing of the stent. A second 6 × 18-mm stent is already in place (*arrows*).

Final Complication Management.

The patient was prepared for diagnostic angiography (DA), again, as for the index procedure, via the left-side transbrachial access route, and was ready for any further intervention. After verifying the moderate ISR, which might have been caused by circumferential stent strut fracture of the aorta-protruding proximal stent part, an 0.014-inch guidewire was threaded through the stent into the distal renal artery. A direct stenting procedure with a second 6 × 18-mm balloon-expandable stent was performed in order to treat the ISR and to fix the fractured part of the stent (**Figs. 4.514** and **4.515**).

Complication Analysis

Stent strut fracture without any dislodgement of stent parts, but causing ISR. A stent fracture in

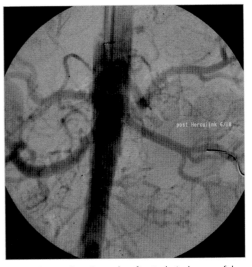

Fig. 4.515 Final angiography after technical successful restenting without any signs of remaining stenosis.

this position is unpredictable. This event might be related to permanent movement (compression forces in axial and lateral projection) during inspiration/expiration.

Prevention Strategies and Take-home Message

The editors know of no strategies to prevent a stent strut fracture of a renal artery stent.

Further Reading

Bessias N, Sfyroeras G, Moulakakis KG, Karakasis F, Ferentinou E, Andrikopoulos V. Renal artery thrombosis caused by stent fracture in a single kidney patient. J Endovasc Ther 2005;12(4):516–520

Best IM. Percutaneous repair of a disrupted left renal artery after rapid stabilization. Clin Pract 2011;1(4):e116

Boufi M, Orsini B, Bianca D, Hartung O, Brunet P, Alimi YS. Renal artery thrombosis caused by stent fracture: the risk of undiagnosed renal artery entrapment. Ann Vasc Surg 2010;24(7):954

Chua SK, Hung HF. Renal artery stent fracture with refractory hypertension: a case report and review of the literature. Catheter Cardiovasc Interv 2009;74(1):37–42

Cohen DE. Re: "Right renal artery in vivo stent fracture." J Vasc Interv Radiol 2008;19(9):1391–1392

Kinney TB. Update on inferior vena cava filters. J Vasc Interv Radiol 2003;14(4):425–440

Nallusamy A, Sundaram V, Abraham G, Mathew M, Das L. Recurrent hypertension from stent fracture. Kidney Int 2008;73(12):1446

Raju MG, Bajzer CT, Clair DG, Kim ES, Gornik HL. Renal artery stent fracture in patients with fibromuscular dysplasia: a cautionary tale. Circ Cardiovasc Interv 2013;6(3):e30–e31

Robertson SW, Jessup DB, Boero IJ, Cheng CP. Right renal artery in vivo stent fracture. J Vasc Interv Radiol 2008;19(3):439–442

Sahin S, Memiş A, Parildar M, Oran I. Fracture of a renal artery stent due to mobile kidney. Cardiovasc Interv Radiol 2005;28(5):683–685

Schuurman JP, De Vries JP, Vos JA, Wille J. Renal artery pseudoaneurysm caused by a complete stent fracture: a case report. J Vasc Surg 2009;49(1):214–216

Tanaka A, Takahashi S, Saito S. Migration of fractured renal artery stent. Catheter Cardiovasc Interv 2011;77(2):305–307

High common femoral artery puncture: prone to retroperitoneal bleeding?

Patient History

An 85-year-old man suffering from lifestyle-limiting claudication was scheduled for diagnostic angiography (DA). DA showed a moderate stenosis of the proximal left-side external iliac artery (EIA) (**Fig. 4.516**). Upon interdisciplinary consensus, direct stenting (8 × 60-mm self-expanding stent) was performed (**Fig. 4.517**).

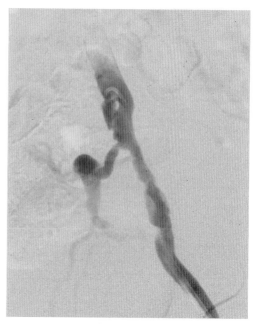

Fig. 4.516 Angiography of the severely stenosed left-side EIA.

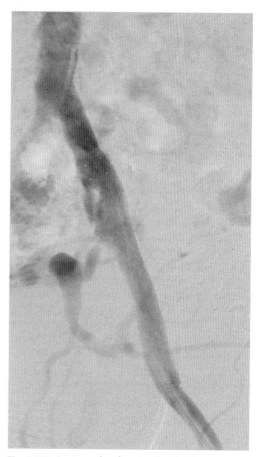

Fig. 4.517 Angiography after stenting the EIA.

Initial Treatment Received

DA and stenting of an EIA stenosis.

Problems Encountered during Treatment

Instead of common femoral artery puncture, re-evaluation of DA showed that the EIA was punctured proximal to the origin of the inferior epigastric artery (**Fig. 4.518**).

Imaging Plan

Careful image interpretation of last angiography; no further imaging is warranted.

Resulting Complication

EIA puncture, followed by 6F sheath placement for stent positioning (**Fig. 4.519**).

Possible Strategies for Complication Management

- Long-term percutaneous transluminal angioplasty at the level of puncture site using crossover technique in order to seal the puncture site, while removing the sheath.

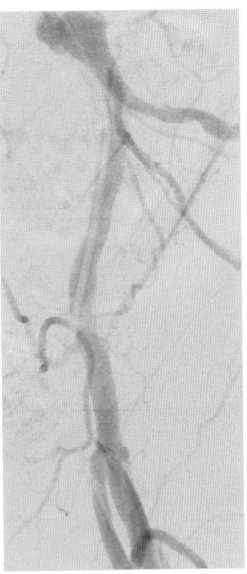

Fig. 4.519 Magnified angiography showing the exact level of sheath entrance proximal the inferior epigastric artery.

- Removal of the sheath during surgical groin cut-down for further sewing of the vessel.
- Evaluating whether the sheath passed the ligament; if the ligament is not penetrated, a vascular closure device is suitable.

Final Complication Management

Evaluation of the exact course of the ligament. In the current case the ligament was not passed,

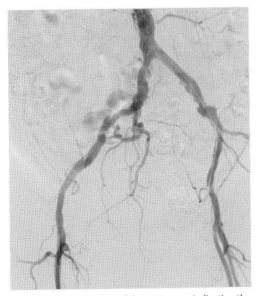

Fig. 4.518 Re-evaluation of the angiogram indicating the high-level puncture at left groin at the distal part of the external iliac artery.

therefore the operator successfully closed the groin with a 6F Angio-Seal (St. Jude Medical) closure device.

Complication Analysis

High retrograde groin puncture (EIA) bearing the risk of unrealized (retroperitoneal) bleeding during external, manual compression.

Prevention Strategies and Take-home Message

- Plan your access route carefully, meaning evaluate anatomical landmarks such as anterior superior iliac spine and mons pubis in order to check the course of the ligament.
- In the case of any uncertainty of the puncture level of the common femoral artery, for example, in obese patients, perform puncture under ultrasound guidance.

Further Reading

Gabriel M, Pawlaczyk K, Waliszewski K, Krasiński Z, Majewski W. Location of femoral artery puncture site and the risk of postcatheterization pseudoaneurysm formation. Int J Cardiol 2007;120(2):167–171

Huggins CE, Gillespie MJ, Tan WA, et al. A prospective randomized clinical trial of the use of fluoroscopy in obtaining femoral arterial access. J Invasive Cardiol 2009;21(3):105–109

5 Suggested Further Reading

For further information, this chapter presents a collection of books and articles not referred to in the case studies.

Books

Ansell G, Bettmann MA, Kaufman JA, Wilkins AR, eds. Complications in diagnostic imaging and interventional radiology. 3rd ed. Oxford, UK: Blackwell Science; 1996

Ben She Yi M. Interventional radiology and clinical complications. Chinese ed. Beijing: People's Health Publishing House; 2000

Butman SM, ed. Complications of percutaneous coronary interventions. London: Springer; 2006

Earnshaw JJ, Wyatt MG eds. Complications in vascular and endovascular surgery: how to avoid them and how to get out of trouble. 1st ed. Shrewsbury, UK: TFM Publishing Ltd; 2011

Moscucci M. Complications of cardiovascular procedures: risk factors, management, and bailout techniques. Philadelphia, PA: Lippincott Williams &Wilkins; 2010

Ouriel K, BT Katzen, Rosenfield K, eds. Complications in endovascular therapy. Boca Raton, FL: CRC Press; 2005

Ratnam L, Patel U, Belli, A-M eds. Managing common interventional radiology complications. A case based approach. London: Springer; 2014

Schillinger M, Minar E, eds. Complications in peripheral vascular interventions. Boca Raton, FL: CRC Press; 2007

Articles

Biopsy, Chest

Lorenz J, Blum M. Complications of percutaneous chest biopsy. Semin Intervent Radiol 2006;23(2):188–193

Chemoembolization, Hepatic

Clark TWI. Complications of hepatic chemoembolization. Semin Intervent Radiol 2006;23(2):119–125

Drainage

Lorenz J, Thomas, JL. Complications of percutaneous fluid drainage. Semin Intervent Radiol 2006;23(2):194–204

Embolization

Bilbao JI, Martínez-Cuesta A, Urtasun F, Cosín O. Complications of embolization. Semin Intervent Radiol 2006; 23(2):126–142

Embolization, AV Fistula

Funaki B, Tepper JA. Embolization of an iatrogenic renal arteriovenous fistula. Semin Intervent Radiol 2006;23(2): 209–212

Embolization, Uterine Fibroid

Schirf BE, Vogelzang RL, Chrisman HB. Complications of uterine fibroid embolization. Semin Intervent Radiol 2006;23(2): 143–149

Endovascular Repair of Abdominal Aortic Aneurysms

Grande W, Stavropoulos SW. Treatment of complications following endovascular repair of abdominal aortic aneurysms. Semin Intervent Radiol 2006;23(2):156–164

Foreign Body Retrieval

Hopf-Jensen S, Hensler HM, Preiss M, Mueller-Huelsbeck S. Solitaire® stent for endovascular coil retrieval. J Clin Neurosci 2013;20(6):884–886

Rossi M, Citone M, Krokidis M, Varano G, Orgera G. Percutaneous retrieval of a guidewire fragment with the use of an angioplasty balloon and an angiographic catheter: the sandwich technique. Cardiovasc Intervent Radiol 2013;36(6): 1707–1710

General

Funaki B. Editorial: Tools, techniques, and cats. Semin Intervent Radiol 2006;23(2):117–118

Savader SJ, Venbrux AC, Savader BL, et al. Complications of interventional radiology: an imaging overview 1993;17(4): 282–291

Infection

Halpenny DF, Torreggiani WC. The infectious complications of interventional radiology based procedures in gastroenterology and hepatology. J Gastrointestin Liver Dis 2011;20(1): 71–75

Inferior Vena Caval Filters

Van Ha TG. Complications of inferior vena caval filters. Semin Intervent Radiol 2006;23(2):150–155

Radiofrequency Ablation

Nemcek AA Jr. Complications of radiofrequency ablation of neoplasms. Semin Intervent Radiol 2006;23(2):177–187

Transjugular Intrahepatic Portosystemic Shunt

Ripamonti R, Ferral H, Alonzo M, Patel NH. Transjugular intrahepatic portosystemic shunt-related complications and practical solutions. Semin Intervent Radiol 2006;23(2):165–176

Index

Note: Page numbers in *italics* indicate illustrations.